VOLUME ONE HUNDRED AND FORTY FOUR

ADVANCES IN IMMUNOLOGY

Advances in Immunology in China - Part A

ASSOCIATE EDITORS

VOLUME ONE HUNDRED AND FORTY FOUR

ADVANCES IN IMMUNOLOGY

Advances in Immunology in China - Part A

Edited by

CHEN DONG
Institute for Immunology and School of Medicine, Tsinghua University; Beijing Key Lab for Immunological Research on Chronic Diseases, Beijing, China

ZHENGFAN JIANG
Key Laboratory of Cell Proliferation and Differentiation of the Ministry of Education, School of Life Sciences, Peking University, Beijing, China

ELSEVIER

ACADEMIC PRESS
An imprint of Elsevier

Academic Press is an imprint of Elsevier
50 Hampshire Street, 5th Floor, Cambridge, MA 02139, United States
525 B Street, Suite 1650, San Diego, CA 92101, United States
The Boulevard, Langford Lane, Kidlington, Oxford OX5 1GB, United Kingdom
125 London Wall, London, EC2Y 5AS, United Kingdom

First edition 2019

Notices
Knowledge and best practice in this field are constantly changing. As new research and experience broaden our understanding, changes in research methods, professional practices, or medical treatment may become necessary.

Practitioners and researchers must always rely on their own experience and knowledge in evaluating and using any information, methods, compounds, or experiments described herein. In using such information or methods they should be mindful of their own safety and the safety of others, including parties for whom they have a professional responsibility.

To the fullest extent of the law, neither the Publisher nor the authors, contributors, or editors, assume any liability for any injury and/or damage to persons or property as a matter of products liability, negligence or otherwise, or from any use or operation of any methods, products, instructions, or ideas contained in the material herein.

ISBN: 978-0-12-817708-2
ISSN: 0065-2776

For information on all Academic Press publications
visit our website at https://www.elsevier.com/books-and-journals

Publisher: Zoe Kruze
Acquisition Editor: Ashlie M. Jackman
Editorial Project Manager: Joanna Collett
Production Project Manager: Vijayaraj Purushothaman
Cover Designer: Alan Studholme

Typeset by SPi Global, India

Contents

Contributors

Lanfen Chen
State Key Laboratory of Cellular Stress Biology, Innovation Center for Cell Signaling Network, School of Life Sciences, Xiamen University, Xiamen, Fujian, China

Chen Dong
Institute for Immunology and School of Medicine, Tsinghua University; Beijing Key Lab for Immunological Research on Chronic Diseases, Beijing, China

Jun Guo
State Key Laboratory of Molecular Biology, Shanghai Science Research Center, CAS Center for Excellence in Molecular Cell Science, Shanghai Institute of Biochemistry and Cell Biology, Chinese Academy of Sciences, University of Chinese Academy of Sciences, Shanghai, China

Kabeer Haneef
Center for life sciences, MOE Key Laboratory of Protein Sciences, Collaborative Innovation Center for Diagnosis and Treatment of Infectious Diseases, Beijing Key Lab for Immunological Research on Chronic Diseases, School of Life Sciences, Institute for Immunology, Tsinghua University, Beijing, China

Qizhao Huang
Cancer Center, The General Hospital of Western Theater Command, Chengdu, China

Yu Jiang
Institute for Immunology and School of Medicine, Tsinghua University, Beijing, China

Wang Jing
Center for life sciences, MOE Key Laboratory of Protein Sciences, Collaborative Innovation Center for Diagnosis and Treatment of Infectious Diseases, Beijing Key Lab for Immunological Research on Chronic Diseases, School of Life Sciences, Institute for Immunology, Tsinghua University, Beijing, China

Hua Li
State Key Laboratory of Molecular Biology, Shanghai Science Research Center, CAS Center for Excellence in Molecular Cell Science, Shanghai Institute of Biochemistry and Cell Biology, Chinese Academy of Sciences, University of Chinese Academy of Sciences, Shanghai, China

Ru Li
Department of Rheumatology & Immunology, Peking University People's Hospital; Beijing Key Laboratory for Rheumatism Mechanism and Immune Diagnosis (BZ0135), Beijing, China

Zhanguo Li
Department of Rheumatology & Immunology, Peking University People's Hospital; Beijing Key Laboratory for Rheumatism Mechanism and Immune Diagnosis (BZ0135), Beijing, China

Wanli Liu
Center for life sciences, MOE Key Laboratory of Protein Sciences, Collaborative Innovation Center for Diagnosis and Treatment of Infectious Diseases, Beijing Key Lab for Immunological Research on Chronic Diseases, School of Life Sciences, Institute for Immunology, Tsinghua University, Beijing, China

Xu Liu
Department of Rheumatology & Immunology, Peking University People's Hospital; Beijing Key Laboratory for Rheumatism Mechanism and Immune Diagnosis (BZ0135), Beijing, China

Linrong Lu
Institute of Immunology; Department of Dermatology and Rheumatology in Sir Run Run Shaw Hospital, Zhejiang University School of Medicine, Hangzhou; Zhejiang University-University of Edinburgh Institute, Zhejiang University, Haining, China

Jun Lyu
Institute of Immunology, Zhejiang University School of Medicine, Hangzhou, China

Xianwen Ren
Beijing Advanced Innovation Centre for Genomics, Peking-Tsinghua Centre for Life Sciences, Biomedical Pioneering Innovation Center (BIOPIC), School of Life Sciences, Peking University, Beijing, China

Samina Shaheen
Center for life sciences, MOE Key Laboratory of Protein Sciences, Collaborative Innovation Center for Diagnosis and Treatment of Infectious Diseases, Beijing Key Lab for Immunological Research on Chronic Diseases, School of Life Sciences, Institute for Immunology, Tsinghua University, Beijing, China

Xing Sun
Department of Rheumatology & Immunology, Peking University People's Hospital; Beijing Key Laboratory for Rheumatism Mechanism and Immune Diagnosis (BZ0135), Beijing, China

Zhengpeng Wan
Center for life sciences, MOE Key Laboratory of Protein Sciences, Collaborative Innovation Center for Diagnosis and Treatment of Infectious Diseases, Beijing Key Lab for Immunological Research on Chronic Diseases, School of Life Sciences, Institute for Immunology, Tsinghua University, Beijing, China

Lie Wang
Institute of Immunology, Zhejiang University School of Medicine, Hangzhou, China

Xiaohu Wang
Institute for Immunology and School of Medicine, Tsinghua University, Beijing, China

Chenqi Xu
State Key Laboratory of Molecular Biology, Shanghai Science Research Center, CAS Center for Excellence in Molecular Cell Science, Shanghai Institute of Biochemistry and Cell Biology, Chinese Academy of Sciences, University of Chinese Academy of Sciences; School of Life Science and Technology, ShanghaiTech University, Shanghai; Fountain-Valley Institute for Life Sciences, Guangzhou, China

Lifan Xu
Institute of Immunology, Third Military Medical University, Chongqing, China

Chengsong Yan
State Key Laboratory of Molecular Biology, Shanghai Science Research Center, CAS Center for Excellence in Molecular Cell Science, Shanghai Institute of Biochemistry and Cell Biology, Chinese Academy of Sciences, University of Chinese Academy of Sciences, Shanghai, China

Yue Yang
Department of Rheumatology & Immunology, Peking University People's Hospital; Beijing Key Laboratory for Rheumatism Mechanism and Immune Diagnosis (BZ0135), Beijing, China

Lilin Ye
Institute of Immunology, Third Military Medical University, Chongqing, China

Yingyue Zeng
Center for life sciences, MOE Key Laboratory of Protein Sciences, Collaborative Innovation Center for Diagnosis and Treatment of Infectious Diseases, Beijing Key Lab for Immunological Research on Chronic Diseases, School of Life Sciences, Institute for Immunology, Tsinghua University, Beijing, China

Zemin Zhang
Beijing Advanced Innovation Centre for Genomics, Peking-Tsinghua Centre for Life Sciences, Biomedical Pioneering Innovation Center (BIOPIC), School of Life Sciences, Peking University, Beijing, China

CHAPTER ONE

Thymocyte selection: From signaling to epigenetic regulation

Jun Lyu[a], Lie Wang[a], Linrong Lu[a,b,c,*]
[a]Institute of Immunology, Zhejiang University School of Medicine, Hangzhou, China
[b]Zhejiang University-University of Edinburgh Institute, Zhejiang University, Haining, China
[c]Department of Dermatology and Rheumatology in Sir Run Run Shaw Hospital, Zhejiang University School of Medicine, Hangzhou, China
*Corresponding author: e-mail address: lu_linrong@zju.edu.cn

Contents

Abstract

During thymocyte development at the double positive stage, thymocytes are subjected to a TCR quality check process termed "thymocyte selection." TCRs with proper binding capabilities to MHC molecules (with self-peptide) are able to transduce cell survival signals and allow the continuing of development to single positive T cells. It has been known that TCRs in DP cells can transduce signals with higher efficiency than peripheral mature T cells, even though they share most of the signaling components. Recent studies have revealed some thymocyte-specific signaling modulators including Themis and Tespa1. The activation of TCR signaling during positive selection results in the activation of several key transcription factors and extensive gene expression change, which has been revealed by newly developed systemic transcriptome analysis tools, and could be used for the evaluation of positive selection process. The fate determination postpositive selection is also governed on the epigenetic level including both DNA methylation and histone modifications.

Advances in Immunology, Volume 144
ISSN 0065-2776
https://doi.org/10.1016/bs.ai.2019.08.005

Abbreviations

DP double positive
IP_3 inositol 1,4,5-trisphosphate
IP_3R inositol 1,4,5-trisphosphate receptor
MHC major histocompatibility complex
SHIP1 Src homology 2-containing inositol-5′-phosphatase 1
SP single positive
TCR T-cell receptor
Tespa1 thymocyte-expressed, positive selection-associated 1
Themis thymocyte-expressed molecule involved in selection

1. Introduction

T-cells are developed in the thymus. T-cell precursors enter the thymus through blood vessels in the medullar and cortex junction. They first migrate to the cortex, go through the double negative stage ($CD4^- CD8^-$), in which they need to finish the V-D-J recombination and successfully express the T-Cell Receptor (TCR) on their surface to proceed to the double positive stage ($CD4^+ CD8^+$,DP). T and B-cells are the most important cells that mediate adaptive immune responses. Unlike B-cells which recognize antigen structures directly through the B-cell receptor, the recognition of antigens by the T-cell receptor is restricted to peptides epitopes presented by MHC molecules. This ability is ensured by a developmental step called positive selection during the development of T-cells, in which TCRs expressed on every single DP cell are assessed for their ability to bind self-peptide MHC complexes expressed on the surface of thymic epithelial cells. The selection process is controlled by the affinity of their TCRs for self-peptides bound to self-MHC molecules that are presented to the DP thymocytes. Only cells expressing a TCR that can bind to MHC-self-peptide above a certain affinity threshold can result in the transduction of a TCR-induced survival signal in DP thymocytes and allow further transition to the SP stage (positive selection). While if the expressed TCR on a DP cell fails to engage self-peptide MHC or does so below the required affinity threshold, the cell will not generate a sufficient signal for survival and thus undergo apoptosis, which is also referred as "death by neglect." This selection process also determines the lineage choices of those cells. Self-peptides bound to class I or class II MHC complexes engage the TCR on DP thymocytes together with coreceptor CD8 or CD4, respectively. If the TCR recognizes MHC-II, the cells will retain CD4 expression and downregulate CD8 expression, thus becoming a $CD4^+$ Single positive (SP) cell. On the contrary, if a cell carries a TCR which recognizes MHC I, then it retains

CD8 expression and becomes a CD8 single positive cell. Single positive thymocytes will then migrate to the medulla. During both the SP and DP stages, thymocytes expressing TCRs that can bind self-peptide MHC with high affinity will transduce strong signals that induce cell death by apoptosis. This event, termed negative selection is a necessary mechanism of central tolerance to ensure the deletion of high affinity self-reactive T-cells. The outcome of thymocyte selection (including both positive selection and negative selection) is to generate a mature MHC-restricted TCR repertoire that is capable of binding to foreign peptides with sufficient affinity but also self-tolerant. Only around 5% of thymocytes survive the selection process and progress to the periphery to mediate adaptive immune responses (Fig. 1).

2. TCR signaling during thymocyte selection

During positive and negative selection of thymocytes, cell fate is determined by the TCR-induced intracellular signals triggered upon the binding of peptide–MHC complex. The engagement of TCRs to ligands with different affinities transduces different signaling cascades that result

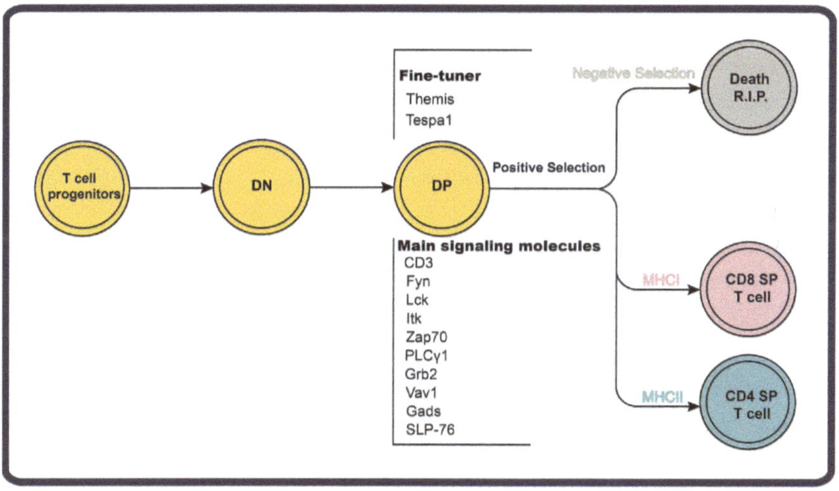

Fig. 1 Selected signaling molecules play critical roles during thymocyte positive selection: After successful V-D-J recombination and the expression of a mature T-cell receptor on the cell surface, DP cells undergo positive selection. This process relies on the sufficient TCR-induced intracellular signals, which is triggered by the binding of TCR to self-peptide/MHC complex on the surface of thymic stromal cells with proper affinity. Earlier studies revealed the critical roles of the major TCR signaling molecules in positive selection. While recent studies uncovered the essential roles of two new signaling modulators Themis and Tespa1 in fine-tuning TCR signaling and ensuring the high efficiency of TCR signaling in DP thymocytes.

in transcription factor activation in the nucleus and determine the cell survival/death as well as other effector events including cytoskeleton remodeling, motility change and lineage choices.

2.1 Traditional TCR signaling components

Upon ligand engagement, nonreceptor tyrosine kinases, including Lck, Zap70, Itk and Fyn will be activated at the proximal region of the TCR, leading to the phosphorylation of tyrosine residues in the immunoreceptor tyrosine-based activation motifs (ITAMs) of the invariant signaling protein CD3 complex by Src-family kinases. Phosphorylated ITAMs will next serve as docking sites to recruit and activate kinase Zap70. Activated Zap70 phosphorylates the adaptor protein Lat, resulting in the formation of the multimolecular signalosome complex known as the "Lat signalosome," which includes PLC-γ1, Grb2, Vav, Gads, SLP-76, and the newly identified adaptor proteins Themis and Tespa1. Recruitment to the Lat signalosome activates these signaling molecules, leading to the activation of downstream of signaling cascades. Activated PLC-γ1 catalyzes the hydrolysis of the membrane lipid component PIP_2 and generates IP_3 and DAG. Both serve as messengers to activate subsequent intracellular signaling pathways. IP_3 can bind to its receptor, calcium channel IP_3Rs on ER membrane, and thus trigger the flux of calcium from ER to cytoplasm. Increased calcium levels activate calcineurin and the transcription factor NFAT. DAG, on the other hand, is able to activate the PKC pathway and leads to the activation of transcription factor NF-κB. The assembly of the LAT signalosome also enables the activation of the mitogen-activation protein kinase Erk pathway and downstream transcription factor AP-1. TCR signaling is critical for the survival, differentiation and maturation of thymocytes. Thus, deletion or manipulation of many known TCR intracellular signaling components often causes defects in thymocyte selection. For example, Targeted disruption of Lck kinase results in diminished TCR signaling and greatly reduced thymus cellularity (~5–10% of normal) and numbers of DP cells (Molina et al., 1992). Mice lacking ZAP-70 have profound defects in thymocyte TCR signaling and have neither CD4 nor CD8 single-positive T cells (Negishi et al., 1995). It is now known that weak but sustained signaling through the Ras-Erk MAP kinase (MAPK) pathway is required for positive selection. Erk deficiency causes substantial reduction of mature SP thymocytes in mice (Fischer, Katayama, Pages, Pouyssegur, & Hedrick, 2005).

Unlike peripheral T cells, which can only be activated by high affinity specific antigen, it is known that relatively weak ligands for the TCR (often very weak agonists or antagonists of the natural antigen for that TCR) induce positive selection. At the same time, developing DP thymocyte express lower levels of the TCR receptor on the cell surface. In both cases, higher signaling transduction efficiency is necessary for a developing thymocyte. The strength of regulation is also critical in discrimination between positive and negative selection because thymocytes that express strongly self-reactive TCRs undergo negative selection (apoptosis) rather than cell survival according to the affinity model of thymocyte selection. From this point of the view, thymocyte-specific regulation of T cell receptor signaling is critical in this process and this is not likely to be achieved by the previously discovered main signaling molecules, since most of them also play critical roles in mediating TCR signaling in peripheral mature T cells (Sebzda et al., 1999). Recently, we have begun to identify molecules with more subtle roles that can distinguish TCR signal strength, including the newly defined signaling molecules Thymocyte-expressed molecule involved in selection (Themis) and Thymocyte-expressed, positive selection-associated 1 (Tespa1) (Fu et al., 2009; Johnson et al., 2009; Kakugawa et al., 2009; Lesourne et al., 2009; Patrick et al., 2009; Wang et al., 2012). Unlike the situation of other molecules, one intriguing observation is that in both *Tespa1*$^{-/-}$ thymocytes and *Themis*$^{-/-}$ thymocytes, despite the obvious defect in positive selection and clear involvement of Tespa1 and Themis in the Lat signalosome, the proximal TCR signaling cascade is essentially unaffected in both knockout cells, followed by relatively mild (Wang et al., 2012) or undetectable (Johnson et al., 2009; Lesourne et al., 2009; Patrick et al., 2009) decreases in distal signaling defects (for example, calcium flux and phosphorylation of Erk), indicating the important role of the fine-tuning of TCR signaling in this affinity sensitive selection process.

2.2 Themis as a fine-tuner of TCR signaling threshold

Themis is a newly identified adaptor protein expressed exclusively in the T cell lineage, with the highest expression level in DP thymocytes (Fu et al., 2009; Johnson et al., 2009; Kakugawa et al., 2009; Lesourne et al., 2009; Patrick et al., 2009). It belongs to a small gene family conserved throughout vertebrate evolution. Three different labs simultaneously reported the essential role of Themis in thymocyte positive selection in 2009, which was later followed by works from several other labs (Kakugawa et al., 2009; Patrick et al., 2009). Although identified through different methods, a similar thymic development phenotype was observed upon the knockout of Themis gene in mice, which were unaffected in early development until the intermediate double positive stage where a strong defect in DP thymocyte selection was noted, resulting in fewer mature CD4 and CD8 SP thymocytes.

Themis is a signaling component of the LAT multimolecular signaling complex. It is recruited to the LAT signaling complex upon TCR activation. It was found that Themis coimmunoprecipitates with molecules in the LAT/SLP76 signaling module and is tyrosine-phosphorylated immediately after TCR crosslinking (Fu et al., 2009). Themis also binds constitutively to adapter molecule growth factor receptor-bound protein 2 (GRB2) through the direct interaction of its polyproline region to the C-terminal SH3 domain of GRB2 (Paster et al., 2013). This association is indispensable for Themis recruitment to the immunological synapse via LAT or for its phosphorylation by Lck and ZAP-70. Two major sites of tyrosine phosphorylation are found in a YY-motif close to a proline-rich region of Themis and are crucial for GRB2 binding, suggesting that this region of Themis might control local phosphorylation-dependent conformational changes important for Themis function. Although Themis can be recruited to the TCR signaling complex and phosphorylated upon TCR activation, unlike other major players previously reported in TCR signaling whose deficiencies cause profound defects in TCR downstream signaling, no clear defect or only very mild changes in TCR signaling were found in the initial screens of Themis$^{-/-}$ thymocytes. The minor defects appeared to be insufficient to explain the severe thymocyte developmental block.

Two working models of Themis were later presented by two different groups: through the using of OT1 TCR transgenic thymocyte and a series of peptide/MHC-tetramer ligands with different affinities to OT1 TCR, Gascoigne and colleagues carefully studied the function of Themis in transducing TCR signaling in the context of different ligand affinities. They found that Themis acts early in the TCR signaling cascade, reducing signal strength through the activation of phosphatase SHP-1 in response to low-affinity, but not high-affinity MHC/peptide ligands. This allows Themis to control the threshold between positive and negative selection of thymocytes (Fu et al., 2013). Without Themis, TCR signaling in response to low-affinity MHC proteins ligands mimics normal signaling responses to negative or agonist-selecting ligands, generating stronger signals that redirect the selection outcome. Thus the defective thymocyte selection in Themis KO thymocytes results from incorrect discrimination between weak and strong MHC-peptide (MHCp) ligands. Under a different experimental setting, a study from Love and colleagues proposed a second model. Instead of reducing TCR signaling, they have shown that Themis is able to promote TCR signaling in DP cells through the inhibition of SHP-1 activity, particularly in the presence of reactive oxygen species (ROS), thus leading to the enhancement of TCR signaling in DP thymocytes and allowing a sufficient signal for thymocytes to proceed positive selection with low-affinity ligands. In stimulated *Themis*$^{-/-}$ thymocytes, SHP-1 recruited to LAT is in its active state. The subsequent dephosphorylation of initiating kinases ZAP-70 and Lck dampens TCR signaling (Choi et al., 2017). TCR–self-pMHC interactions then fail to produce sufficient signals for positive selection of DP thymocytes, leading to death by neglect and reduced SP cells. Thus, the developmental defect in *Themis*$^{-/-}$ thymocytes is secondary to reduced TCR signaling responses, rather than enhanced responses.

The puzzling and seemingly contradictory results observed from these different assays of TCR signaling in *Themis*$^{-/-}$ thymocytes by different groups indicate that the effects of Themis deficiency on TCR signaling responses are more complicated than can be explained by current models. Both models include the role of SHP-1 but propose opposite roles for Themis with respect to SHP-1 (activating or inhibitory, respectively) in different experimental settings. But in fact, conditional deletion of the *Ptpn6* gene which encodes SHP-1 led to unimpaired positive selection and very subtle defects of cell survival in postselection SP thymocytes, very likely due to enhanced negative selection (Martinez, Morris, Neeld, & Evavold, 2016). The defects in thymocyte maturation is observed at the first stage of positive selection (TCR^{int}CD69^{int}) in *Themis*$^{-/-}$ mice, whereas *Ptpn6*$^{-/-}$ mice do not exhibit a developmental defect until the later TCR^{hi}CD69^{hi} postselection stage and demonstrate a lesser CD4 SP cell reduction. This could be due to the functional redundancy between Shp1 and other phosphatases like Shp2 in the T cell lineage, or more likely, because of other as yet undiscovered mechanisms which differ from the current models.

Nevertheless, the stage-specific expression of Themis and its ability to regulate TCR-driven cell activation during T cell development, provides a means to explain the unusual sensitivity of DP thymocytes to TCR stimulation, a property that is essential for positive selection.

2.3 Tespa1: A thymic-specific regulator of Ca^{2+} signaling during positive selection

Although not completely T cell specific, another adaptor protein Tespa1 (thymocyte-expressed, positive selection–associated 1) has been recently discovered to play an important role in regulating TCR signal strength in DP thymocytes. Tespa1 gene deletion in mice leads to significant inhibition of DP-to-SP transition and displays all the hallmarks of a defect in positive selection. There are fewer than normal SP thymocytes in *Tespa1*$^{-/-}$ thymus. The defect is noticeable at the CD4^{+} CD8^{int} stage, at which DP cells start to express the activation marker CD69 when TCR begins to signal. Initial analysis revealed substantial decreases of TCR-induced Ca^{2+} and Erk activation, indicating a positive regulatory role of Tespa1 in TCR signaling (Wang et al., 2012).

Tespa1 is also a signaling molecule which can be recruited to the LAT signaling complex upon TCR stimulation in DP thymocytes through its direct interaction with PLCγ1. However, the precise domain or structural motif responsible for the interaction has not been identified. It has notable homology to a protein termed Ki-Ras-induced actin-interacting protein (Krap), particularly in the region that controls Krap's binding to the inositol-1,4,5-trisphosphate (IP_3) receptor on the endoplasmic reticulum (ER) in epithelial cells (Gascoigne & Fu, 2012). Indeed, recent work showed that the Tespa1 protein constitutively binds to IP_3R, the calcium channel on the ER membrane. The interaction between Tespa1 and IP3Rs is independent of its binding to its upstream binding partner PLCγ1 and requires the conserved F187 and F188 sites homologous to Krap IP_3R binding sites. It has been shown that this direct binding between the two molecules allows the recruitment of IP_3R to the TCR proximal region upon TCR activation in thymocytes (Fujimoto, Matsuzaki, Tanaka, & Shirasawa, 2013; Liang et al., 2017; Matsuzaki et al., 2012). The Tespa1-mediated translocation of IP_3R facilitates the phosphorylation of IP_3R by the TCR proximal protein kinase Fyn, which has been previously reported to enhance calcium flux efficiency upon TCR stimulation (Cui et al., 2004). More importantly, the Tespa1-induced relocation of IP_3R to the TCR-proximal region brings IP_3R and PLCγ1 together. Interestingly, IP_3R uses IP_3 as a ligand to activate its calcium channel activity, while IP_3 is generated by activated PLCγ1 through the hydrolysis of membrane phospholipid component PIP_2. This then enables the prompt use of IP_3 locally immediately after its generation. Similar to autocrine stimulation, IP_3Rs on the ER membrane are now able to access higher concentrations of its ligand and respond in a faster and stronger manner. In Tespa1 KO thymocytes, or when the IP_3R binding site is mutated, IP_3R relocation is not observed. Although TCR stimulation is still able to activate a calcium flux signal, it happens in a much weaker and slower manner, since the IP_3Rs on the ER membrane are now far away from PLCγ1, the IP_3 generation site, and will only be able to respond after IP_3 molecules reach their ER locations through diffusion (Fig. 2).

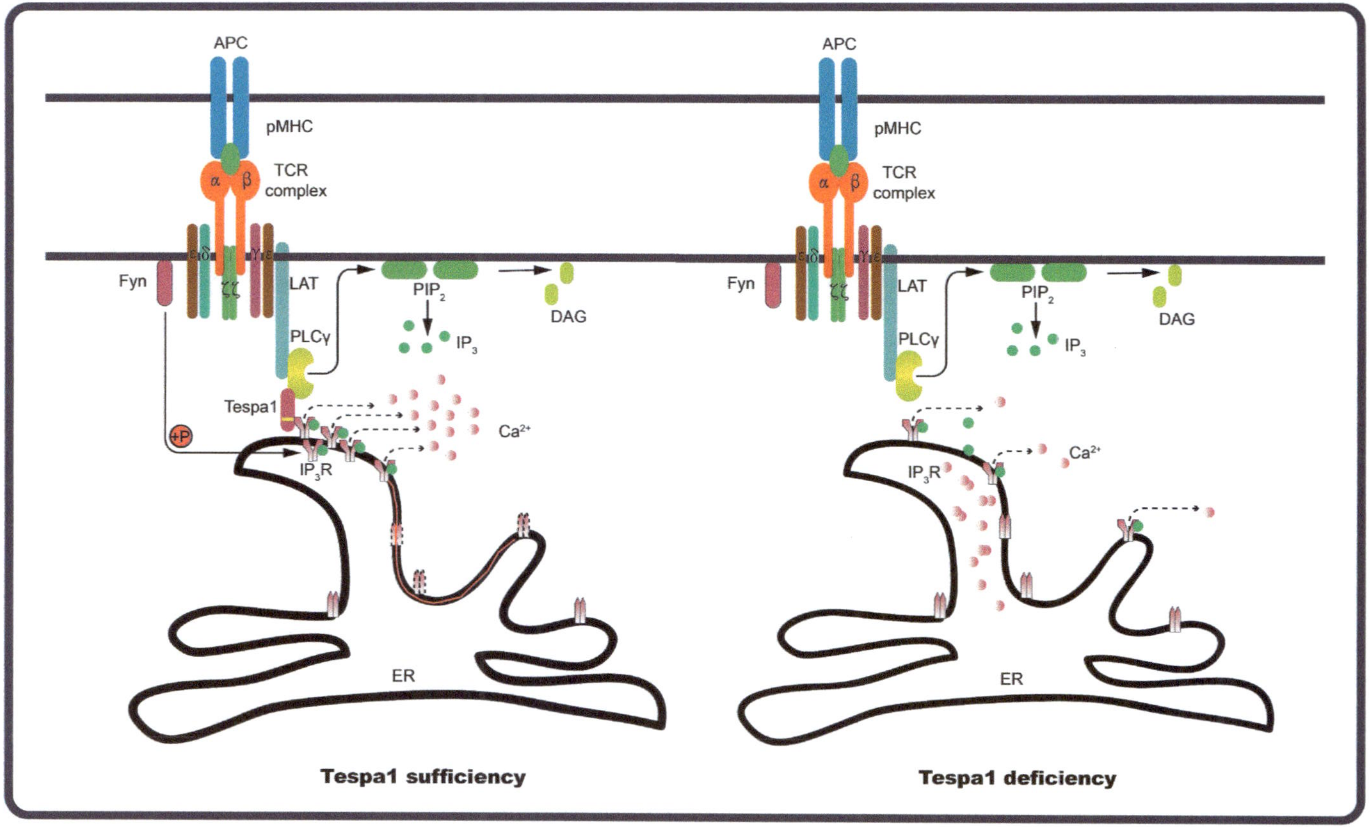

Fig. 2 Model of TCR signaling and the function of Tespa1 during positive selection: During thymocyte selection, TCRs on DP cells recognize self-peptide/MHC ligand, which transmits signal via the Lat signaling complex, resulting in the recruitment and activation of PLCγ1 and production of diacylglycerol (DAG) and IP_3. IP_3 bind to the calcium channels IP_3Rs on the ER membrane to trigger calcium flux. Tespa1, as an adaptor protein, is able to recruit IP_3R to the TCR signaling complex through direct binding to both PLCγ1 and IP_3R. The translocation of IP_3R to the proximal region of TCR signaling complex allows more efficient use of IP_3 and enables faster and more robust calcium flux signal. In Tespa1 knockout DP cells or in mature T cells in which Tespa1 expression level has been decreased. The triggering of calcium flux signal is not as efficient since IP_3 need to reach the IP_3R sites through diffusion.

Newly generated *Tespa1-FFAA* mice which carry a Tespa1 mutation that cannot bind to IP_3R enabled us to assess whether the Tespa1-IP_3R1 axis is the major mechanism by which Tespa1 regulates TCR signaling and thymocyte development. The defective TCR downstream signaling in *Tespa1-FFAA* thymocytes was identical to that of Tespa1-knockout cells. The *Tespa1-FFAA* mutation severely impaired the maturation of CD4 and CD8 SP thymocytes. The reductions in both CD4 and CD8 SP thymocyte mirrors the thymic selection defect in *Tespa1*$^{-/-}$ mice.

Despite the substantial reductions of single positive $CD4^+$ and $CD8^+$ SP thymocytes, *Tespa1* knockout mice were able to restore peripheral $CD4^+$ and $CD8^+$ cell numbers gradually with aging, which suggests a restricted role of Tespa1 during positive selection but not in peripheral T cells. We have recently compared the relative contributions and stage-specificity of Themis and Tespa1 during thymocyte development by comparing the transcriptome of WT, *Themis*$^{-/-}$ and *Tespa1*$^{-/-}$ thymocytes at different developmental stages (P2: $CD69^{neg}TCRb^{lo\text{-}int}$, preselection DP cells; P3: $CD69^{int}TCRb^{int\text{-}hi}$, under-selection cells; P4: $CD69^{hi}TCRb^{hi}$, post-selection cells). We found that Tespa1 deficiency specifically influences a group of genes in P3 thymocytes, culminating in cells undergoing positive selection, while Themis deletion has a broader influence on gene expression in all three groups of cells. In BM chimeras composed of *Tespa1*$^{-/-}$ and *Themis*$^{-/-}$ bone marrow, *Tespa1*$^{-/-}$ cells achieved better peripheral T-cell recovery through homeostatic proliferation instead of the more severe developmental defect seen in thymus when compared with *Themis*$^{-/-}$ cells. Moreover, Tespa1 downregulates its expression substantially in peripheral T cells. Conditional knockout of Tespa1 in peripheral T-cells did not show any defects in TCR signaling and TCR-induced proliferation, indicating the dominant stage-specific function of Tespa1 in regulation TCR signaling during positive selection.

A Themis and Tespa1 double knockout mouse line has been generated recently. The DKO mice have an additive impairment in thymocyte development, shown by an additive reduction in both $CD4^+$ and $CD8^+$ single positive thymocytes. Peripheral $CD4^+$ and $CD8^+$ T-cell numbers in both spleen and lymph nodes were also further reduced in DKO mice. Consistent with an additive defect in thymocyte development, TCR signaling in DKO thymocytes resulting from both Themis and Tespa1 deficiency. The DKO thymocytes also displayed the lowest levels of CD69 and CD5 at $CD4^+CD8^{int}$ stage during the initiation of positive selection. Thus, Themis and Tespa1 are two functionally independent adaptor proteins capable of regulating TCR signal strength during thymocyte selection, suggesting the use of multiple mechanisms during positive selection to ensure TCR sensitivity in developing thymocytes during selection.

2.4 Other signaling components which facilitate thymocyte selection

Some other signaling regulators involved in positive development have also been reported recently, showing a thymic-specific role in regulating TCR signaling in DP thymocytes.

The serine/threonine kinase LKB1 is a multifunctional tumor suppressor which is critical in regulating cell growth, polarity, and proliferation in many different cell types. It has recently been shown to be involved in thymocyte positive selection through regulation of T cell receptor (TCR) signaling (Cao et al., 2011; MacIver et al., 2011). LKB1 is phosphorylated by Lck and predominately interacts with LAT and PLCγ1 following TCR stimulation. Deletion of LKB1 results in impaired recruitment of PLCγ1 to the LAT signalosome and attenuated PLCγ1 activity followed by significant defect in the generation of mature CD4 and CD8 single positive SP thymocytes (Cao et al., 2011).

Upon TCR activation, calcium flux from ER will lead to further influx of extracellular calcium through calcium channels on the cell membrane. It is known that sustained entry of Ca^{2+} into $CD4^+CD8^+$ double-positive thymocytes is required for positive selection of $CD4^+$ T cells. Despite the fact that genetic deletion of its two key components (ORAI and STIM) has no effect on the positive selection of $CD4^+$ and $CD8^+$ T cells, a new calcium channel voltage-gated Na^+ channel (VGSC) was shown to be responsible for inducing the sustained calcium signal in positive selection (Lo, Donermeyer, & Allen, 2012). Both the pharmacological inhibition of VGSC activity, or the genetic disruption of the VGSC encoding genes Scn5a or Scn4b, inhibited the sustained Ca^{2+} influx induced by positively selecting ligands and the positive selection of $CD4^+$ T cells (Lo et al., 2012). Thus, active VGSCs in thymocytes provide a mechanism by which a weak positive selection signal can induce sustained Ca^{2+} signals required for $CD4^+$ T cell development. Scn5a is not expressed in mature $CD4^+$ T cells. Thus, stage-specific expression of VGSC empowers DP thymocytes to respond to positively selecting ligands, whereas no expression in peripheral T cells avoids autoreactivity.

During positive selection, DP thymocytes survey the MHC-self peptide ligands expressed in the thymic cortex, sufficient interaction time between

DP cells and thymic cortex epithelial cells is critical for positive selection. It has been shown that the deletion of a G protein-coupled receptor kinase-interactor 2 (GIT2) led to enhanced migration ability of DP cells, which resulted in a compromised ability of thymocytes to scan antigen in cortex and defects in positive selection (Phee et al., 2010).

On the contrary, tightening the interactions between DP cells and cells with self-ligands would be beneficial for enhancing signals for positive selection. Claudins are crucial constituents of tight-junction strands in epithelial cells. Claudin protein Cldn4 has been unexpectedly found to be expressed on DP thymocytes (Kawai et al., 2011). Cldn4 showed a potent T-cell receptor costimulatory activity. It was strongly recruited to the immunological synapse upon T-cell receptor engagement through antigen-presenting cells. Functionally, knockdown of Cldn4 resulted in reduced generation of CD4/CD8 single-positive cells from DP cells in in vitro thymic differentiation assays (Kawai et al., 2011).

When examined, the expression pattern of these newly defined regulators, VGSC and Cldn4 are expressed highly in DP thymocytes but are down regulated in peripheral T cells, indicating possible roles in tuning TCR signaling in a thymic-specific manner.

3. Gene expression profiling during positive selection

Upon the receiving of proper TCR signaling, DP thymocytes then initiate a series of cellular events including defending against cell apoptosis, enhancing cell survival, promoting cell migration to the medulla, committing to the $CD4^+$ or $CD8^+$ T lineage, closure of TCR rearrangement, etc. The initiation of these different cellular programing processes requires the translation of intracellular signals to different patterns of gene expression through the activation of multiple transcriptional factors. Many transcription factors have been reported to play critical roles in thymocyte development. Early studies focusing on thymocyte survival have identified several transcription factors that are critical for DP cell survival, including the TCR-1 downstream of Wnt/β-catenin pathway, RORγt (Retinoid-related orphan nuclear factor γt), c-myb (myeloblastosis oncogene), and HEB (also called TCF-12, transcription factor 12) (Douglas, Jacobs, Bothwell, & Hayday, 2001; He et al., 2000; Jones & Zhuang, 2007; Xie, Huang, Sadim, & Sun, 2005). However, most of these TFs start to function before the activation of TCR at the preselection stage, thus are not considered as TCR-activated transcription factors. Some transcription factors, however, act as direct targets of TCR positive selection signaling. They are present in the cytoplasm and are able to translocate to the nucleus to exert transcriptional activity after receiving TCR signals. Some of them are also regulated at the transcriptional level themselves, these have low initial expression levels and are significantly up-regulated after TCR activation.

3.1 Transcriptional factors downstream of TCR signaling

NFAT (Nuclear Factor of Activated T-cells) is the primary transcription factor activated downstream of the calcium signal. It exists in the cytoplasm in a phosphorylated form in the absence of TCR stimulation. After TCR is stimulated, phosphatase calcineurin activated by calcium ions is able to activate NFAT through dephosphorylation. The activated NFAT then translocates into the nucleus and functions as a gene transcriptional factor. The immunosuppressant cyclosporin A (CsA) works through the inhibition calcineurin activity and inhibits NFAT translocation into the nucleus. Studies have shown that treatment of thymocytes with CsA prevents the occurrence of positive selection, while overexpression of an activated form of calcineurin enhances the activity of NFAT and is able to promote positive selection of thymocytes (Hayden-Martinez, Kane, & Hedrick, 2000; Hodge et al., 1996; Jenkins, Schwartz, & Pardoll, 1988).

Multifunctional Transcriptional factor NF-κB is also activated upon TCR activation and is involved in thymocyte selection as a downstream target of PKC and CD28 costimulation. NF-κB present in the cytoplasm binds to its inhibitory protein IκB. After TCR activation, phosphorylation-induced degradation of IκB allows the release and activation of sequenced cytoplasmic NF-κB. It then translocates into the nucleus to initiate downstream gene transcription. The NF-κB family has five members, and due to redundant function, NF-κB knockout mice do not clearly reveal its effects on positive selection. However, by using a genetic modification of IκB, which cannot be degraded and results in inhibited NF-κB activation, it has been shown that NF-κB activity is essential for $CD8^+$ T lymphocyte positive selection. This mutated IκB causes a substantial decrease in $CD8^+$ T lymphocytes, but only a very small percentage decrease in $CD4^+$ T lymphocyte number (Boothby, Mora, Scherer, Brockman, & Ballard, 1997; Hettmann & Leiden, 2000).

Egr (early growth response) protein is a class of transcription factors containing zinc finger structures (Swirnoff & Milbrandt, 1995). All three Egr members Egr1, Egr2 and Egr3 are expressed in thymocytes, and their expression levels are increased after TCR activation (Shao, Kono, Chen, Rubin, & Kaye, 1997). The effects of Egr2 and Egr3 on positive selection have not been extensively studied, but there is clear evidence showing that Egr1 is involved in positive selection (Miyazaki & Lemonnier, 1998). TCR transgenic mice with Egr1 overexpression exerted more efficient positive selection (Bettini, Xi, Milbrandt, & Kersh, 2002). While the Egr1-deficient TCR transgenic mice showed a three to fourfold decrease of SP cell numbers after positive selection. Egr1 expression itself is upregulated by ERK activation induced upon TCR activation (Basson et al., 2000). Activated ERK phosphorylates the downstream substrates Elk-1 and SAP-1a, both of which bind to the promoter region of Egr1 to drive Egr1 expression (Xi & Kersh, 2003).

Twist2 (Twist Family BHLH Transcription Factor 2) is another transcription factor that can be induced during thymocyte selection. In particular, positive selection TCR signals induce *Twist2* expression via the Ca^{2+}–Calcineurin–NFATc3-dependent pathway. Twist2 then functions to retain histone deacetylase 7 (HDAC7) in the nucleus and recruits it to the *Nur77* promoter region to repress *Nur77* expression in positively selected thymocytes, thus preventing cellular apoptosis. In *Twist2*-deficient mice, loss of Twist2 increases TCR sensitivity to thymocyte apoptosis in DP cells undergoing positive selection (Oh et al., 2016).

Transcription factors that play a negative role in thymocyte selection have also been discovered. Ikaros (Ikzf1) is a member of nuclear zinc-finger protein family that includes Aiolos and Helios in T cells. Ikaros was originally identified as a T lineage-specific transcription factor involved in TCR regulation, and Ikaros deficiency resulted in impaired T-cell development/activation both in vitro and in vivo. A role for Ikaros downstream of TCR signaling was further reported in Ikaros null mice, which displayed enhanced positive selection, even with reduced TCR signal strength (Oh et al., 2016).

Another example comes from the study of another transcription factor Tox (Thymocyte selection-associated high mobility group box factor). Tox is highly expressed in DP thymocytes upon TCR stimulation (Wilkinson et al., 2002). It has been shown that more DP thymocytes develop into $CD8^+$ T cells during positive selection in Tox transgenic mice. Moreover, Tox overexpression is capable of promoting $CD8^+$ T cell development in MHC class II-restricted TCR transgenic mice, suggesting that Tox overexpression may impair the TCR signal intensity which is necessary for the lineage differentiation of CD4 single positive T cells. In support of this idea, decreased thymocyte CD5 expression was observed in Tox transgenic mice during positive selection, suggesting an attenuated TCR signal (Azzam et al., 1998). Therefore, Tox may negatively regulate positive selection by diminishing the TCR signal.

3.2 Signature genes of positive selection

With technological advances in transcriptome analysis, exploring the activities of cells from the perspective of their transcriptomes has become a widely accepted means of characterizing cells subtypes or developmental stages. In 2008, under the support of the National Institutes of Health, the Immunological Genome Project (ImmGen) was launched by a number of immunologists and computational biologists across the United States. This project has now finished the transcriptome analysis of more than 250 immune cell subpopulations by using gene chip microarray analysis. The ImmGen data, as well as the specialized data browsers are now available to the public on www.immgen.org (Heng et al., 2008). In our recent study, we have analyzed the transcriptome of mouse thymocytes at different developmental stages including $CD69^{-}$ and $CD69^{int}$ DP thymocytes by using second-generation high-throughput sequencing technology. $CD69^{-}$ and $CD69^{int}$ DP thymocytes represent cells that do not receive a positive selection signal and cells that have received a positive selection signal, respectively. We found that the positive selection signal leads to expression level changes (i.e. more than twofold) of more than 2000 genes in DP cells. By analyzing this data together with gene expression changes from the same population from ImmGen ($CD69^{-}$ DP and $CD69^{+}$ DP T cell transcriptome data), we were able to create a list of conservative genes whose expression levels changed during positive selection. In the ImmGen data sets provided by the Benoist-Mathis Lab (Joslin Diabetes Center of Harvard Medical School) and the Joonsoo Kang Lab (University of Massachusetts Medical School,) we identified genes with more than twofold changes in expression levels during positive selection. By merging the microarray data sets from ImmGen and the RNAseq data from our laboratory, we obtained a positive selection gene set with 381 genes which simultaneously appeared in all three data sets. Among these genes, about 50% are up-regulated, and about 50% are down-regulated. Up-regulated genes include some known marker genes of positive selection, including *Cd53*, *Itm2a*, *Sema4a*, *H2-K1*, *Pdcd1*, with the most significant down-regulated genes *Rag1* and *Rag2* (Mick, Starr, McCaughtry, McNeil, & Hogquist, 2004). We also found genes that can indicate TCR signal intensity, such as *Cd69*, *Cd5*, and *Nr4a1* (Mingueneau et al., 2013). Transcriptional factor genes downstream of the TCR signal such as *Nfat*,

Nfkb, *Rel*, *Egr1*, *Erg2* and *Tox*, survival related genes such as *Bcl2* and *Bcl2l1*, and the migration related gene *Ccr7* were also be found in this gene set. Therefore, we named the gene set consisting of 381 genes as "positive selection signature gene set."

As discussed above, our previous work revealed the critical role of Tespa1 in promoting thymocyte positive selection through enhancing TCR-induced calcium flux signaling. Therefore, transcriptome analysis of Tespa1-deficient thymocytes under positive selection would help to reveal how TCR signaling during positive selection regulates subsequent biological events. We determined the transcriptomes of Tespa1-deficient thymocytes at the preselective (P2), under-selection (P3), and postselection (P4) stages and compared them to wild type cells at the same stages. Analysis of transcriptome data of WT and Tespa1-deficient mice by the GSEA algorithm (developed by the Broad Institute) revealed that our "positive selection signature gene set" was specifically affected at the P3 stage upon the deletion of Tespa1. Compared with WT cells, genes such as Ccr7, H2-K1, Rel, Il-7r, Bcl-2, and Nfkb2 were down-regulated, and genes such as Rag1, Rag2, and Rorc were up-regulated. In the earlier P2 stage, the absence of Tespa1 only affected the expression levels of approximately 300 genes, in which the positive selection signature genes were not present. However, at the P3 stage, along with the emerging expression of positive selection signature genes, the affected gene number by Tespa1 deficiency also increases to more than 2000. Thus the stage-specific effects of Tespa1 deficiency are also reflected in the biological processes measurable at the transcriptional level and support the previously described hypothesis that Tespa1 is a stage-specific regulator during positive selection. Hallmark gene sets are also widely used in transcriptome analysis. This consists of 50 sub-gene sets that summarize and represent well-studied biological states and processes, which are based on calculated correlations and repetitive filtering of previous data (Liberzon et al., 2015). GSEA analysis showed that, in P2 phase, Tespa1 deletion only affected three subsets of Hallmark gene sets, while in P3 phase, Tespa1 deletion negatively regulated 13 subsets. Besides the gene sets with clear functions in thymocyte selection, depletion affected some gene sets related to cytokine signaling, including the IL-2 signaling pathway, IL-6 signaling pathway, TGFβ signaling pathway and TNFα-mediated NFκB signaling pathway. Both TNFα and IFNα signals have been recently reported to be involved in thymocyte maturation. Further studies are required to verify and illuminate how TCR signaling coordinates with cytokine signaling to regulate positive selection (Xing, Wang, Jameson, & Hogquist, 2016).

4. Epigenetic regulation

Gene expression patterns are preserved through cell division by heritable modifications of DNA and chromatin, which termed as epigenetic modifications and expand the Watson–Crick base pairing information content of the genome. Two of the most characterized epigenetic modifications are DNA methylation and histone modification. T cell development, especially the lineage commitment to CD4 and CD8 SP cells during positive selection, is tightly regulated by such epigenetic mechanisms.

4.1 DNA methylation in T cell development

DNA methylation is frequently described as a "silencing" epigenetic mark and occurs in different genomic contexts: at transcriptional start sites with or without CpG islands, in gene bodies, at regulatory elements and at repeat sequences. While DNA demethylation is the process of removal of a methyl group from nucleotides in DNA, and is linked to transcriptional activation and gene expression. Genome-wide DNA methylation profiling has revealed the gain and loss of methylation occurs during human thymocyte differentiation. It has been shown that DNA demethylation was much more frequent than de novo methylation, which strongly correlates with the activation of gene expression closely associated with T-cell differentiation and TCR function (Rodriguez et al., 2015). DNA methyltransferases are needed to maintain gene silencing in T cells. For example, DNA methyltransferase I (encoded by Dnmt1) is a key factor for *Cd4* gene silencing and required for the proper expression of genes that define cell fate during thymocyte development. It has been shown that the deletion of Dnmt1 in double-positive thymocytes impaired activation-induced proliferation (Lee et al., 2001; Sellars et al., 2015). Following positive selection, DP thymocytes give rise to both $CD4^+$ and $CD8^+$ mature single-positive (SP) thymocytes. Ten-Eleven-Translocation (TET) proteins are a family of a-ketoglutarate and Fe^{2+}-dependent enzymes that alter the methylation status of DNA by converting ^{5m}C into ^{5hm}C. During positive selection, TET1 and TET3 can be recruited to E4p (a cis-acting proximal enhancer) and E4m (maturity enhancer) of the *Cd4* gene locus to orchestrate DNA demethylation, and the following removal of 5mC is required for subsequent maintenance of *Cd4* transcription after selection (Issuree et al., 2018).

4.2 Histone modification in T cell development

Histone posttranslational modifications are covalent residue modifications of histone proteins, including phosphorylation on serine or threonine, methylation on lysine or arginine, acetylation on lysine, ubiquitylation on lysine and sumolation on lysine. Histone modifications are critical epigenetic processes as they can alter chromatin structure to allow or prevent the recruitment of transcription activators or repressors.

Histone acetylation at lysine residues mediated by histone acetyltransferases is a well-studied form of modification. Histone deacetylase 1 and 2 (HDAC1/2) regulate chromatin structure as the catalytic core of the Sin3A, NuRD and CoREST corepressor complexes, and mice with reduced HDAC1/2 activity (Hdac1 deleted and a single Hdac2 allele) develop a lethal pathology by 3-months of age, caused by neoplastic transformation of immature T cells in the thymus (Dovey et al., 2013). HDAC1 and HDAC2 maintain integrity of the CD4 lineage by repressing Runx-CBFβ complexes that otherwise induces a $CD8^+$ effector T cell-like program in $CD4^+$ T cells (Boucheron et al., 2014). HDAC3 is also required for efficient T cell development, and is needed to restrain CD8-lineage genes in DP thymocytes for the generation of CD4 T cells, thus HDAC3-deficient DP thymocytes are biased towards the CD8 lineage prior to positive selection (Philips et al., 2019; Stengel et al., 2015). HDAC7 is a regulator of Nur77 and cell apoptosis in developing thymocytes (Dequiedt et al., 2003). HDAC7 represses the expression of Nur77 by interacting with MEF2D in the nucleus and plays an important role in the regulation of Nur77 expression and apoptosis in response to T cell activation. In addition, the Histone acetyltransferase complex Brd1 is crucial in activating CD8 expression in thymocytes (Mishima et al., 2014).

For histone methylation, there are also several well-known regulators. Cxxc1, an important component of the H3K4 methyltransferase complex Setd1, directly regulates promoter-associated H3K4me3 and the expression of genes that are essential for thymocyte survival and TCR signaling (Cao et al., 2016). Loss of Cxxc1 leads to a 99% reduction in the thymic cellularity, with very few DP left and almost 100% depletion of SP cells. The peripheral $CD4^+$ and $CD8^+$ T cells were also abolished due to thymocyte development inability. Cxxc1 controlls T-cell differentiation by modifying the promoter-associated H3K4me3 levels, which in turn leads to broad gene expression regulation in DP thymocytes. Cxxc1 promotes survival of thymocytes through regulating RORγt expression. Cxxc1 directly binds to Rorc gene locus and coordinates histone modifications (including H3K4me3, H3K9ac, and H3K27ac) to maintain active expression of RORγt in thymocytes. TRIM28 is required for the formation of H3K4me3 and mediates chromatin modifications at the TCRα enhancer and regulates the development of T and natural killer T cells (Zhou et al., 2012). H3K27me3 demethylase Jmjd3 and Utx, are required for $CD4^+$ T-cell differentiation in the thymus via directly regulating the expression of sphingosine phosphate receptor S1pr1 (Manna et al., 2015).

Acknowledgments

This work was supported in part by research grants to L.L from the National Natural Science Foundation of China (31770954 and 31530019). We thank Richard Sloan for assistance with language editing.

References

Azzam, H. S., Grinberg, A., Lui, K., Shen, H., Shores, E. W., & Love, P. E. (1998). CD5 expression is developmentally regulated by T cell receptor (TCR) signals and TCR avidity. *The Journal of Experimental Medicine*, *188*, 2301–2311.

Basson, M. A., Wilson, T. J., Legname, G. A., Sarner, N., Tomlinson, P. D., Tybulewicz, V. L., et al. (2000). Early growth response (Egr)-1 gene induction in the thymus in response to TCR ligation during early steps in positive selection is not required for CD8 lineage commitment. *The Journal of Immunology*, *165*, 2444–2450.

Bettini, M., Xi, H., Milbrandt, J., & Kersh, G. J. (2002). Thymocyte development in early growth response gene 1-deficient mice. *Journal of Immunology*, *169*, 1713–1720.

Boothby, M. R., Mora, A. L., Scherer, D. C., Brockman, J. A., & Ballard, D. W. (1997). Perturbation of the T lymphocyte lineage in transgenic mice expressing a constitutive repressor of nuclear factor (NF)-κB. *Journal of Experimental Medicine*, *185*, 1897–1907.

Boucheron, N., Tschismarov, R., Goeschl, L., Moser, M. A., Lagger, S., Sakaguchi, S., et al. (2014). CD4(+) T cell lineage integrity is controlled by the histone deacetylases HDAC1 and HDAC2. *Nature Immunology*, *15*, 439–448.

Cao, W., Guo, J., Wen, X., Miao, L., Lin, F., Xu, G., et al. (2016). CXXC finger protein 1 is critical for T-cell intrathymic development through regulating H3K4 trimethylation. *Nature Communications*, *7*, 11687.

Cao, Y., Li, H., Liu, H., Zhang, M., Hua, Z., Ji, H., et al. (2011). LKB1 regulates TCR-mediated PLCgamma1 activation and thymocyte positive selection. *The EMBO Journal*, *30*, 2083–2093.

Choi, S., Warzecha, C., Zvezdova, E., Lee, J., Argenty, J., Lesourne, R., et al. (2017). THEMIS enhances TCR signaling and enables positive selection by selective inhibition of the phosphatase SHP-1. *Nature Immunology*, *18*, 433–441.

Cui, J., Matkovich, S. J., deSouza, N., Li, S., Rosemblit, N., & Marks, A. R. (2004). Regulation of the type 1 inositol 1,4,5-trisphosphate receptor by phosphorylation at tyrosine 353. *The Journal of Biological Chemistry*, *279*, 16311–16316.

Dequiedt, F., Kasler, H., Fischle, W., Kiermer, V., Weinstein, M., Herndier, B. G., et al. (2003). HDAC7, a thymus-specific class II histone deacetylase, regulates Nur77 transcription and TCR-mediated apoptosis. *Immunity*, *18*, 687–698.

Douglas, N. C., Jacobs, H., Bothwell, A. L., & Hayday, A. C. (2001). Defining the specific physiological requirements for c-Myc in T cell development. *Nature Immunology*, *2*, 307–315.

Dovey, O. M., Foster, C. T., Conte, N., Edwards, S. A., Edwards, J. M., Singh, R., et al. (2013). Histone deacetylase 1 and 2 are essential for normal T-cell development and genomic stability in mice. *Blood*, *121*, 1335–1344.

Fischer, A. M., Katayama, C. D., Pages, G., Pouyssegur, J., & Hedrick, S. M. (2005). The role of Erk1 and Erk2 in multiple stages of T cell development. *Immunity*, *23*, 431–443.

Fu, G., Casas, J., Rigaud, S., Rybakin, V., Lambolez, F., Brzostek, J., et al. (2013). Themis sets the signal threshold for positive and negative selection in T-cell development. *Nature*, *504*, 441–445.

Fu, G., Vallee, S., Rybakin, V., McGuire, M. V., Ampudia, J., Brockmeyer, C., et al. (2009). Themis controls thymocyte selection through regulation of T cell antigen receptor-mediated signaling. *Nature Immunology*, *10*, 848–856.

Fujimoto, T., Matsuzaki, H., Tanaka, M., & Shirasawa, S. (2013). Tespa1 protein is phosphorylated in response to store-operated calcium entry. *Biochemical and Biophysical Research Communications*, *434*, 162–165.

Gascoigne, N. R., & Fu, G. (2012). Tespa1: Another gatekeeper for positive selection. *Nature Immunology*, *13*, 530–532.

Hayden-Martinez, K., Kane, L. P., & Hedrick, S. M. (2000). Effects of a constitutively active form of calcineurin on T cell activation and thymic selection. *The Journal of Immunology*, *165*, 3713–3721.

He, Y. W., Beers, C., Deftos, M. L., Ojala, E. W., Forbush, K. A., & Bevan, M. J. (2000). Down-regulation of the orphan nuclear receptor ROR gamma t is essential for T lymphocyte maturation. *Journal of Immunology*, *164*, 5668–5674.

Heng, T. S. P., Painter, M. W., & Project, I. G (2008). The immunological genome project: Networks of gene expression in immune cells. *Nature Immunology*, *9*, 1091–1094.

Hettmann, T., & Leiden, J. M. (2000). NF-κB is required for the positive selection of CD8+ thymocytes. *The Journal of Immunology*, *165*, 5004–5010.

Hodge, M. R., Ranger, A. M., de la Brousse, F. C., Hoey, T., Grusby, M. J., & Glimcher, L. H. (1996). Hyperproliferation and dysregulation ofIL-4 expression in NF-ATp-deficient mice. *Immunity*, *4*, 397–405.

Issuree, P. D., Day, K., Au, C., Raviram, R., Zappile, P., Skok, J. A., et al. (2018). Stage-specific epigenetic regulation of CD4 expression by coordinated enhancer elements during T cell development. *Nature Communications*, *9*, 3594.

Jenkins, M. K., Schwartz, R. H., & Pardoll, D. M. (1988). Effects of cyclosporine A on T cell development and clonal deletion. *Science*, *241*, 1655–1658.

Johnson, A. L., Aravind, L., Shulzhenko, N., Morgun, A., Choi, S. Y., Crockford, T. L., et al. (2009). Themis is a member of a new metazoan gene family and is required for the completion of thymocyte positive selection. *Nature Immunology*, *10*, 831–839.

Jones, M. E., & Zhuang, Y. (2007). Acquisition of a functional T cell receptor during T lymphocyte development is enforced by HEB and E2A transcription factors. *Immunity*, *27*, 860–870.

Kakugawa, K., Yasuda, T., Miura, I., Kobayashi, A., Fukiage, H., Satoh, R., et al. (2009). A novel gene essential for the development of single positive thymocytes. *Molecular and Cellular Biology*, *29*, 5128–5135.

Kawai, Y., Hamazaki, Y., Fujita, H., Fujita, A., Sato, T., Furuse, M., et al. (2011). Claudin-4 induction by E-protein activity in later stages of CD4/8 double-positive thymocytes to increase positive selection efficiency. *Proceedings of the National Academy of Sciences of the United States of America*, *108*, 4075–4080.

Lee, P. P., Fitzpatrick, D. R., Beard, C., Jessup, H. K., Lehar, S., Makar, K. W., et al. (2001). A critical role for Dnmt1 and DNA methylation in T cell development, function, and survival. *Immunity*, *15*, 763–774.

Lesourne, R., Uehara, S., Lee, J., Song, K. D., Li, L., Pinkhasov, J., et al. (2009). Themis, a T cell-specific protein important for late thymocyte development. *Nature Immunology*, *10*, 840–847.

Liang, J., Lyu, J., Zhao, M., Li, D., Zheng, M., Fang, Y., et al. (2017). Tespa1 regulates T cell receptor-induced calcium signals by recruiting inositol 1,4,5-trisphosphate receptors. *Nature Communications, 8*, 15732.

Liberzon, A., Birger, C., Thorvaldsdóttir, H., Ghandi, M., Mesirov, J. P., & Tamayo, P. (2015). The molecular signatures database hallmark gene set collection. *Cell Systems, 1*, 417–425.

Lo, W.-L., Donermeyer, D. L., & Allen, P. M. (2012). A voltage-gated sodium channel is essential for the positive selection of CD4+ T cells. *Nature Immunology, 13*, 880.

MacIver, N. J., Blagih, J., Saucillo, D. C., Tonelli, L., Griss, T., Rathmell, J. C., et al. (2011). The liver kinase B1 is a central regulator of T cell development, activation, and metabolism. *Journal of Immunology, 187*, 4187–4198.

Manna, S., Kim, J. K., Bauge, C., Cam, M., Zhao, Y., Shetty, J., et al. (2015). Histone H3 Lysine 27 demethylases Jmjd3 and Utx are required for T-cell differentiation. *Nature Communications, 6*, 8152.

Martinez, R. J., Morris, A. B., Neeld, D. K., & Evavold, B. D. (2016). Targeted loss of SHP1 in murine thymocytes dampens TCR signaling late in selection. *European Journal of Immunology, 46*, 2103–2110.

Matsuzaki, H., Fujimoto, T., Ota, T., Ogawa, M., Tsunoda, T., Doi, K., et al. (2012). Tespa1 is a novel inositol 1,4,5-trisphosphate receptor binding protein in T and B lymphocytes. *FEBS Open Bio, 2*, 255–259.

Mick, V. E., Starr, T. K., McCaughtry, T. M., McNeil, L. K., & Hogquist, K. A. (2004). The regulated expression of a diverse set of genes during thymocyte positive selection in vivo. *Journal of Immunology, 173*, 5434–5444.

Mingueneau, M., Kreslavsky, T., Gray, D., Heng, T., Cruse, R., Ericson, J., et al. (2013). The transcriptional landscape of alphabeta T cell differentiation. *Nature Immunology, 14*, 619–632.

Mishima, Y., Wang, C., Miyagi, S., Saraya, A., Hosokawa, H., Mochizuki-Kashio, M., et al. (2014). Histone acetylation mediated by Brd1 is crucial for Cd8 gene activation during early thymocyte development. *Nature Communications, 5*, 5872.

Miyazaki, T., & Lemonnier, F. A. (1998). Modulation of thymic selection by expression of an immediate-early gene, early growth response 1 (Egr-1). *Journal of Experimental Medicine, 188*, 715–723.

Molina, T. J., Kishihara, K., Siderovski, D. P., van Ewijk, W., Narendran, A., Timms, E., et al. (1992). Profound block in thymocyte development in mice lacking p56lck. *Nature, 357*, 161–164.

Negishi, I., Motoyama, N., Nakayama, K., Nakayama, K., Senju, S., Hatakeyama, S., et al. (1995). Essential role for zap-70 in both positive and negative selection of thymocytes. *Nature, 376*, 435–438.

Oh, S., Oh, J., Lee, C., Oh, S., Jeon, S., Choi, J., et al. (2016). Expression of Twist2 is controlled by T-cell receptor signaling and determines the survival and death of thymocytes. *Cell Death and Differentiation, 23*, 1804–1814.

Paster, W., Brockmeyer, C., Fu, G., Simister, P. C., de Wet, B., Martinez-Riano, A., et al. (2013). GRB2-mediated recruitment of THEMIS to LAT is essential for thymocyte development. *Journal of Immunology, 190*, 3749–3756.

Patrick, M. S., Oda, H., Hayakawa, K., Sato, Y., Eshima, K., Kirikae, T., et al. (2009). Gasp, a Grb2-associating protein, is critical for positive selection of thymocytes. *Proceedings of the National Academy of Sciences of the United States of America, 106*, 16345–16350.

Phee, H., Dzhagalov, I., Mollenauer, M., Wang, Y., Irvine, D. J., Robey, E., et al. (2010). Regulation of thymocyte positive selection and motility by GIT2. *Nature Immunology, 11*, 503–511.

Philips, R. L., Lee, J. H., Gaonkar, K., Chanana, P., Chung, J. Y., Romero Arocha, S. R., et al. (2019). HDAC3 restrains CD8-lineage genes to maintain a bi-potential state in CD4(+)CD8(+) thymocytes for CD4-lineage commitment. *eLife, 8*, e43821.

Rodriguez, R. M., Suarez-Alvarez, B., Mosen-Ansorena, D., Garcia-Peydro, M., Fuentes, P., Garcia-Leon, M. J., et al. (2015). Regulation of the transcriptional program by DNA methylation during human alphabeta T-cell development. *Nucleic Acids Research*, *43*, 760–774.

Sebzda, E., Mariathasan, S., Ohteki, T., Jones, R., Bachmann, M. F., & Ohashi, P. S. (1999). Selection of the T cell repertoire. *Annual Review of Immunology*, *17*, 829–874.

Sellars, M., Huh, J. R., Day, K., Issuree, P. D., Galan, C., Gobeil, S., et al. (2015). Regulation of DNA methylation dictates Cd4 expression during the development of helper and cytotoxic T cell lineages. *Nature Immunology*, *16*, 746–754.

Shao, H., Kono, D. H., Chen, L. Y., Rubin, E. M., & Kaye, J. (1997). Induction of the early growth response (Egr) family of transcription factors during thymic selection. *Journal of Experimental Medicine*, *185*, 731–744.

Stengel, K. R., Zhao, Y., Klus, N. J., Kaiser, J. F., Gordy, L. E., Joyce, S., et al. (2015). Histone deacetylase 3 is required for efficient T cell development. *Molecular and Cellular Biology*, *35*, 3854–3865.

Swirnoff, A. H., & Milbrandt, J. (1995). DNA-binding specificity of NGFI-A and related zinc finger transcription factors. *Molecular and Cellular Biology*, *15*, 2275–2287.

Wang, D., Zheng, M., Lei, L., Ji, J., Yao, Y., Qiu, Y., et al. (2012). Tespa1 is involved in late thymocyte development through the regulation of TCR-mediated signaling. *Nature Immunology*, *13*, 560–568.

Wilkinson, B., Chen, J. Y.-F., Han, P., Rufner, K. M., Goularte, O. D., & Kaye, J. (2002). TOX: An HMG box protein implicated in the regulation of thymocyte selection. *Nature Immunology*, *3*, 272.

Xi, H., & Kersh, G. J. (2003). Induction of the early growth response gene 1 promoter by TCR agonists and partial agonists: Ligand potency is related to sustained phosphorylation of extracellular signal-related kinase substrates. *The Journal of Immunology*, *170*, 315–324.

Xie, H., Huang, Z., Sadim, M. S., & Sun, Z. (2005). Stabilized β-catenin extends thymocyte survival by up-regulating Bcl-xL. *The Journal of Immunology*, *175*, 7981–7988.

Xing, Y., Wang, X., Jameson, S. C., & Hogquist, K. A. (2016). Late stages of T cell maturation in the thymus involve NF-kappaB and tonic type I interferon signaling. *Nature Immunology*, *17*, 565–573.

Zhou, X. F., Yu, J., Chang, M., Zhang, M., Zhou, D., Cammas, F., et al. (2012). TRIM28 mediates chromatin modifications at the TCRalpha enhancer and regulates the development of T and natural killer T cells. *Proceedings of the National Academy of Sciences of the United States of America*, *109*, 20083–20088.

CHAPTER TWO

B cell mechanosensing: A mechanistic overview

Samina Shaheen, Zhengpeng Wan, Kabeer Haneef, Yingyue Zeng, Wang Jing, Wanli Liu*
Center for life sciences, MOE Key Laboratory of Protein Sciences, Collaborative Innovation Center for Diagnosis and Treatment of Infectious Diseases, Beijing Key Lab for Immunological Research on Chronic Diseases, School of Life Sciences, Institute for Immunology, Tsinghua University, Beijing, China
*Corresponding author: e-mail address: liulab@tsinghua.edu.cn

Contents

Abstract

B cells are essential to the adaptive immune system for providing the humoral immunity against cohorts of pathogens. The presentation of antigen to the B cell receptor (BCR) leads to the initiation of B cell activation, which is a process sensitive to the stiffness

Advances in Immunology, Volume 144
ISSN 0065-2776
https://doi.org/10.1016/bs.ai.2019.08.003

features of the substrates presenting the antigens. Mechanosensing of the B cells, potentiated through BCR signaling and the adhesion molecules, efficiently regulates B cell activation, proliferation and subsequent antibody responses. Defects in sensing of the antigen-presenting substrates can lead to the activation of autoreactive B cells in autoimmune diseases. The use of high-resolution, high-speed live-cell imaging along with the sophisticated biophysical materials, has uncovered the mechanisms underlying the initiation of B cell activation within seconds of its engagement with the antigen presenting substrates. In this chapter, we reviewed studies that have contributed to uncover the molecular mechanisms of B cell mechanosensing during the initiation of B cell activation.

1. The initiation of B cell activation

B lymphocytes (B cells) generate protective antibodies upon recognition of pathological antigens. Following the recognition of antigen, B cell activation leads to subsequent cellular responses that include their proliferation and differentiation into plasma and memory B cells (Pierce & Liu, 2010; Rajewsky, 1996). Extracellular matrix (ECM) of the cells is highly complex and enriched with diverse antigenic information including antigen density (Fleire et al., 2006; Liu, Meckel, Tolar, Sohn, & Pierce, 2010a; Tang et al., 2016; Wang et al., 2016), affinity (Fleire et al., 2006; Liu, Meckel, et al., 2010a), valency (Bachmann et al., 1993; Liu et al., 2004; Liu & Chen, 2005) and their Brownian mobility (Wan & Liu, 2012). B cells and T cells use their surface expressed antigen receptors to sense wide arrays of external antigens (Saitakis et al., 2017; Shaheen et al., 2017; Wan et al., 2013; Zeng et al., 2015). B cell receptor (BCR) is composed of a membrane-bound entity of immunoglobulin (Ig) and an Igα–Igβ heterodimer in a 1:1 stoichiometry (Pierce & Liu, 2010). Engagement of the BCR and antigen leads to the initiation of B cell activation, the representative feature is that discrete puncta rich with BCR molecules (referred as BCR microclusters) are formed between the interface of B cells and antigen presenting substrate (Pierce & Liu, 2010). In the case of T cell, TCR microclusters are also formed in the initiation of TCR activation (Bachmann & Jennings, 2010; Carrasco & Batista, 2007). Typically, *in vivo*, lymphocytes encounter antigens presented on the antigen presenting cells (APC) which harbor multitudes of diverse stiffness features (Junt et al., 2007). For example, viruses and immune complexes are mainly presented to B cells by macrophages, dendritic cells lining the subcapsular sinuses, and the well-appreciated follicular dendritic cells (Phan, Grigorova, Okada, & Cyster, 2007; Qi, Egen, Huang, & Germain, 2006). It has been proved that the degree of stiffness of the substrates presenting the antigens efficiently regulates the activation of both B and T cells (Bashour et al., 2014; Dustin & Groves, 2012; Judokusumo, Tabdanov, Kumari, Dustin, & Kam, 2012; O'Connor et al., 2012; Saitakis et al., 2017; Shaheen et al., 2017; Tesniere et al., 2008; Wan et al., 2013; Zeng et al., 2015). While investigating the activation of B cells upon recognition of these types of membrane-bound antigens, the stiffness features of both APCs and B cells cannot be neglected due to the formation of complex membrane structures involving multiple receptors, ligands, and signaling molecule interactions, referred to as the immunological synapse, between the membrane interface of APCs and B cells (Schaefer, 2010). Thus, the formation of BCR microclusters and the B cell immunological synapse are two key early events in the initiation of B cell activation (Fleire et al., 2006; Liu et al., 2004; Liu, Meckel, et al., 2010a; Pierce & Liu, 2010).

2. Mechanosensing

Cells interact with the complex mechanical environments by sensing the physical perturbations and using the surface receptors to generate chemical signals to initiate subsequent cellular responses through a process named mechanotransduction (Gasiorowski, Murphy, & Nealey, 2013; Guillou et al., 2016; Ingber, 2006; Liu, Chen, & Zhu, 2015; Orr, Helmke, Blackman, & Schwartz, 2006; Sun, Chen, & Fu, 2012; Uffmann et al., 2004). Mechanosensing is essential for various phenomena, ranging from cell movements and tissue structure rearrangements to cell differentiation and the immune responses (Discher, Janmey, & Wang, 2005; Pelham & Wang, 1997). Cells of the adaptive immune system including B lymphocytes and T lymphocytes, use their surface receptors (BCRs and TCRs) to sense the exogenous antigenic information. Physical cues from the antigen not only can regulate B cell activation by applying a mechanical force on the BCR but can also have diverse effects on different B cell subsets (Nowosad, Spillane, & Tolar, 2016; Spillane & Tolar, 2017; Upadhyaya, 2017). During the last decade, the ability of the cells to sense and acquire information from their surroundings has been proven. The information is subsequently utilized to initiate the corresponding signaling pathways and alter the gene expression and their fate.

2.1 Substrate stiffness/rigidity

Stiffness or rigidity is one of the particular parameters of mechanosensing. Interestingly, cells and tissues show diversity in stiffness values. For example, human T cells, with a range of 0.1 kPa, are considered very soft in nature (Bufi et al., 2015; Guillou et al., 2016). Furthermore, stiffness of skeletal muscle and calcified bone reaches to 10 kPa and GPa, respectively (Oakes et al., 2009; Trappmann et al., 2012). Stiffness is considered to influence several processes, including cell survival, migration, growth and differentiation of many type of cells (Asano et al., 2017; Bangasser et al., 2017; Hassanisaber et al., 2019; Hui, Balagopalan, Samelson, & Upadhyaya, 2015; Huse, 2017; Husson, Chemin, Bohineust, Hivroz, & Henry, 2011; Judokusumo et al., 2012; Mennens et al., 2017; O'Connor et al., 2012; Tabdanov et al., 2015; Xia et al., 2018; Zhao et al., 2018). It also plays a key role in regulating the activation of cell receptors, and their signaling and intracellular communications (Huse, 2017). Substrate stiffness can affect the activation of T and B cells (Husson et al., 2011; Judokusumo et al., 2012; O'Connor et al., 2012; Saitakis et al., 2017; Shaheen et al., 2017; Tabdanov et al., 2015; Wan et al., 2013; Zeng et al., 2015), the forces they delivered to lymphocytes (Hui et al., 2015; Husson et al., 2011), as well as the cytotoxicity of T lymphocytes (Basu et al., 2016).

2.2 Tools employed for B cell mechanical sensing

Recent advancements in the live cell imaging and biophysical techniques (Table 1) have enabled the observation and analysis of the fundamental aspects of B cell responses toward different substrates presenting the antigen (Davey, Liu, Sohn, Brzostowski, & Pierce, 2012; Pierce, 2009). Through these approaches, it became possible to elucidate the underlying molecular mechanism by which B cells can discriminate the differences in stiffness of the antigen presenting substrates. It has now become possible to study the mechanical sensing regulation of different autoimmune diseases like rheumatoid arthritis (RA) (Shaheen et al., 2017; Wang et al., 2018).

Polyacrylamide (PA) and polydimethylsiloxane (PDMS) gel systems, with variety of stiffness range, have been widely used in force related studies (Hassanisaber et al., 2019; Huang et al., 2009; Mennens et al., 2017; O'Connor et al., 2012; Qin, Huang, Xiong, Zhang, & Fang, 2007; Shaheen et al., 2017; Tamzalit et al., 2019; Wan et al., 2013; Wang et al., 2018; Xia et al., 2018; Xing et al., 2014; Zeng et al., 2015; Zhao et al., 2018). PA gels belong to the class of biocompatible hydrogels which have

Table 1 Tools employed for measuring mechanical force.

Technique	Principle
PA, PDMS elastomers	Biocompatible nature of polyacrylamide (PA) and polydimethylsiloxane (PDMS) gel systems, with variety of stiffness range, have enabled their use in force related studies. PA/PDMS forms a planar surface with highly hydrophobic features that can easily tether proteins through adsorption. Confocal microscopy can be used to image the cells
Atomic force microscopy	This approach (AFM) is utilized for the measurements of minute forces to a calibrated and flexible cantilever. Typically, it involves pressing the cantilever tip into the sample from top for generating positive deflections to mimic the physical properties of samples or coating of cantilever tip and surface of the sample with interacting proteins. Subsequent, contact and withdrawal of the tip induces negative deflections used for measurement of binding strength (Noy, 2011)
Traction force microscopy	TFM uses deformable substrates to image the cells. The substrates contain fluorescent fiducially probes that are used for the measurement of force produced due to the cells (Dembo & Wang, 1999). Alternatively, synthetic micropillars (Tan et al., 2003) can also be used to attach the cells and measurement of force using the known parameters of the pillars i.e. height, width and composition
Biomembrane force probe	In this technique, red blood cells (RBCs) attached with a stimulatory bead and immobilized at the end of micropipette, are used as force transducers. This system offers to mimic stiffness of a broader range and measurement of force ranging from 0.01 pN to 1 nN (Chen, Zarnitsyna, Sarangapani, Huang, & Zhu, 2008; Evans, Ritchie, & Merkel, 1995)
Tension-gauge tether	This method involves immobilization of ligands using DNA duplexes to target specific receptors (Wang & Ha, 2013). The sequences, their lengths and junction points with the attached ligand determine the rupture force (Liu, Blanchfield, et al., 2016; Zhang, Ge, Zhu, & Salaita, 2014). Real time detection of single molecule pulling events is achievable by second-generation tension gauge tethers
Intracellular tension sensors	Here, the Forster resonance energy transfer (FRET) donor and acceptor are used for the detection of force above certain threshold and visualization of intracellular forces at subcellular levels. The donor and acceptor are typically separated by a folded peptide (Borghi et al., 2012; Conway et al., 2013; Grashoff et al., 2010)
Magnetic and optical trapping	In these approaches, magnetic field or focused laser beams are used for optical trapping of particles under piconewton-scale restoring forces. The subject particle under investigation can be fixed to surface by biomolecular linkage and used for measuring the pulling force (Moffitt, Chemla, Smith, & Bustamante, 2008; Sarkar & Rybenkov, 2016)

been used for bacterial cell culture and have been proven instrumental in studying the effect of substrate stiffness on the morphology of mammalian cells (Engler, Griffin, et al., 2004; Engler, Richert, Wong, Picart, & Discher, 2004; Rehfeldt, Engler, Eckhardt, Ahmed, & Discher, 2007; Tuson, Renner, & Weibel, 2012). Interestingly, the physical properties of PA gels including the stiffness can be modified (Baker, Murff, & Milam, 2010). PDMS is a biocompatible organosilicon elastomer that has been used as an anticaking or antibloating agent. These unique features make it ideal for long-term cell culture based experiments and *in vivo* immunization experiments. PDMS forms a planar surface with highly hydrophobic features that can easily tether proteins through adsorption (Mateu, 2012). It is known that stiffer and softer PDMS might differ in their microarchitecture, although such an effect is much milder than that on a PA gel system (Hui et al., 2015). In T cell studies, PDMS substrate with softer (20 kPa) or stiffer (1100 kPa) stiffness were used (Engler, Griffin, et al., 2004; Mateu, 2012). Whereas in B cell studies, PDMS substrates have been used to evaluate the effects of substrate stiffness on B-cell activation, proliferation, class-switch differentiation *in vitro* and T cell-independent antibody responses *in vivo* (Shaheen et al., 2017; Wan et al., 2013; Zeng et al., 2015). Furthermore, Tension gauge tethered (TGT) system based on double stranded DNA (dsDNA) specifically nitrophenol-conjugated TGT (NP-TGT) was employed to study the mechanical threshold sense by B cells (Wan et al., 2015, 2018). DNA molecule shows an excellent force application geometry which has been accurately calculated by an *in vitro* single molecular force measurements (Albrecht et al., 2003; Lang, Fordyce, Engh, Neuman, & Block, 2004).This system was developed by Ha and colleagues (Wang & Ha, 2013), in which they used these TGT sensors to probe the tension on a single integrin-ECM ligand named cyclic RGDfK bond which is required for cell adhesion. However, we have modified this system by conjugating these TGTs with 4-Hydroxy-3-nitrophenylacetyl (NP) to the ligand chain which are known as NP-TGTs. We acquired 8TGT sensors with their predefined mechanical force of 12, 16, 23, 33, 43, 50, 54 and 56 pN. High resolution high speed live cell imaging techniques *via* total internal reflection fluorescence microscopy (TIRFM) was used to analyze the activation of BCRs in response to these TGTs (Wan et al., 2015, 2018).

3. Substrate stiffness regulates B cell activation

Immune cells get activated when the membrane receptors engage with cognate antigens on the surface of APCs. It has been illustrated that

B and T cell signaling is responsive toward the physical and mechanical signals (Upadhyaya, 2017). One of the obvious but unanswered question is that how likely it is that antigen presenting substrates can have different stiffness features *in vivo*? Or is it possible that the B cells encounter a microenvironment of variable stiffness? The answer to the question is probably yes. The *in vivo* presentation of B cells to the substrates of variable stiffness remained understudied for many years (Bachmann & Jennings, 2010; Junt et al., 2007). The term stiffness refers to the rigidity, which shows the extent of that object to resist the deformations after application of force on it. Young's modulus is commonly used to describe the stiffness of an elastic substrate. For instance, the Young's modulus value of different viral particles ranges from 45 to 1000 MPa (Mateu, 2012), while most of the mammalian cells show medium stiffness features ranging from 0.01 to 1000 kPa (Phan et al., 2007). Secreted soluble pathogen antigens in our plasma only exhibit very low stiffness of no more than 100 Pa (Araujo Gde et al., 2012). Thus, substrates presenting the antigens on rigid virus capsid vesicles exhibit high stiffness features; those on the membrane of the virus-infected host cells show medium level stiffness; while those in a soluble form, as in the case of secreted pathogen antigens in body fluid, only exhibit extremely low stiffness. Likewise, the ECM associated antigens acquired by B cells in the antigen and BCR contact manner (Ciechomska et al., 2014), have the stiffness in the range from 0.012 kPa to 20 kPa in the tissues (Bao & Suresh, 2003; Engler, Griffin, et al., 2004; Nemir & West, 2010; Paszek et al., 2005). The impact of stiffness features of antigen presenting substrates on the activation of B cells after the engagement of BCR to the antigen has been highlighted in limited studies. Tolar and colleagues have demonstrated that B cells use the mechanical energy to examine the strength of antigen binding which lead to the B cell capability to discriminate the antigen affinity (Natkanski et al., 2013). By employing the advance live cell imagining technologies, it has been shown that the initiation of B cell activation depends on the formation of BCR microclusters and the immunological synapse immediately after the recognition of antigen by the BCR (Xu et al., 2014). Using PA gel substrates with stiffness feature ranging from a 2.6 to 22.1 kPa Young's modulus, we observed that the initiation of B cell activation immediately after BCR-antigen recognition is very sensitive to the stiffness feature of the substrates presenting the antigens (Wan et al., 2013).

3.1 Effect of stiffness on BCR microcluster formation

BCR microcluster is a basic platform in B cell activation, allowing the efficient assembly of the membrane-proximal BCR signalosome

(Harwood & Batista, 2010; Liu, Meckel, et al., 2010a). Although BCR microcluster is not a steady-state membrane structure, unlike TCR microcluster which exists in the absence of ligands (Campi, Varma, & Dustin, 2005; Liu, Wang, & Xu, 2016; Saito & Yokosuka, 2006; Xu et al., 2019). Evidences have suggested that TCR exists in the monomeric and nanocluster form independent of antigen ligand (Molnár et al., 2012) but BCR also forms nanocluster in the resting lymphocytes (Liu, Wang, et al., 2016). Upon antigen biding nanocluster of both the antigen receptors i.e. TCR and BCR along with the nanocluster of signaling molecules form microcluster (Liu, Wang, et al., 2016). Several lines of studies demonstrated that during their formation, BCR microclusters exhibit morphological changes (Batista, Treanor, & Harwood, 2010; Weber et al., 2008; Xu et al., 2014). BCR microclusters grow both in the number of BCRs within each microcluster and in the geometric dimensions (size) of each microcluster, providing a mechanism to amplify signaling (Liu, Meckel, et al., 2010a; Wang et al., 2016; Xu et al., 2017). Moreover, the BCR microcluster growth is subjected to the fine regulation by the BCR-activating coreceptor CD19 and inhibitory coreceptor FcγRIIB (Liu, Won Sohn, Tolar, Meckel, & Pierce, 2010; Xu et al., 2014, 2016). BCR microcluster growth also provides explanations for some of the basic aspects of B cell responses, including antigen affinity discrimination and the value of class switching, as well as insights into the underlying causes of B cell tumorigenesis (Pierce & Liu, 2010; Thauland & Parker, 2010; Wang et al., 2017; Xu et al., 2016). BCR microclusters with growth features can be formed after the antigen recognition by BCR (Wang et al., 2017). Evidences suggested that antigen-binding induced the dynamic growth feature of BCR microclusters was affected by stiffness (Wan et al., 2013). The integrated fluorescence intensity (FI) of each individual BCR microcluster induced by antigens tethered to stiffer *versus* softer PDMS substrates was quantified. Following a 2D Gaussian function-based mathematical fitting of each BCR microcluster (Liu, Meckel, et al., 2010a). Integrated FI was accurately quantified for hundreds of such BCR microclusters that were induced by antigens in these two types of conditions. Prominent and larger BCR microclusters were observed on the substrate with higher stiffness presenting the antigen (Wan et al., 2013). Likewise, Pearson's correlation index analysis showed the enhanced colocalization of pTyr and pSyk with the BCR microclusters on the antigen presenting stiffer substrate (Wan et al., 2013). These findings suggest that BCR microcluster formation can be greatly influenced by the stiffness features of the substrates presenting the antigen.

3.2 Effect of mechanosensing on immunological synapse formation

Evenly distributed BCRs on the cell surface at resting stage become polarized and accumulate into the contact area between the cell and the planar antigen-presenting surface which eventually leads to the formation of a typical immunological synapse (Liu, Won Sohn, et al., 2010; Pierce & Liu, 2010). Evidences have shown the formation of immunological synapse (highly organized 3D structure made up of surface and cytoplasmic molecules) at the interface of APC and the T cell during the antigen recognition which modulates the immune responses and effector responses in the event of T cell activation (Carroll-Portillo et al., 2015; Gupta et al., 2006; Kumari et al., 2015; Milone & Kam, 2013; Rodriguez-Fernandez, Riol-Blanco, & Delgado-Martin, 2010; Thauland & Parker, 2010). Targeting the synapse has helped to establish immunotherapy as a mainstream element in cancer treatment (Dustin, 2014).

The B cell immunological synapse is a critical structure for the initiation of signaling, the acquisition and subsequent internalization of foreign antigens. It would be interesting to know how the formation of the B cell immunological synapse is affected by antigen tethered to the substrates with different stiffness features. B cells and T cells recognize their cognate antigens on the surfaces of other cells, either as immobilized whole protein in the case of B cells or as short peptides bound to MHC molecules in the case of T cells. The engagement of antigenic ligands by the B cell receptor or T cell receptor rapidly induces robust intracellular signaling responses, which lead within minutes to the formation of an immunological synapse between the lymphocyte and the antigen-presenting cell. Classical immunological synapses are defined by a stereotyped concentric architecture in which a central cluster of antigen receptors is surrounded by concentric, annular accumulations of integrin and F-actin molecules (Carroll-Portillo et al., 2015; Gupta et al., 2006; Kumari et al., 2015). According to these observations, this organization promotes strong adhesion to and cytoskeletal polarization toward the APC, and it also excludes inhibitory molecules such as the phosphatase CD45. Immunological synapses can persist for dozen of minutes to hours, and they represent the cell-biological context in which T cells and B cells undergo activation and mount effector responses.

Zeng et al. investigated that the formation of B cell immunological synapse on the PDMS surface with different stiffness through TIRFM. First to compare the effect on more physiological surface, planer lipid bilayer (PLB)

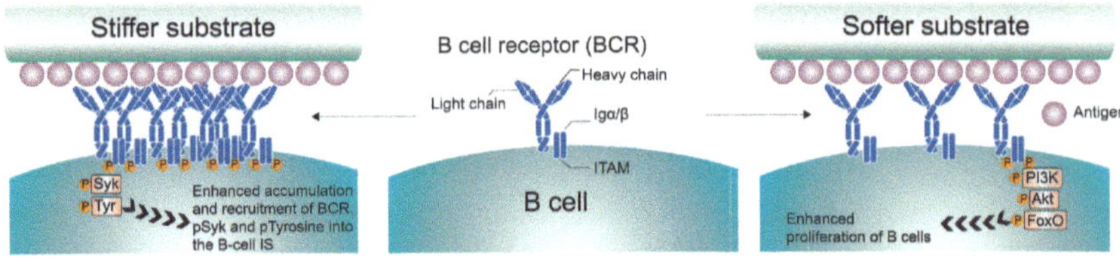

Fig. 1 B cell responses toward different substrates. The formation of BCR microclusters and the B cell immunological synapse are two key early events in the initiation of B cell activation. B cells show enhance recruitment of pSyk and pTyr into B cell IS on the stiffer substrate in the event of its activation. However, B cells show enhanced expansion on softer substrates. This is well supported by the enhanced phosphorylation of PI3K, Akt and FoxO1 molecules of B cells on the softer substrate.

on PDMS was employed and was subsequently quantified for the amount of the presented Alexa 568 and biotin-conjugated NP8-BSA to make sure that comparable density of NP8-BSA were tethered to the PLBs in the case of stiffer vs softer PDMS (Zeng et al., 2015). More BCR pTyr and pSyk molecules were accumulated to the immunological synapse of B1–8 primary B cells when encountering antigens tethered to stiffer substrates (Fig. 1). Likewise, by using confocal fluorescence microscopy, we observed the formation of a typical B cell immunological synapse with the accumulation of BCR and signaling molecule microclusters into the contact interface between the B cells and the antigen-containing planar gels (Liu, Meckel, Tolar, Sohn, & Pierce, 2010b; Wan et al., 2013). Accumulation of BCR, pSyk, and pTyr molecules into the B cell immunological synapse was significantly enhanced on the substrate presenting the antigen with the higher stiffness compared to antigen presented on the substrate with the lower stiffness (Wan et al., 2013; Zeng et al., 2015). These observations are also consistent with a study by Kam and colleagues investigating the mechanosensing capability of T cells using a PA gel based experimental system, showing that the activation of T cells was obviously enhanced upon encountering stiffer substrate, as quantified by the recruitment of pSFK and pZAP70 into immunological synapse (Judokusumo et al., 2012).

3.3 BCR isotypes activation exhibit distinct mechanical force threshold

BCR and signaling molecule microclusters induced by antigen on substrates with high stiffness are much more prominent and show enhanced colocalization as compared with substrates of low stiffness (Zeng et al., 2015). A multithreshold effect of mechanical force was observed during the analysis of generated IgM-BCR microclusters on different TGTs (Wan et al., 2015). Quantifying the microclusters of the signaling molecule pSyk, pPLCγ2, and pTyr demonstrated that the volume of these signaling molecule microclusters produced by different NP-TGT molecules is also dependent on mechanical force with a multithreshold effect (Wan et al., 2015). Thus the evidence supported that BCR signaling is highly dependent on the strength of the mechanical force, but different type of BCRs have different activation thresholds of mechanical force. Wan et al. have examined the mechanical force induced activation of all the five types of isotypes of membrane bound BCRs including IgM, IgD, IgA, IgG and IgE (Wan et al., 2018). Evidence suggests that IgM-, IgD- and IgA-BCR shared the same multithreshold. For example BCR accumulation was higher on high-mechanical force (56 pN) NP-TGTs while it was found moderate on the medium level of mechanical force NP-TGTs and was very weak on the lower level of mechanical force threshold (12 pN). In contrast, IgG- and IgE-BCRs preferred low threshold of mechanical force for their activation as the recruitment of the BCRs was equal on all of the NP-TGT surfaces (12, 43 and 56 pN) (Wan et al., 2018). It was found that IgM-BCR requires a multithreshold effect of mechanical force during its activation. While, the isotype-switched IgG- or IgE-BCR requires a low level of mechanical threshold. Low threshold of IgG-BCR activation *via* mechanical force crucially dependent on the cytoplasmic tail of the IgG-BCR heavy chain i.e. IgG-tail tethered to the plasma membrane (Wan et al., 2018). Mechanistically, Wan et al. have elucidated that in the IgG tail, positively charged residues play significant role by highly enriching phosphatidylinositol (4,5)-bisphosphate (PI(4,5)P2) into the membrane microdomains of IgG-BCRs. Manipulating the amount of (PI(4,5)P2) within the membrane microdomains of IgG-BCR have significantly altered the threshold and the sensitivity of activation of IgG-BCR. Thus we revealed a lipid-dependent mechanism for determining the mechanical force threshold for IgG-BCR activation (Wan et al., 2018).

4. B cells exert and sense the mechanical forces

It is now well established that lymphocyte activation is a mechanosensitive process. This property was initially documented by experiments in which T cells and B cells were stimulated on deformable matrices that were coated with activating ligands (Douglass & Vale, 2005; Judokusumo et al., 2012; Pore et al., 2013; Saitakis et al., 2017;

Treanor, Depoil, Bruckbauer, & Batista, 2011). Recent work has revealed that the mechanical activity of the synapse also has a crucial role in potentiating cytotoxicity. This discovery was enabled by the adaptation of single-cell biophysical approaches to measure synaptic forces. Using both standard gel based traction force microscopy (TFM) and a higher-resolution approach in which cells were imaged on arrays of deformable micropillars (Table 1), it was found that T cells exert nano-newton scale forces against antigen-presenting surfaces (Hu & Butte, 2016). Similar observations were made by a study in which individual T cells are presented with stimulatory beads attached to long, mechanically calibrate micropipettes (Basu et al., 2016). Available data suggest that after encountering membrane-bound antigen, B cells first exhibit a substantial spreading response on the antigen presenting surface followed by contraction responses (Depoil et al., 2009). This indicate that dynamic traction forces can be generated between the B cell and the surface presenting antigens. However, B cell exert traction force was poorly characterized. Wang et al. have used TFM to profile the origin, dynamics and the function of traction force generation within the B cell immunological synapse during B cell activation. We observed that B cells generate 10–20 nN of traction force upon encountering with the antigen presented on the substrate with stiffness of 0.5–1 kPa (Wang et al., 2018). Notably, studies have demonstrated that this stiffness value mimic the stiffness of antigen presenting cells *in vivo* (Bufi et al., 2015; Rosenbluth, Lam, & Fletcher, 2006; Spillane & Tolar, 2017).

As cells strain against adhesions to move forward, they exert force against the underlying matrix. TFM has been employed to measure the forces directly. These studies have revealed intriguing differences between leukocyte cell types. In neutrophils, force exertion concentrates at the rear, near the boundary between the cell body and the uropod (Califano & Reinhart-King, 2010; Ghibaudo et al., 2008). Extended, fully activated integrins also cluster in this region (Schnyder et al., 2011; Treanor et al., 2010). The same pattern of integrin activation is seen in migrating T cells (Keren et al., 2008), implying that T cells have a similar force profile to that of neutrophils. By contrast, in macrophages and DCs, peak traction forces are observed near the front of the advancing cell (Chen, Irianto, et al., 2012; Natkanski et al., 2013). This suggests a profile similar to fibroblasts and endothelial cells, which form strong integrin-mediated adhesions at the base of their lamellipodia (Balestrini & Billiar, 2006; Isenberg & Tranquillo, 2003). Antigen presented on substrates with high stiffness, substantially facilitates the formation of the B cell immunological synapse and the initiation of B cell activation compared with antigens presented on the substrates with low stiffness (Shaheen et al., 2017; Wan et al., 2013; Zeng et al., 2015). In general, lymphocytes exhibited stronger signaling responses and cytokine secretion on stiff surfaces than they do on softer surfaces, which is consistent with the idea that antigen receptors pull against their ligands to achieve an optimal signaling capacity (Huse, 2017). Interestingly, peak ligand-induced proliferation was observed at intermediate, rather than high, levels of substrate stiffness. Although the basis for this discrepancy remains unclear, it is possible that the robust signaling observed for high-stiffness substrates triggers activation-induced cell death, which could adversely affect lymphocyte expansion. Nevertheless, these studies made it clear that the mechanical properties of antigen-presenting surfaces strongly influence lymphocyte activation (Huse, 2017).

5. Regulation of B cell mechanosensing through motor proteins

In the case of adherent cells and lymphocytes, they require myosin-based contractility to sense extracellular matrix stiffness (Assoian & Klein, 2008; Engler, Sen, Sweeney, & Discher, 2006; Judokusumo et al., 2012; Trichet et al., 2012). Additionally, to match their matrix properties, these cells modulate their contractile forces by exerting stronger forces on the stiffer surfaces and exert weaker forces on the softer surfaces (Califano & Reinhart-King, 2010; Elosegui-Artola et al., 2016; Ghibaudo et al., 2008; Hui et al., 2015; Saez, Buguin, Silberzan, & Ladoux, 2005). Therefore, the mechanical life of a cell particularly depends on the continuous cytoskeletal remodeling and the signal transduction (Huse, 2017). Successive studies have demonstrated that the organization of B cell cytoskeleton provides crucial support in the event of B cell activation by maintaining the dynamic growth features of microclusters of BCR and signaling molecules (Schnyder et al., 2011; Treanor et al., 2010, 2011). The importance of actin cytoskeleton in the B cell activation coupled with BCR signaling has been also demonstrated in detail (Tolar, 2017). Furthermore, in the B cell immunological synapse, the centripetal movement of BCR microclusters has been shown to be coordinated by the cytoskeleton, motor proteins and the BCR signaling molecules (Schnyder et al., 2011). Several lines of studies have shown that the membrane cytoskeleton and the motor proteins play a key role in the morphology changes and the cell mechanics (Chen, Irianto, et al., 2012; Keren et al., 2008; Kozlov & Mogilner, 2007).

Considering these observations, it is valid to speculate that BCR might have this capability to sense the substrate presenting antigens. This property of BCR may allow it to coordinate the molecular events during the initiation of B cell activation. This speculation is very well supported by the two contemporary studies on T cell mechanosensing (Judokusumo et al., 2012; O'Connor et al., 2012), with the pharmaceutical approach. Using several cytoskeletal inhibitors, we determined that the B cell mainly depend on the microtubules for discrimination of the substrate with various stiffnesses while, it only mildly links to the actin cytoskeleton in this event (Zeng et al., 2015). Motor proteins including myosin IIA and dynein are known to play important roles in B cell activation. Evidences have supported that the B cells utilize the contraction forces generated by myosin IIA to rupture the interaction between the BCR and antigen molecules (Natkanski et al., 2013).While dynein is required for the retrograde motile feature of the BCR microclusters into the center of B cell immunological synapse (Schnyder et al., 2011). We also assessed the contribution of these two motor proteins in NP-TGT sensors to see their dependence on the multithreshold force during the activation of B cells. Unexpectedly, the inactivation of myosin IIA did not dramatically change the dependence on mechanical forces, however we observed a significant drop in the strength of the synaptic accumulation of the BCRs for the high threshold NP-TGT sensor and no drop was observed for the medium-level threshold NP-TGT sensor, nor the low threshold NP-TGT sensor (Wan et al., 2015). On the other hand, when inactivating dynein, we did not observe significant changes in the BCR accumulations compared to DMSO controls. These evidences suggest that the breakthroughs of the high end but not the medium-level and low-end thresholds of mechanical forces are supported by myosin IIA (Wan et al., 2015). On the other hand, generation of traction force in B cells after recognizing the antigen relied on the remodeling of microfilament and motor proteins including dynein and the myosin. Moreover, we also observed that the requirement of membrane-proximal BCR signaling molecules and the adaptor molecules linking BCR microclusters and motor proteins to sustain traction force generation (Wang et al., 2018).

6. Substrate stiffness regulates B cell proliferation, differentiation and antibody responses

The microenvironment B cells will likely encounter *in vivo* is quite divers in stiffness. More importantly, it is known that the substrate stiffness can regulate the proliferation and differentiation of mesenchymal stem cells (MSCs) and embryonic stem (ES) cells (Discher, Mooney, & Zandstra, 2009; Sun et al., 2012). For example, softer substrates (0.1–1 kPa) tend to cause MSCs to differentiate into neuronal cells, whereas stiffer substrates (8–17 kPa) give rise to myocyte-like cells and the stiffest substrate (Liao, Huang, Zhu, Xiong, & Fang, 2010) (25–40 kPa) results in osteoblast-like cells (Engler et al., 2006). Matrix stiffness also modulates phenotypes of cancer cells. Tissue stiffness, determined mainly by the ECM, increases during progression of breast and other (though not all) cancers; breast cancer cells in stiff 3D matrices show more aggressive behavior such as luminal filling, invasion, and epithelial-mesenchymal transition (EMT) (Levental et al., 2009; Provenzano, Inman, Eliceiri, & Keely, 2009). By contrast, growing the same cells in soft matrix typical of normal tissue promotes a differentiated, epithelial, less invasive phenotype (Levental et al., 2009; Provenzano et al., 2009). These results strongly suggest that mechanical consequences of matrix remodeling are a causal factor in cancer progression. They also concord with the general notion that the mesenchymal phenotype is associated with a higher force regime than the epithelial cells. This information suggests that the downstream proliferation and differentiation of B cells following the initiation of their activation might also be subjected to the regulation of substrate stiffness. It will also be interesting to elucidate the potential of stiffness feature of the substrates presenting the antigens in affecting the antibody responses *in vivo*.

6.1 Proliferation and class switch

B cell proliferation can be driven by the Lipopolysaccharide (LPS) stimuli, cognate antigen or CD40. Interestingly, bacteria are also known to possess quite diverse range of stiffness ranging from 50 kPa to 769 MPa (Tuson, Auer, et al., 2012). Therefore, it is very likely that B cells can encounter stiffer or softer bacterial cells *in vivo*. Nevertheless, the available data indicate that softer substrate coated with antigen showed enhanced proliferation of mouse primary B cell. While, anti-CD40 antibody tethered stiffer substrates have shown mildly enhanced proliferation of mouse primary B cells compared to the case of softer substrates (Zeng et al., 2015). On the other hand, the effect of coating antigen and anti-CD40 on the substrates was similar. This fact support the idea that BCR and CD40 co-ordinate and balance the force sensing dependent proliferation responses of B cells. Conclusively, B cell proliferation by using force sensing ability is also regulated by the co-ordination of TLR4, CD40 and BCR (O'Connor et al., 2012; Zeng et al., 2015). Likewise in the T cells, force sensing ability is strongly associated with CD3 rather with CD28 (Bashour et al., 2014; Judokusumo et al., 2012). In the case of *in vitro* evidence, it is indicated that class-switch differentiation of B cell through LPS and IL-4 have similar effects on softer or stiffer substrate as were indicated *in vivo* (Zeng et al., 2015). In the meantime, it is also the evident that B cell shows enhance recruitment of pSyk and pTyr into B cell immunological synapse on the stiffer substrate in the event of its activation (Zeng et al., 2015). It cannot be neglected that T cells have the same preference of T cell expansion on softer substrate (Bashour et al., 2014), while they also show enhance recruitment of pSFK and pZAP70 on stiffer substrate in T cell activation (Judokusumo et al., 2012). We speculate that B and T cell proliferation efficiencies can be determined by multisignaling pathways among which the activation of PI3K-Akt-FoxO1 plays an important role (Fruman et al., 1999; Okkenhaug, Bilancio, Emery, & Vanhaesebroeck, 2004; Okkenhaug & Vanhaesebroeck, 2003). This speculation is well supported by Weiss and colleagues that there is a sharp TCR signaling (measured as Zap70) threshold for the proof of cell division *in vivo* and *in vitro* (Au-Yeung et al., 2014). To the notice, this threshold is a fixed value that is actually independent of the magnitude of TCR stimulus. On the contrary, they identified a temporal threshold of TCR signaling which is required for the proliferation of T cell. Upon reaching this temporal threshold, T cell will undergo proliferation independent of Zap70 kinase (Au-Yeung et al., 2014). We have observed that the phosphorylation of PI3K, Akt and FoxO1 molecules of B cells is enhanced significantly on the softer substrate (Fig. 1). Hence the above point provides an explanation mechanistically for the enhanced activation of B cell on the softer substrate which we believe can also explain the similar situation in the case of T cells. Furthermore, Reth and his colleague showed that cre-mediated Syk deletion in $Syk^{flox/Zap\text{-}70}$ mouse primary B cells reduced the phosphorylation of Erk but not the phosphorylation of Akt (Konigsberger et al., 2015). This observation suggests that it is not likely that B cell activation has to require the coupled signaling of Syk and Akt molecules (Konigsberger et al., 2015).

6.2 Softer substrate enhances antibody responses in vivo

Evidences have supported that the stiffness features of the substrate presenting the antigen will dramatically affect the mutagenicity of those antigens and will enhance B cell expansion. For example, it is observed that anti-Ig (anti-IgM antibody as a surrogate antigen) conjugated with dextran will be potent up to 1000 folds to drive the B cell expansion *in vitro* as compared to the unconjugated soluble anti-Ig (Brunswick et al., 1989). Next in line evidence has also suggested that T cell independent type 1 and type 2 have different antibody responses by immunizing the mice with TNP (Trinitrophenyl) conjugated with different type of carriers including dextran, brucella and ficoll (Mond et al., 1983; Yaffe, Mond, Ahmed, & Scher, 1983). We have also found that antibody response in mice immunized with T cell independent antigen NP67-ficoll coated on softer substrate was significantly higher compared to the stiffer substrate coated with the same antigen (Zeng et al., 2015).

7. Integrin as a potential mechanosensor

The major types of integrin molecules expressed by B cells are leukocyte function-associated antigen-1 (LFA-1) (αLβ2) and very late antigen-4 (VLA-4) (α4β1) (Arana, Harwood, & Batista, 2008). The ligands of LFA-1 and VLA-4 are adhesion molecules i.e. intercellular adhesion molecules (ICAM-1/2) and vascular cell adhesion molecule-1 (VCAM-1), respectively (Arana, Harwood, et al., 2008) which are also widely expressed on other type of cells like DCs and follicular dendritic cells (FDCs) (Freedman et al., 1990; Koopman et al., 1991; Kushnir, Liu, & MacPherson, 1998). It is well established that the cells are capable of sensing the mechanical signals from the microenvironment by the conventional mechanosensor i.e. integrin (Ross et al., 2013; Sun, Guo, & Fässler, 2016). As discussed by Campbell and Humphries, integrins undergo complex conformational rearrangements that govern both affinity for extracellular matrix proteins and associations with cytoskeletal proteins (Calvete, 2004; Campbell & Humphries, 2011; Wegener & Campbell, 2008). Reconstitution with β1-class integrins promotes myosin-II-independent formation of small peripheral adhesions and cell protrusions, whereas expression of αv-class integrins induces the formation of large focal adhesions. Co-expression of both integrin classes leads to full myosin activation and traction-force development on stiff fibronectin-coated substrates (Schiller et al., 2013). Experimental data supports the idea that integrin conformation can be modulated by the applied force (Friedland, Lee, & Boettiger, 2009; Puklin-Faucher, Gao, Schulten, & Vogel, 2006). Studies of the leukocyte integrin LFA-1 also suggest a role of force in integrin conformation (Jin, Andricioaei, & Springer, 2004; Xie et al., 2010; Zhu et al., 2008). Integrins play an important role in mediating the effects of mechanical force and growth factors on blood vessels in hypertension (Chao & Davis, 2011).The data also suggested that integrin adhesion receptors can modulate the attachment of breast cancer cells to bone matrix molecules (van der Pluijm et al., 1997). Application of tension to cells through their integrin-mediated adhesions, often by stretching cells on elastic substrata, regulates a wide range of signaling pathways, downstream genes and differentiation programs. These effects are of considerable physiological and pathological significance because the experimental system mimics stretching of tissues *in vivo*. Cardiac hypertrophy and remodeling of the smooth muscle layers in arteries represent two examples of integrin-dependent processes that are of particular clinical relevance (Brancaccio et al., 2006; Heerkens, Izzard, & Heagerty, 2007; Heerkens, Quinn, Withers, & Heagerty, 2014).

7.1 Bidirectional regulation of integrins

Integrins are known to receive two signals for their regulation. Inside-out activation of integrin depends on the signal initiate from inside of the cell. While the outside-in activation of integrin depends on the interaction with the ligand which induces the signal from membrane and allow the cell to sense the information from extracellular environment (Mehrbod, Trisno, & Mofrad, 2013; Shen, Delaney, & Du, 2012; Ye, Kim, & Ginsberg, 2011). LFA1 is the predominant integrin on T and B cells, and it binds tightly to the intercellular adhesion molecule 1 (ICAM-1) and ICAM-2. LFA1 has an essential role in lymphocyte activation as it mediates tight adhesion to the target cell and then transduces outside-in signals that promote effector responses (Pribila, Quale, Mueller, & Shimizu, 2004; Yi, Wu, Crites, & Hammer, 2012). Interaction between LFA-1 and ICAM-1 in germinal center B cells (GCBs) prevents apoptosis (Koopman et al., 1994). As the results showed that the CD98hc as an integrin binding domain may be important for the B cell proliferation (Cantor et al., 2009).

7.2 Integrin mediated B cell mechanosensing

ICAM-1, an adhesion molecule present on the surface of activated APCs and endothelial cells, is the ligand of the integrin LFA-1 and a key regulator of T cell migration and activation (Altmann, Hogg, Trowsdale, & Wilkinson, 1989; Van Seventer, Shimizu, Horgan, & Shaw, 1990). Following ICAM-1 binding, LFA-1 can be modulated by mechanical forces (Chen & Zhu, 2013; Springer & Dustin, 2012) and promote T cell migration (Jacobelli, Bennett, Pandurangi, Tooley, & Krummel, 2009; Morin et al., 2008). In the experimental system by Kam and colleagues or by Milone and colleagues, no adhesive molecules were used but anti-CD3 and/or anti-CD28 surrogate antigens (Bashour et al., 2014; Judokusumo et al., 2012; O'Connor et al., 2012). These T cell studies, in addition to the B cell studies presented in this chapter, show that mechanosensing by lymphocyte cells may not solely function through direct interaction between ICAM-1 and the well-characterized mechanosensor LFA-1 (Chen, Lou, Evans, & Zhu, 2012; Chen, Lou, & Zhu, 2010). However, direct ICAM-1 and LFA-1 interactions may still be required to maintain and regulate the mechanosensing ability of lymphocyte cells as other studies have shown that they can fine-tune the activation of both B and T cells (Arana, Harwood, et al., 2008; Arana, Vehlow, et al., 2008; Carrasco, Fleire, Cameron, Dustin, & Batista, 2004; McLeod, Shum, Lee, Takei, & Gold, 2004; Spaargaren et al., 2003). Considering this, Shaheen et al. observed that the presence of adhesion molecules (ICAM-1 or VCAM-1) greatly enhanced the B cells' capability to discriminate between the degrees of stiffness (Shaheen et al., 2017). At the molecular level, several different experimental approaches involving ligand valency indicated that crosslinking of three or more integrins was crucial for the sensing and signaling of surface rigidity (Coussen, Choquet, Sheetz, & Erickson, 2002). Thus, to confirm this conclusion we used splenic primary B cells from CD11a (ITGAL) knockout (KO) mice, which lack the lymphocyte function-associated antigen 1 (LFA-1) (Shaheen et al., 2017). Interestingly, recent studies indicate that germinal center B cells recognize antigens on antigen presenting cells through a specialized immune synapse architecture that is distinct from that of mature naïve B cells (Nowosad et al., 2016). Moreover, it has also been reported that specialized APC such as FDCs, are usually stiff cells that can promote the efficient antigen extraction and stringent affinity discrimination of GCBs, while regular dendritic cells that are mainly responsible for the antigen presentation for mature naïve B cells are mostly soft (Spillane & Tolar, 2017). Based on the published studies, we propose that adhesion molecules on antigen-presenting cells in germinal centers play an important role in enhancing the activation of GCBs. Indeed, this is supported by a recent study showing that integrin-ligand interaction within the germinal center B cells and the antigen presenting follicular dendritic cells (FDCs) are important for the responses in GC (Wang, Rodda, Bannard, & Cyster, 2014). PA-gels have also been used with three different Young's modulus values i.e. 0.5, 6.4 and 100 kPa for respectively mimicking the typical stiffness range reported for human monocyte-derived dendritic cells (Bufi et al., 2015), human endothelial cells (Kataoka et al., 2002; Mathur, Collinsworth, Reichert, Kraus, & Truskey, 2001) and tendon tissue or bone (Gasiorowski et al., 2013; Oakes et al., 2009). PA-gels, which do not allow for nonspecific adsorption of serum proteins, were coated with recombinant biotinylated ICAM-1/Fc chimeric molecules. Stiffness affects the ICAM-1-dependent migration of human CD4+ T lymphoblast. Indeed, mean instantaneous velocities and traveled distances are increased for T cells on ICAM-1 coated 100kPa gels as compared to 0.5 and 6.4kPa gels (Jacobelli et al., 2009). These results correlate with the fact that mechanically induced transitions of LFA-1/ICAM-1-binding promoted T cell migration (Jacobelli et al., 2009; Morin et al., 2008) and APC scanning (Comrie, Li, Boyle, & Burkhardt, 2015). Since the adhesion and activation of lymphocytes requires integrin and adhesion molecules *in vivo* under physiological conditions (Arana, Vehlow, et al., 2008). It could follow that the capability of B cells to discern substrate stiffness is also regulated by the direct activation of integrins with external adhesion molecules (Shaheen et al., 2017). The addition of ICAM-1 dramatically enhanced the synaptic accumulation of the BCRs, suggesting the increased sensitivity to antigen stimulation in the initiation of B cell activation, consistent with the published studies in both the BCR (Carrasco et al., 2004) and TCR system (Bachmann et al., 1997; Dustin, 2009). However, it was clear that the outside-in activation of integrin did not change the fact that B cell activation is dependent on mechanical forces with a similar multithreshold effect (Wan et al., 2015).

8. BCR signaling dependent B cell mechanosensing

Shaheen et al. investigated the molecular nature of the mechanosensor machinery used by the B cells to distinguish substrate stiffness in the absence of adhesion molecule-triggered integrin activation. The screening of a library of chicken DT40 B cell lines deficient for specific signaling molecules (Kurosaki, 1999; Kurosaki, Shinohara, & Baba, 2010), including Lyn, Syk, PLCγ2, Btk, BLNK, PKCβ and Carma-1, was performed to dissect the underlining molecular mechanism. The first striking observation was that only BCR signaling dependent, not independent, accumulation of BCRs into the B cell immunological synapse is subjected to strict regulation by the mechanosensing capability of B cells. It is also indicated that the BCR signaling-independent accumulation of BCRs and/or antigens was likely induced by the passive trapping of BCRs and antigens into the B cell immunological synapse, since both types of molecules exhibit free Brownian thermal diffusion before recognition (Liu, Meckel, et al., 2010a, 2010b; Tolar, Hanna, Krueger, & Pierce, 2009; Weber et al., 2008). Furthermore, it is also indicated that both signaling-independent signaling-dependent mechanisms account for the accumulation of BCRs into the BCR microclusters. These two steps are not mutually exclusive, but are instead closely related in a sequential and synergistic way to maximize efficient BCR clustering. Specifically, signaling-independent BCR clustering initiates the earliest signaling upon antigen and BCR recognition, which further enhances BCR clustering in a signaling-dependent manner. Furthermore, the initial signaling-independent accumulation of BCRs into the BCR microclusters is not sensitive to the stiffness features of the substrates whereas the subsequent signaling-dependent accumulation of BCRs into the BCR microclusters is. Therefore, it is reasonable to conclude that the thermal diffusion-mediated and BCR signaling-independent passive trapping of BCR molecules is not sensitive to substrate stiffness since the Brownian diffusion of BCRs on the plasma membrane would not be affected by the stiffness of the substrates.

Through major efforts, the role of BCR signaling transduction in enabling the B cells to discriminate between substrate stiffness during the initiation of B cell activation was elucidated. PKCβ is the most downstream signaling molecule among Lyn, Syk, PLCγ2, Btk, and BLNK (Shinohara et al., 2005). A canonical function of PKCβ in B cell activation is to directly phosphorylate the downstream signaling molecule Carma-1 at Ser-559, Ser-644 and Ser-652, which induces the association of Carma1 with Bcl10 and Malt1. The formation of Carma1, Bcl10 and Malt1 (CBM) signaling complexes leads to the activation of NF-κB (Shinohara et al., 2005; Su et al., 2002). However, the activation of NF-κB leads to a downstream gene expression signature in B cells at a late time point, usually hours after the initial BCR and antigen recognition, whereas substrate stiffness discrimination in B cells occurs within the few minutes following interaction between the BCR and antigen. Therefore, it was speculated that the PKCβ-mediated NF-κB activation would not contribute to the capabilities of B cells to discriminate substrate stiffness. Indeed, it was found that Carma1-KO DT-40 B cells effectively maintained their discrimination capability (Shaheen et al., 2017). The initiation of B cell activation is dependent on the adhesion of B cells to the surface of the substrate presenting the antigen. We thus assessed the potential requirement of PKCβ in the discrimination capability of B cells through its function in regulating B cell adhesion responses. Our hypothesis was based on published studies showing that PKC family members play key roles in mediating the adhesion responses of many types of mammalian cells through "inside–out" activation of integrin molecules (Besson, Wilson, & Yong, 2002; Buensuceso et al., 2005; Disatnik, Boutet, Lee, Mochly-Rosen, & Rando, 2002; Haller et al., 1998). Mechanistically, these results indicated that PKCβ functions downstream of Btk and PLCγ2, since PMA (phorbol myristate acetate) induced activation of PKCβ can bypass the requirements of Btk and PLCγ2 for discriminating substrate stiffness, demonstrating the vital importance of PKCβ in mediating the capability of B cells to discriminate between substrate stiffness (Shaheen et al., 2017). The involvement for PKCβ-mediated NF-κB activation was excluded by showing that Carma1-KO B cells still managed to maintain their discrimination capability. This result makes sense since the activation of NF-κB leads to alterations in gene expression profiles in B cells at a later time point (on the scale of hours), while the substrate stiffness discrimination capability of B cells kicks in minutes after the initial BCR and antigen interaction. Then, the next question becomes which molecular mechanisms determine this dependence of PKCβ and other upstream BCR signaling molecules for the substrate stiffness discrimination of B cells? Some interesting insights were provided by the observation that the membrane proximal BCR signaling molecules including Btk, PLCγ2, BLNK and PKCβ are essential for the inside–out activation of integrin molecules (Arana, Harwood, et al., 2008; Arana, Vehlow, et al., 2008; Spaargaren et al., 2003). With these findings that the outside-in activating signal of integrin significantly enhanced the capability of B cells to discriminate substrate stiffness, the hypothesis that PKCβ-dependent FAK activation accounts for the substrate stiffness discrimination capability of B cells was validated.

9. Role of FAK in B cell mechanical force sensing

Focal adhesion kinase (FAK) considered to be a key player in the cell adhesion responses mediated by mechanosensing (Avraham, Park, Schinkmann, & Avraham, 2000; Bashour et al., 2014; Slack-Davis et al., 2007; Yu, Fay, Smoligovets, Wu, & Groves, 2012). As one of the important regulator of integrin activation, FAK is a member of non-receptor tyrosine kinase family that was first identified as a focal contact in 1970. Focal contact is a multiprotein structure having integrin at its center providing the mechanical link to the extracellular matrix regulating the inside-out and outside-in signaling (Abercrombie, Heaysman, & Pegrum, 1971; Curtis, 1964; Izzard & Lochner, 1976). By the analysis of molecular regulation of force-dependent reinforcement of cell–matrix contacts, several proteins involved in mechanosensing were identified (Galbraith, Yamada, & Sheetz, 2002; Giannone, Jiang, Sutton, Critchley, & Sheetz, 2003; Sawada et al., 2006; von Wichert et al., 2003). Stretching of the exposed cytoskeletons following Triton X-100 treatment revealed force-dependent binding of several adhesion proteins to the cytoskeleton, including FAK (also known as PTK2) (Sawada & Sheetz, 2002; Sawada et al., 2006). FAK is expressed in almost all tissues, notably, increased expression and activation of Pyk2 and FAK has been found in a number of metastatic cancers (Alexopoulou et al., 2014; Behmoaram et al., 2008; Lark et al., 2003, 2005; Munshi, Ganju, Avraham, Mesri, & Groopman, 1999; Owens et al., 1995, 1996; Tremblay et al., 1996). Their correlation with invasive phenotype in cancer cells together with their contribution to cell adhesion, motility, and cell cycle regulation have positioned FAK as potential targets for disease modulation, particularly in cancer cell metastasis (Brunton & Frame, 2008).

Mechanical forces also regulate cell migration. Cells grown on flexible substrates show enhanced rates of cell migration compared with rigid substrates (Pelham & Wang, 1997). On matrices that have boundaries between regions of different elasticities, cells migrate toward areas of higher substrate rigidity, a process termed durotaxis (Wang, Dembo, Hanks, & Wang, 2001). This effect requires expression of FAK suggesting that this molecule is involved in sensing forces (Lo, Wang, Dembo, & Wang, 2000). Moreover, it has also been reported that FAK is required for the chemoattractant-induced migration and adhesion response in B cells (Tse et al., 2012).

FAK plays a key role in the activation of integrin signaling pathways by providing a key docking site for Src family kinases, which in turn phosphorylate downstream signaling molecules (Bashour et al., 2014; Slack-Davis et al., 2007; Yu et al., 2012). Specifically, early biochemical studies demonstrated that FAK phosphorylation at Tyr-925 regulates cross-talk between focal adhesion turnover and cell protrusion in embryonic fibroblasts (Deramaudt et al., 2011). Indeed, FAK inactivation completely blunted the capability of the B cells to discriminate substrate stiffness, which could be rescued by the exogenous expression of FAK-WT but not the inactivated mutant at Tyr-925 (Shaheen et al., 2017). Mechanistically, FAK activation is triggered by BCR engagement in a PKCβ-dependent manner (Shaheen et al., 2017). These findings suggest that integrin-induced FAK phosphorylation can be blocked by inhibiting PKC, and that the PKC activator, PMA, drastically enhanced the phosphorylation, and thus activation, of FAK (Disatnik & Rando, 1999). Further colocalization analyses indicated that pFAK is mainly localized to the peripheral region of the B cell immunological synapse, and highly colocalized with F-actin, strongly suggesting that FAK activation supported B cell spreading and adhesion responses (Shaheen et al., 2017). Indeed, additional analyses demonstrated that PKCβ-dependent FAK activation accounts for B cell discrimination of stiffness by potentiating B cell spreading and adhesion responses (Shaheen et al., 2017). These findings in B cells show that the spreading and adhesion responses of B cells are regulated by typical PKC-mediated FAK activation. A similar observation was reported in muscle cells and also in the case of snail defense cells from *Lymnaea stagnalis* (Disatnik & Rando, 1999; Walker, Lacchini, Sealey, Mackintosh, & Davies, 2010). In short, we have demonstrated that PKCβ-dependent FAK activation accounts for B cell discrimination of stiffness during the initiation of B cell activation (Fig. 2).

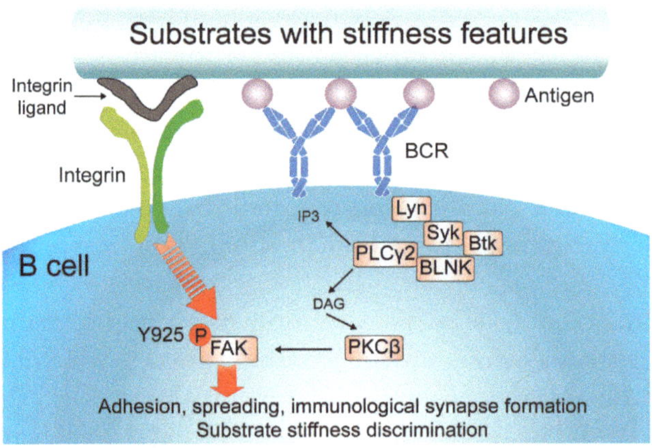

Fig. 2 Molecular mechanism of B cell mechanical sensing of different substrates. B cells have the capability to discriminate substrate stiffness through BCR signaling and integrin activation dependent mechanism. Membrane proximal signaling cascade of BCR including Lyn, Syk, PLCγ2 and PKCβ are crucial player of B cell mechanical sensing. Activation of integrin through ligand binding is important in the regulation of B cell activation through adhesion. PKCβ-dependent FAK activation accounts for B cell discrimination of stiffness by spreading and adhesion responses during the initiation of B cell activation.

10. Pathological significance of mechanosensing

Evidences suggest that cells or tissues can greatly modify their stiffness in pathological situations. Inflammation usually cause increase in the stiffness, on the other hand, tumors become stiffer than normal tissues during metastasis (Bufi et al., 2015; Mathur et al., 2001; Paszek et al., 2005). Some other groups have reported that infection and the tumor necrosis factor mediated signaling also become the cause of stiffness of the arteries (Dulai et al., 2012; Evani & Ramasubramanian, 2016; Park & Lakatta, 2012). This kind of pathological situation might modulate the efficiency of T cell scanning by tissue stiffening. Furthermore, transformation and malignancy are associated with cellular softening (Birge, Kalodimos, Inagaki, & Tanaka, 2009; Schwickert et al., 2011; Tolar & Spillane, 2014). It has been revealed that the leukemic cells and the metastatic cancer cells are generally softer in the range of 0.05–0.2 kPa (Rosenbluth et al., 2006), thus showing another type of mechanism of immune evasion. Therefore, stiffness of the environment is probably a key regulator of T cell migration and antigen detection *in vivo*. Hence, it is unlikely that B cell mechanosensing will not contribute toward the disease environment.

11. Role of B cell mechanosensing in autoimmune disease

Abnormal recognition of self-antigen by B and T cells leads to the production of autoantibodies in autoimmune diseases. B cells are known to be involved in the pathogenesis of autoimmune diseases like systemic lupus erythematosus (SLE) or RA and diabetes type1 (Martin & Chan, 2006; Shlomchik, 2009; Yanaba et al., 2008). In these diseases the mechanism of initiation of inflammatory process includes the loss of tolerance and hyperactivation leads to the production of autoantibodies, self-antigen presentation to the T cell and cytokine production (Carroll-Portillo et al., 2015; Liu, Meckel, et al., 2010b). B cells acquire ECM associated antigens in a BCR and contact-dependent manner (Ciechomska et al., 2014), in the presence of a considerable range of stiffness of ECM in the tissue, from 0.012 kPa to 20 kPa (Bao & Suresh, 2003; Engler, Griffin, et al., 2004; Nemir & West, 2010; Paszek et al., 2005). The ECM-associated microenvironment is an abundant source of antigens (Knight, 2015; Schaefer, 2010; Tesniere et al., 2008).The capability of B cells to sense the stiffness features of antigen-presenting surfaces may be related to the pathological activation of auto-reactive B cells in autoimmune disease patients. For example, in patients with RA, reduced cartilage stiffness leads to the activation of auto-antigen reactive B cells, which subsequently causes the production of autoantibodies (Mauri & Ehrenstein, 2007). These clinical reports strongly suggest that the altered stiffness properties of the ECM are linked to the aberrant activation of auto-antigen reactive B cells. However, it is unknown whether the primary B cells in RA patients maintain their capability to discriminate the stiffness of the substrates presenting antigens, and if so, how such capabilities differ from primary B cells derived from healthy individuals. We have demonstrated that RA patients exhibit disordered or weaker mechanosensing capability as compared to the healthy controls (Fig. 3) (Shaheen et al., 2017). Likewise, RA patients generated higher traction forces compared to healthy donors (Wang et al., 2018). These findings have obvious clinical relevance as there is a diverse range in stiffness features of the antigen presenting substrates as well as changes in substrate stiffness at the physiological level *versus* pathological conditions which are associated with disease (Knight, 2015). It is also known that the auto-reactive human primary B cells from RA patients can efficiently acquire the autoantigen aggrecan, in a BCR and adhesion-dependent manner (Ciechomska et al., 2014) and RA patients usually exhibit highly enriched B cells in the synovia (Nakken et al., 2011). It is speculated that the altered stiffness properties of the ECM, which displays the autoantigens, can drive the autoreactive B cells to break the energy state and instead undergo aberrant activation. The reduced cartilage stiffness is known to render B cells into auto-antigen presenters in RA patients, which subsequently causes the production of autoantibodies (Mauri & Ehrenstein, 2007). Since the ECM-associated microenvironment provides an abundant source of antigens, it has been proposed that any change in ECM stiffness could be identified as a threatening signal by the immune system and thus trigger the response from immune cells (Knight, 2015; Schaefer, 2010; Tesniere et al., 2008). It is therefore an intriguing hypothesis that the capability of B cells to sense the stiffness features of antigen presenting surfaces may be potentially related to the detection of that danger by the immune system (Knight, 2015).

Our findings shed light on the precise molecular mechanism of how B cells discriminate substrate stiffness through a PKCβ- and FAK-dependent manner during the initiation of B cell activation, improving our understanding of the sophisticated mechanosensing capability of B cells. By employing the more recent technologies like TGTs, 3D culture systems and genetically

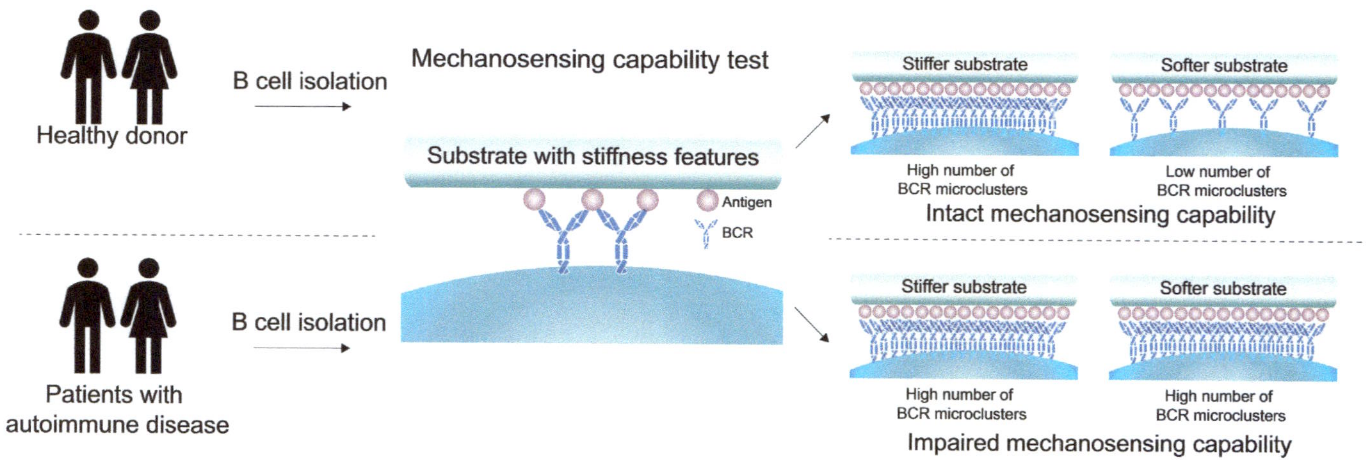

Fig. 3 Altered B cell mechanosensing in RA patients. B cells from healthy controls preferentially enhanced the synaptic accumulation of BCR microclusters on stiffer substrates. In marked contrast, B cells from RA patients exhibited a different preference of enhancing the accumulation on softer substrates.

encoded tension sensor modules and the patterned surfaces along with the development of the new methods to measure the force and investigate the underlying mechanism should be the direction for the future. We also propose that the mechanosensing and mechanotransducing abilities of immune cells deserve further investigation as these studies can enhance our understanding of immune cell activation upon antigen recognition and may help build better vaccines to ultimately cure autoimmune diseases.

Acknowledgments

This work is supported by funds from National Science Foundation China (81825010, 81730043, 81621002 and 31811540397).

Conflict of interest disclosure

The authors declare no financial or commercial conflict of interest.

References

Abercrombie, M., Heaysman, J. E., & Pegrum, S. M. (1971). The locomotion of fibroblasts in culture. IV. Electron microscopy of the leading lamella. *Experimental Cell Research*, *67*(2), 359–367.

Albrecht, C., Blank, K., Lalic-Mülthaler, M., Hirler, S., Mai, T., Gilbert, I., et al. (2003). DNA: A programmable force sensor. *Science*, *301*(5631), 367–370.

Alexopoulou, A. N., Ho-Yen, C. M., Papalazarou, V., Elia, G., Jones, J. L., & Hodivala-Dilke, K. (2014). Tumour-associated endothelial-FAK correlated with molecular sub-type and prognostic factors in invasive breast cancer. *BMC Cancer*, *14*, 237.

Altmann, D. M., Hogg, N., Trowsdale, J., & Wilkinson, D. (1989). Cotransfection of ICAM-1 and HLA-DR reconstitutes human antigen-presenting cell function in mouse L cells. *Nature*, *338*(6215), 512–514.

Arana, E., Harwood, N. E., & Batista, F. D. (2008). Regulation of integrin activation through the B-cell receptor. *Journal of Cell Science*, *121*(Pt. 14), 2279–2286.

Arana, E., Vehlow, A., Harwood, N. E., Vigorito, E., Henderson, R., Turner, M., et al. (2008). Activation of the small GTPase Rac2 via the B cell receptor regulates B cell adhesion and immunological-synapse formation. *Immunity*, *28*(1), 88–99.

Araujo Gde, S., Fonseca, F. L., Pontes, B., Torres, A., Cordero, R. J., Zancope-Oliveira, R. M., et al. (2012). Capsules from pathogenic and non-pathogenic Cryptococcus spp. manifest significant differences in structure and ability to protect against phagocytic cells. *PLoS One*, 7(1), e29561.

Asano, S., Ito, S., Takahashi, K., Furuya, K., Kondo, M., Sokabe, M., et al. (2017). Matrix stiffness regulates migration of human lung fibroblasts. *Physiological Reports*, *5*(9), e13281.

Assoian, R. K., & Klein, E. A. (2008). Growth control by intracellular tension and extracellular stiffness. *Trends in Cell Biology*, *18*(7), 347–352.

Au-Yeung, B. B., Zikherman, J., Mueller, J. L., Ashouri, J. F., Matloubian, M., Cheng, D. A., et al. (2014). A sharp T-cell antigen receptor signaling threshold for T-cell proliferation. *Proceedings of the National Academy of Sciences of the United States of America*, *111*(35), E3679–E3688.

Avraham, H., Park, S. Y., Schinkmann, K., & Avraham, S. (2000). RAFTK/Pyk2-mediated cellular signalling. *Cellular Signalling*, *12*(3), 123–133.

Bachmann, M. F., & Jennings, G. T. (2010). Vaccine delivery: A matter of size, geometry, kinetics and molecular patterns. *Nature Reviews. Immunology*, *10*(11), 787.

Bachmann, M. F., McKall-Faienza, K., Schmits, R., Bouchard, D., Beach, J., Speiser, D. E., et al. (1997). Distinct roles for LFA-1 and CD28 during activation of naive T cells: Adhesion versus costimulation. *Immunity*, 7(4), 549–557.

Bachmann, M. F., Rohrer, U. H., Kundig, T. M., Burki, K., Hengartner, H., & Zinkernagel, R. M. (1993). The influence of antigen organization on B cell responsiveness. *Science*, *262*(5138), 1448–1451.

Baker, B. A., Murff, R. L., & Milam, V. T. (2010). Tailoring the mechanical properties of polyacrylamide-based hydrogels. *Polymer*, *51*(10), 2207–2214.

Balestrini, J. L., & Billiar, K. L. (2006). Equibiaxial cyclic stretch stimulates fibroblasts to rapidly remodel fibrin. *Journal of Biomechanics*, *39*(16), 2983–2990.

Bangasser, B. L., Shamsan, G. A., Chan, C. E., Opoku, K. N., Tüzel, E., Schlichtmann, B. W., et al. (2017). Shifting the optimal stiffness for cell migration. *Nature Communications*, *8*, 15313.

Bao, G., & Suresh, S. (2003). Cell and molecular mechanics of biological materials. *Nature Materials*, *2*(11), 715–725.

Bashour, K. T., Gondarenko, A., Chen, H., Shen, K., Liu, X., Huse, M., et al. (2014). CD28 and CD3 have complementary roles in T-cell traction forces. *Proceedings of the National Academy of Sciences of the United States of America*, *111*(6), 2241–2246.

Basu, R., Whitlock, B. M., Husson, J., Le Floc'h, A., Jin, W., Oyler-Yaniv, A., et al. (2016). Cytotoxic T cells use mechanical force to potentiate target cell killing. *Cell*, *165*(1), 100–110.

Batista, F. D., Treanor, B., & Harwood, N. E. (2010). Visualizing a role for the actin cytoskeleton in the regulation of B-cell activation. *Immunological Reviews*, *237*(1), 191–204.

Behmoaram, E., Bijian, K., Jie, S., Xu, Y., Darnel, A., Bismar, T. A., et al. (2008). Focal adhesion kinase-related proline-rich tyrosine kinase 2 and focal adhesion kinase are co-overexpressed in early-stage and invasive ErbB-2-positive breast cancer and cooperate for breast cancer cell tumorigenesis and invasiveness. *The American Journal of Pathology*, *173*(5), 1540–1550.

Besson, A., Wilson, T. L., & Yong, V. W. (2002). The anchoring protein RACK1 links protein kinase Cepsilon to integrin beta chains. Requirements for adhesion and motility. *The Journal of Biological Chemistry*, *277*(24), 22073–22084.

Birge, R. B., Kalodimos, C., Inagaki, F., & Tanaka, S. (2009). Crk and CrkL adaptor proteins: Networks for physiological and pathological signaling. *Cell Communication and Signaling: CCS*, 7(1), 13.

Borghi, N., Sorokina, M., Shcherbakova, O. G., Weis, W. I., Pruitt, B. L., Nelson, W. J., et al. (2012). E-cadherin is under constitutive actomyosin-generated tension that is increased at cell-cell contacts upon externally applied stretch. *Proceedings of the National Academy of Sciences of the United States of America*, *109*(31), 12568–12573.

Brancaccio, M., Hirsch, E., Notte, A., Selvetella, G., Lembo, G., & Tarone, G. (2006). Integrin signalling: The tug-of-war in heart hypertrophy. *Cardiovascular Research*, *70*(3), 422–433.

Brunswick, M., June, C. H., Finkelman, F. D., Dintzis, H. M., Inman, J. K., & Mond, J. J. (1989). Surface immunoglobulin-mediated B-cell activation in the absence of detectable elevations in intracellular ionized calcium: A model for T-cell-independent B-cell activation. *Proceedings of the National Academy of Sciences of the United States of America*, *86*(17), 6724–6728.

Brunton, V. G., & Frame, M. C. (2008). Src and focal adhesion kinase as therapeutic targets in cancer. *Current Opinion in Pharmacology*, *8*(4), 427–432.

Buensuceso, C. S., Obergfell, A., Soriani, A., Eto, K., Kiosses, W. B., Arias-Salgado, E. G., et al. (2005). Regulation of outside-in signaling in platelets by integrin-associated protein kinase C beta. *The Journal of Biological Chemistry*, *280*(1), 644–653.

Bufi, N., Saitakis, M., Dogniaux, S., Buschinger, O., Bohineust, A., Richert, A., et al. (2015). Human primary immune cells exhibit distinct mechanical properties that are modified by inflammation. *Biophysical Journal*, *108*(9), 2181–2190.

Califano, J. P., & Reinhart-King, C. A. (2010). Substrate stiffness and cell area predict cellular traction stresses in single cells and cells in contact. *Cellular and Molecular Bioengineering*, *3*(1), 68–75.

Calvete, J. J. (2004). Structures of integrin domains and concerted conformational changes in the bidirectional signaling mechanism of alphaIIbbeta3. *Experimental Biology and Medicine (Maywood, N.J.)*, *229*(8), 732–744.

Campbell, I. D., & Humphries, M. J. (2011). Integrin structure, activation, and interactions. *Cold Spring Harbor Perspectives in Biology*, *3*(3), a004994.

Campi, G., Varma, R., & Dustin, M. L. (2005). Actin and agonist MHC-peptide complex-dependent T cell receptor microclusters as scaffolds for signaling. *The Journal of Experimental Medicine*, *202*(8), 1031–1036.

Cantor, J., Browne, C. D., Ruppert, R., Féral, C. C., Fässler, R., Rickert, R. C., et al. (2009). CD98hc facilitates B cell proliferation and adaptive humoral immunity. *Nature Immunology*, *10*(4), 412.

Carrasco, Y. R., & Batista, F. D. (2007). B cells acquire particulate antigen in a macrophage-rich area at the boundary between the follicle and the subcapsular sinus of the lymph node. *Immunity*, *27*(1), 160–171.

Carrasco, Y. R., Fleire, S. J., Cameron, T., Dustin, M. L., & Batista, F. D. (2004). LFA-1/ICAM-1 interaction lowers the threshold of B cell activation by facilitating B cell adhesion and synapse formation. *Immunity*, *20*(5), 589–599.

Carroll-Portillo, A., Cannon, J. L., te Riet, J., Holmes, A., Kawakami, Y., Kawakami, T., et al. (2015). Mast cells and dendritic cells form synapses that facilitate antigen transfer for T cell activation. *The Journal of Cell Biology*, *210*(5), 851–864.

Chao, J. T., & Davis, M. J. (2011). The roles of integrins in mediating the effects of mechanical force and growth factors on blood vessels in hypertension. *Current Hypertension Reports*, *13*(6), 421–429.

Chen, J., Irianto, J., Inamdar, S., Pravincumar, P., Lee, D. A., Bader, D. L., et al. (2012). Cell mechanics, structure, and function are regulated by the stiffness of the three-dimensional microenvironment. *Biophysical Journal*, *103*(6), 1188–1197.

Chen, W., Lou, J., Evans, E. A., & Zhu, C. (2012). Observing force-regulated conformational changes and ligand dissociation from a single integrin on cells. *The Journal of Cell Biology*, *199*(3), 497–512.

Chen, W., Lou, J., & Zhu, C. (2010). Forcing switch from short- to intermediate- and long-lived states of the alphaA domain generates LFA-1/ICAM-1 catch bonds. *The Journal of Biological Chemistry*, *285*(46), 35967–35978.

Chen, W., Zarnitsyna, V. I., Sarangapani, K. K., Huang, J., & Zhu, C. (2008). Measuring receptor–ligand binding kinetics on cell surfaces: From adhesion frequency to thermal fluctuation methods. *Cellular and Molecular Bioengineering*, *1*(4), 276.

Chen, W., & Zhu, C. (2013). Mechanical regulation of T-cell functions. *Immunological Reviews*, *256*(1), 160–176.

Ciechomska, M., Wilson, C. L., Floudas, A., Hui, W., Rowan, A. D., van Eden, W., et al. (2014). Antigen-specific B lymphocytes acquire proteoglycan aggrecan from cartilage extracellular matrix resulting in antigen presentation and CD4+ T-cell activation. *Immunology*, *141*(1), 70–78.

Comrie, W. A., Li, S., Boyle, S., & Burkhardt, J. K. (2015). The dendritic cell cytoskeleton promotes T cell adhesion and activation by constraining ICAM-1 mobility. *The Journal of Cell Biology*, *208*(4), 457–473.

Conway, D. E., Breckenridge, M. T., Hinde, E., Gratton, E., Chen, C. S., & Schwartz, M. A. (2013). Fluid shear stress on endothelial cells modulates mechanical tension across VE-cadherin and PECAM-1. *Current Biology: CB, 23*(11), 1024–1030.
Coussen, F., Choquet, D., Sheetz, M. P., & Erickson, H. P. (2002). Trimers of the fibronectin cell adhesion domain localize to actin filament bundles and undergo rearward translocation. *Journal of Cell Science, 115*(Pt. 12), 2581–2590.
Curtis, A. S. (1964). The mechanism of adhesion of cells to glass. A study by interference reflection microscopy. *The Journal of Cell Biology, 20*, 199–215.
Davey, A. M., Liu, W., Sohn, H. W., Brzostowski, J., & Pierce, S. K. (2012). Understanding the initiation of B cell signaling through live cell imaging. *Methods in Enzymology, 506*, 265–290. Elsevier.
Dembo, M., & Wang, Y.-L. (1999). Stresses at the cell-to-substrate interface during locomotion of fibroblasts. *Biophysical Journal, 76*(4), 2307–2316.
Depoil, D., Weber, M., Treanor, B., Fleire, S. J., Carrasco, Y. R., Harwood, N. E., et al. (2009). Early events of B cell activation by antigen. *Science Signaling, 2*(63). pt1-pt1.
Deramaudt, T. B., Dujardin, D., Hamadi, A., Noulet, F., Kolli, K., De Mey, J., et al. (2011). FAK phosphorylation at Tyr-925 regulates cross-talk between focal adhesion turnover and cell protrusion. *Molecular Biology of the Cell, 22*(7), 964–975.
Disatnik, M. H., Boutet, S. C., Lee, C. H., Mochly-Rosen, D., & Rando, T. A. (2002). Sequential activation of individual PKC isozymes in integrin-mediated muscle cell spreading: A role for MARCKS in an integrin signaling pathway. *Journal of Cell Science, 115*(Pt. 10), 2151–2163.
Disatnik, M. H., & Rando, T. A. (1999). Integrin-mediated muscle cell spreading. The role of protein kinase c in outside-in and inside-out signaling and evidence of integrin cross-talk. *The Journal of Biological Chemistry, 274*(45), 32486–32492.
Discher, D. E., Janmey, P., & Wang, Y.-L. (2005). Tissue cells feel and respond to the stiffness of their substrate. *Science, 310*(5751), 1139–1143.
Discher, D. E., Mooney, D. J., & Zandstra, P. W. (2009). Growth factors, matrices, and forces combine and control stem cells. *Science, 324*(5935), 1673–1677.
Douglass, A. D., & Vale, R. D. (2005). Single-molecule microscopy reveals plasma membrane microdomains created by protein-protein networks that exclude or trap signaling molecules in T cells. *Cell, 121*(6), 937–950.
Dulai, R., Perry, M., Twycross-Lewis, R., Morrissey, D., Atzeni, F., & Greenwald, S. (2012). The effect of tumor necrosis factor-α antagonists on arterial stiffness in rheumatoid arthritis: A literature review. In *Paper presented at the seminars in arthritis and rheumatism*.
Dustin, M. L. (2009). Modular design of immunological synapses and kinapses. *Cold Spring Harbor Perspectives in Biology, 1*(1), a002873.
Dustin, M. L. (2014). The immunological synapse. *Cancer Immunology Research, 2*(11), 1023–1033.
Dustin, M. L., & Groves, J. T. (2012). Receptor signaling clusters in the immune synapse. *Annual Review of Biophysics, 41*, 543–556.
Elosegui-Artola, A., Oria, R., Chen, Y., Kosmalska, A., Perez-Gonzalez, C., Castro, N., et al. (2016). Mechanical regulation of a molecular clutch defines force transmission and transduction in response to matrix rigidity. *Nature Cell Biology, 18*(5), 540–548.
Engler, A. J., Griffin, M. A., Sen, S., Bonnemann, C. G., Sweeney, H. L., & Discher, D. E. (2004). Myotubes differentiate optimally on substrates with tissue-like stiffness: Pathological implications for soft or stiff microenvironments. *The Journal of Cell Biology, 166*(6), 877–887.
Engler, A. J., Richert, L., Wong, J. Y., Picart, C., & Discher, D. E. (2004). Surface probe measurements of the elasticity of sectioned tissue, thin gels and polyelectrolyte multilayer films: Correlations between substrate stiffness and cell adhesion. *Surface Science, 570*(1–2), 142–154.

Engler, A. J., Sen, S., Sweeney, H. L., & Discher, D. E. (2006). Matrix elasticity directs stem cell lineage specification. *Cell, 126*(4), 677–689.

Evani, S. J., & Ramasubramanian, A. K. (2016). Biophysical regulation of *Chlamydia pneumoniae*-infected monocyte recruitment to atherosclerotic foci. *Scientific Reports, 6,* 19058.

Evans, E., Ritchie, K., & Merkel, R. (1995). Sensitive force technique to probe molecular adhesion and structural linkages at biological interfaces. *Biophysical Journal, 68*(6), 2580–2587.

Fleire, S., Goldman, J., Carrasco, Y., Weber, M., Bray, D., & Batista, F. (2006). B cell ligand discrimination through a spreading and contraction response. *Science, 312*(5774), 738–741.

Freedman, A. S., Munro, J. M., Rice, G. E., Bevilacqua, M. P., Morimoto, C., McIntyre, B. W., et al. (1990). Adhesion of human B cells to germinal centers in vitro involves VLA-4 and INCAM-110. *Science, 249*(4972), 1030–1033.

Friedland, J. C., Lee, M. H., & Boettiger, D. (2009). Mechanically activated integrin switch controls alpha5beta1 function. *Science, 323*(5914), 642–644.

Fruman, D. A., Snapper, S. B., Yballe, C. M., Davidson, L., Yu, J. Y., Alt, F. W., et al. (1999). Impaired B cell development and proliferation in absence of phosphoinositide 3-kinase p85alpha. *Science, 283*(5400), 393–397.

Galbraith, C. G., Yamada, K. M., & Sheetz, M. P. (2002). The relationship between force and focal complex development. *The Journal of Cell Biology, 159*(4), 695–705.

Gasiorowski, J. Z., Murphy, C. J., & Nealey, P. F. (2013). Biophysical cues and cell behavior: The big impact of little things. *Annual Review of Biomedical Engineering, 15,* 155–176.

Ghibaudo, M., Saez, A., Trichet, L., Xayaphoummine, A., Browaeys, J., Silberzan, P., et al. (2008). Traction forces and rigidity sensing regulate cell functions. *Soft Matter, 4*(9), 1836–1843.

Giannone, G., Jiang, G., Sutton, D. H., Critchley, D. R., & Sheetz, M. P. (2003). Talin1 is critical for force-dependent reinforcement of initial integrin-cytoskeleton bonds but not tyrosine kinase activation. *The Journal of Cell Biology, 163*(2), 409–419.

Grashoff, C., Hoffman, B. D., Brenner, M. D., Zhou, R., Parsons, M., Yang, M. T., et al. (2010). Measuring mechanical tension across vinculin reveals regulation of focal adhesion dynamics. *Nature, 466*(7303), 263–266.

Guillou, L., Babataheri, A., Saitakis, M., Bohineust, A., Dogniaux, S., Hivroz, C., et al. (2016). T-lymphocyte passive deformation is controlled by unfolding of membrane surface reservoirs. *Molecular Biology of the Cell, 27*(22), 3574–3582.

Gupta, N., Wollscheid, B., Watts, J. D., Scheer, B., Aebersold, R., & DeFranco, A. L. (2006). Quantitative proteomic analysis of B cell lipid rafts reveals that ezrin regulates antigen receptor-mediated lipid raft dynamics. *Nature Immunology,* 7(6), 625–633.

Haller, H., Lindschau, C., Maasch, C., Olthoff, H., Kurscheid, D., & Luft, F. C. (1998). Integrin-induced protein kinase Calpha and Cepsilon translocation to focal adhesions mediates vascular smooth muscle cell spreading. *Circulation Research, 82*(2), 157–165.

Harwood, N. E., & Batista, F. D. (2010). Early events in B cell activation. *Annual Review of Immunology, 28,* 185–210.

Hassanisaber, H., Jafari, L., Campeau, M. A., Drevelle, O., Lauzon, M. A., Langelier, E., et al. (2019). The effect of substrate bulk stiffness on focal and fibrillar adhesion formation in human abdominal aortic endothelial cells. *Materials Science and Engineering: C, 98,* 572–583.

Heerkens, E. H., Izzard, A. S., & Heagerty, A. M. (2007). Integrins, vascular remodeling, and hypertension. *Hypertension, 49*(1), 1–4.

Heerkens, E. H., Quinn, L., Withers, S. B., & Heagerty, A. M. (2014). Beta integrins mediate FAK Y397 autophosphorylation of resistance arteries during eutrophic inward remodeling in hypertension. *Journal of Vascular Research, 51*(4), 305–314.

Hu, K. H., & Butte, M. J. (2016). T cell activation requires force generation. *The Journal of Cell Biology*, *213*(5), 535–542.
Huang, J., Peng, X., Qin, L., Zhu, T., Xiong, C., Zhang, Y., et al. (2009). Determination of cellular tractions on elastic substrate based on an integral Boussinesq solution. *Journal of Biomechanical Engineering*, *131*(6), 061009.
Hui, K. L., Balagopalan, L., Samelson, L. E., & Upadhyaya, A. (2015). Cytoskeletal forces during signaling activation in Jurkat T-cells. *Molecular Biology of the Cell*, *26*(4), 685–695.
Huse, M. (2017). Mechanical forces in the immune system. *Nature Reviews. Immunology*, *17*(11), 679–690.
Husson, J., Chemin, K., Bohineust, A., Hivroz, C., & Henry, N. (2011). Force generation upon T cell receptor engagement. *PLoS One*, *6*(5), e19680.
Ingber, D. E. (2006). Cellular mechanotransduction: Putting all the pieces together again. *The FASEB Journal*, *20*(7), 811–827.
Isenberg, B. C., & Tranquillo, R. T. (2003). Long-term cyclic distention enhances the mechanical properties of collagen-based media-equivalents. *Annals of Biomedical Engineering*, *31*(8), 937–949.
Izzard, C. S., & Lochner, L. R. (1976). Cell-to-substrate contacts in living fibroblasts: An interference reflexion study with an evaluation of the technique. *Journal of Cell Science*, *21*(1), 129–159.
Jacobelli, J., Bennett, F. C., Pandurangi, P., Tooley, A. J., & Krummel, M. F. (2009). Myosin-IIA and ICAM-1 regulate the interchange between two distinct modes of T cell migration. *Journal of Immunology*, *182*(4), 2041–2050.
Jin, M., Andricioaei, I., & Springer, T. A. (2004). Conversion between three conformational states of integrin I domains with a C-terminal pull spring studied with molecular dynamics. *Structure*, *12*(12), 2137–2147.
Judokusumo, E., Tabdanov, E., Kumari, S., Dustin, M. L., & Kam, L. C. (2012). Mechanosensing in T lymphocyte activation. *Biophysical Journal*, *102*(2), L5–L7.
Junt, T., Moseman, E. A., Iannacone, M., Massberg, S., Lang, P. A., Boes, M., et al. (2007). Subcapsular sinus macrophages in lymph nodes clear lymph-borne viruses and present them to antiviral B cells. *Nature*, *450*(7166), 110.
Kataoka, N., Iwaki, K., Hashimoto, K., Mochizuki, S., Ogasawara, Y., Sato, M., et al. (2002). Measurements of endothelial cell-to-cell and cell-to-substrate gaps and micromechanical properties of endothelial cells during monocyte adhesion. *Proceedings of the National Academy of Sciences of the United States of America*, *99*(24), 15638–15643.
Keren, K., Pincus, Z., Allen, G. M., Barnhart, E. L., Marriott, G., Mogilner, A., et al. (2008). Mechanism of shape determination in motile cells. *Nature*, *453*(7194), 475–480.
Knight, A. M. (2015). B-cell acquisition of antigen: Sensing the surface. *European Journal of Immunology*, *45*(6), 1600–1604.
Konigsberger, S., Weis, V., Prodohl, J., Stehling, M., Hobeika, E., Reth, M., et al. (2015). Suboptimal B-cell antigen receptor signaling activity in vivo elicits germinal center counterselection mechanisms. *European Journal of Immunology*, *45*(2), 603–611.
Koopman, G., Keehnen, R. M., Lindhout, E., Newman, W., Shimizu, Y., Van Seventer, G. A., et al. (1994). Adhesion through the LFA-1 (CD11a/CD18)-ICAM-1 (CD54) and the VLA-4 (CD49d)-VCAM-1 (CD106) pathways prevents apoptosis of germinal center B cells. *The Journal of Immunology*, *152*(8), 3760–3767.
Koopman, G., Parmentier, H. K., Schuurman, H., Newman, W., Meijer, C., & Pals, S. T. (1991). Adhesion of human B cells to follicular dendritic cells involves both the lymphocyte function-associated antigen 1/intercellular adhesion molecule 1 and very late antigen 4/vascular cell adhesion molecule 1 pathways. *Journal of Experimental Medicine*, *173*(6), 1297–1304.
Kozlov, M. M., & Mogilner, A. (2007). Model of polarization and bistability of cell fragments. *Biophysical Journal*, *93*(11), 3811–3819.

Kumari, S., Depoil, D., Martinelli, R., Judokusumo, E., Carmona, G., Gertler, F. B., et al. (2015). Actin foci facilitate activation of the phospholipase C-gamma in primary T lymphocytes via the WASP pathway. *eLife*, *4*, e04953.

Kurosaki, T. (1999). Genetic analysis of B cell antigen receptor signaling. *Annual Review of Immunology*, *17*, 555–592.

Kurosaki, T., Shinohara, H., & Baba, Y. (2010). B cell signaling and fate decision. *Annual Review of Immunology*, *28*, 21–55.

Kushnir, N., Liu, L., & MacPherson, G. G. (1998). Dendritic cells and resting B cells form clusters in vitro and in vivo: T cell independence, partial LFA-1 dependence, and regulation by cross-linking surface molecules. *The Journal of Immunology*, *160*(4), 1774–1781.

Lang, M. J., Fordyce, P. M., Engh, A. M., Neuman, K. C., & Block, S. M. (2004). Simultaneous, coincident optical trapping and single-molecule fluorescence. *Nature Methods*, *1*(2), 133.

Lark, A. L., Livasy, C. A., Calvo, B., Caskey, L., Moore, D. T., Yang, X., et al. (2003). Overexpression of focal adhesion kinase in primary colorectal carcinomas and colorectal liver metastases: Immunohistochemistry and real-time PCR analyses. *Clinical Cancer Research*, *9*(1), 215–222.

Lark, A. L., Livasy, C. A., Dressler, L., Moore, D. T., Millikan, R. C., Geradts, J., et al. (2005). High focal adhesion kinase expression in invasive breast carcinomas is associated with an aggressive phenotype. *Modern Pathology*, *18*(10), 1289–1294.

Levental, K. R., Yu, H., Kass, L., Lakins, J. N., Egeblad, M., Erler, J. T., et al. (2009). Matrix crosslinking forces tumor progression by enhancing integrin signaling. *Cell*, *139*(5), 891–906.

Liao, Q., Huang, J., Zhu, T., Xiong, C., & Fang, J. (2010). A hybrid model to determine mechanical properties of soft polymers by nanoindentation. *Mechanics of Materials*, *42*(12), 1043–1047.

Liu, Y., Blanchfield, L., Ma, V. P.-Y., Andargachew, R., Galior, K., Liu, Z., et al. (2016). DNA-based nanoparticle tension sensors reveal that T-cell receptors transmit defined pN forces to their antigens for enhanced fidelity. *Proceedings of the National Academy of Sciences of the United States of America*, *113*(20), 5610–5615. 201600163.

Liu, W., & Chen, Y. H. (2005). High epitope density in a single protein molecule significantly enhances antigenicity as well as immunogenicity: A novel strategy for modern vaccine development and a preliminary investigation about B cell discrimination of monomeric proteins. *European Journal of Immunology*, *35*(2), 505–514.

Liu, B., Chen, W., & Zhu, C. (2015). Molecular force spectroscopy on cells. *Annual Review of Physical Chemistry*, *66*, 427–451.

Liu, W., Meckel, T., Tolar, P., Sohn, H. W., & Pierce, S. K. (2010a). Antigen affinity discrimination is an intrinsic function of the B cell receptor. *Journal of Experimental Medicine*, *207*(5), 1095–1111.

Liu, W., Meckel, T., Tolar, P., Sohn, H. W., & Pierce, S. K. (2010b). Intrinsic properties of immunoglobulin IgG1 isotype-switched B cell receptors promote microclustering and the initiation of signaling. *Immunity*, *32*(6), 778–789.

Liu, W., Peng, Z., Liu, Z., Lu, Y., Ding, J., & Chen, Y.-H. (2004). High epitope density in a single recombinant protein molecule of the extracellular domain of influenza A virus M2 protein significantly enhances protective immunity. *Vaccine*, *23*(3), 366–371.

Liu, W., Wang, H., & Xu, C. (2016). Antigen receptor nanoclusters: Small units with big functions. *Trends in Immunology*, *37*(10), 680–689.

Liu, W., Won Sohn, H., Tolar, P., Meckel, T., & Pierce, S. K. (2010). Antigen-induced oligomerization of the B cell receptor is an early target of Fc gamma RIIB inhibition. *Journal of Immunology*, *184*(4), 1977–1989.

Lo, C. M., Wang, H. B., Dembo, M., & Wang, Y. L. (2000). Cell movement is guided by the rigidity of the substrate. *Biophysical Journal, 79*(1), 144–152.

Martin, F., & Chan, A. C. (2006). B cell immunobiology in disease: Evolving concepts from the clinic. *Annual Review of Immunology, 24*, 467–496.

Mateu, M. G. (2012). Mechanical properties of viruses analyzed by atomic force microscopy: A virological perspective. *Virus Research, 168*(1–2), 1–22.

Mathur, A. B., Collinsworth, A. M., Reichert, W. M., Kraus, W. E., & Truskey, G. A. (2001). Endothelial, cardiac muscle and skeletal muscle exhibit different viscous and elastic properties as determined by atomic force microscopy. *Journal of Biomechanics, 34*(12), 1545–1553.

Mauri, C., & Ehrenstein, M. R. (2007). Cells of the synovium in rheumatoid arthritis. B cells. *Arthritis Research & Therapy, 9*(2), 205.

McLeod, S. J., Shum, A. J., Lee, R. L., Takei, F., & Gold, M. R. (2004). The Rap GTPases regulate integrin-mediated adhesion, cell spreading, actin polymerization, and Pyk2 tyrosine phosphorylation in B lymphocytes. *The Journal of Biological Chemistry, 279*(13), 12009–12019.

Mehrbod, M., Trisno, S., & Mofrad, M. R. K. (2013). On the activation of integrin αIIbβ3: Outside-in and inside-out pathways. *Biophysical Journal, 105*(6), 1304–1315.

Mennens, S. F. B., Bolomini-Vittori, M., Weiden, J., Joosten, B., Cambi, A., & van den Dries, K. (2017). Substrate stiffness influences phenotype and function of human antigen-presenting dendritic cells. *Scientific Reports*, 7(1), 17511.

Milone, M. C., & Kam, L. C. (2013). Investigative and clinical applications of synthetic immune synapses. *Wiley Interdisciplinary Reviews. Nanomedicine and Nanobiotechnology, 5*(1), 75–85.

Moffitt, J. R., Chemla, Y. R., Smith, S. B., & Bustamante, C. (2008). Recent advances in optical tweezers. *Annual Review of Biochemistry*, 77, 205–228.

Molnár, E., Swamy, M., Holzer, M., Beck-García, K., Worch, R., Thiele, C., et al. (2012). Cholesterol and sphingomyelin drive ligand-independent T-cell antigen receptor nanoclustering. *The Journal of Biological Chemistry, 287*(51), 42664–42674.

Mond, J. J., Farrar, J., Paul, W. E., Fuller-Farrar, J., Schaefer, M., & Howard, M. (1983). T cell dependence and factor reconstitution of in vitro antibody responses to TNP-B. Abortus and TNP-Ficoll: Restoration of depleted responses with chromatographed fractions of a T cell-derived factor. *Journal of Immunology, 131*(2), 633–637.

Morin, N. A., Oakes, P. W., Hyun, Y. M., Lee, D., Chin, Y. E., King, M. R., et al. (2008). Nonmuscle myosin heavy chain IIA mediates integrin LFA-1 de-adhesion during T lymphocyte migration. *The Journal of Experimental Medicine, 205*(1), 195–205.

Munshi, N., Ganju, R. K., Avraham, S., Mesri, E. A., & Groopman, J. E. (1999). Kaposi's sarcoma-associated herpesvirus-encoded G protein-coupled receptor activation of c-jun amino-terminal kinase/stress-activated protein kinase and lyn kinase is mediated by related adhesion focal tyrosine kinase/proline-rich tyrosine kinase 2. *The Journal of Biological Chemistry, 274*(45), 31863–31867.

Nakken, B., Munthe, L. A., Konttinen, Y. T., Sandberg, A. K., Szekanecz, Z., Alex, P., et al. (2011). B-cells and their targeting in rheumatoid arthritis—Current concepts and future perspectives. *Autoimmunity Reviews, 11*(1), 28–34.

Natkanski, E., Lee, W.-Y., Mistry, B., Casal, A., Molloy, J. E., & Tolar, P. (2013). B cells use mechanical energy to discriminate antigen affinities. *Science (New York, N.Y.), 340*(6140), 1587–1590.

Nemir, S., & West, J. L. (2010). Synthetic materials in the study of cell response to substrate rigidity. *Annals of Biomedical Engineering, 38*(1), 2–20.

Nowosad, C. R., Spillane, K. M., & Tolar, P. (2016). Germinal center B cells recognize antigen through a specialized immune synapse architecture. *Nature Immunology, 17*(7), 870–877.

Noy, A. (2011). Force spectroscopy 101: How to design, perform, and analyze an AFM-based single molecule force spectroscopy experiment. *Current Opinion in Chemical Biology*, *15*(5), 710–718.

Oakes, P. W., Patel, D. C., Morin, N. A., Zitterbart, D. P., Fabry, B., Reichner, J. S., et al. (2009). Neutrophil morphology and migration are affected by substrate elasticity. *Blood*, *114*(7), 1387–1395.

O'Connor, R. S., Hao, X., Shen, K., Bashour, K., Akimova, T., Hancock, W. W., et al. (2012). Substrate rigidity regulates human T cell activation and proliferation. *Journal of Immunology*, *189*(3), 1330–1339.

Okkenhaug, K., Bilancio, A., Emery, J. L., & Vanhaesebroeck, B. (2004). Phosphoinositide 3-kinase in T cell activation and survival. *Biochemical Society Transactions*, *32*(Pt. 2), 332–335.

Okkenhaug, K., & Vanhaesebroeck, B. (2003). PI3K in lymphocyte development, differentiation and activation. *Nature Reviews. Immunology*, *3*(4), 317–330.

Orr, A. W., Helmke, B. P., Blackman, B. R., & Schwartz, M. A. (2006). Mechanisms of mechanotransduction. *Developmental Cell*, *10*(1), 11–20.

Owens, L. V., Xu, L., Craven, R. J., Dent, G. A., Weiner, T. M., Kornberg, L., et al. (1995). Overexpression of the focal adhesion kinase (p125FAK) in invasive human tumors. *Cancer Research*, *55*(13), 2752–2755.

Owens, L. V., Xu, L., Dent, G. A., Yang, X., Sturge, G. C., Craven, R. J., et al. (1996). Focal adhesion kinase as a marker of invasive potential in differentiated human thyroid cancer. *Annals of Surgical Oncology*, *3*(1), 100–105.

Park, S., & Lakatta, E. G. (2012). Role of inflammation in the pathogenesis of arterial stiffness. *Yonsei Medical Journal*, *53*(2), 258–261.

Paszek, M. J., Zahir, N., Johnson, K. R., Lakins, J. N., Rozenberg, G. I., Gefen, A., et al. (2005). Tensional homeostasis and the malignant phenotype. *Cancer Cell*, *8*(3), 241–254.

Pelham, R. J., Jr., & Wang, Y. (1997). Cell locomotion and focal adhesions are regulated by substrate flexibility. *Proceedings of the National Academy of Sciences of the United States of America*, *94*(25), 13661–13665.

Phan, T. G., Grigorova, I., Okada, T., & Cyster, J. G. (2007). Subcapsular encounter and complement-dependent transport of immune complexes by lymph node B cells. *Nature Immunology*, *8*(9), 992.

Pierce, S. K. (2009). Understanding B cell activation: From single molecule tracking, through Tolls, to stalking memory in malaria. *Immunologic Research*, *43*(1–3), 85–97.

Pierce, S. K., & Liu, W. (2010). The tipping points in the initiation of B cell signalling: How small changes make big differences. *Nature Reviews Immunology*, *10*(11), 767.

Pore, D., Parameswaran, N., Matsui, K., Stone, M. B., Saotome, I., McClatchey, A. I., et al. (2013). Ezrin tunes the magnitude of humoral immunity. *Journal of Immunology*, *191*(8), 4048–4058.

Pribila, J. T., Quale, A. C., Mueller, K. L., & Shimizu, Y. (2004). Integrins and T cell-mediated immunity. *Annual Review of Immunology*, *22*(1), 157–180.

Provenzano, P. P., Inman, D. R., Eliceiri, K. W., & Keely, P. J. (2009). Matrix density-induced mechanoregulation of breast cell phenotype, signaling and gene expression through a FAK-ERK linkage. *Oncogene*, *28*(49), 4326–4343.

Puklin-Faucher, E., Gao, M., Schulten, K., & Vogel, V. (2006). How the headpiece hinge angle is opened: New insights into the dynamics of integrin activation. *The Journal of Cell Biology*, *175*(2), 349–360.

Qi, H., Egen, J. G., Huang, A. Y., & Germain, R. N. (2006). Extrafollicular activation of lymph node B cells by antigen-bearing dendritic cells. *Science*, *312*(5780), 1672–1676.

Qin, L., Huang, J., Xiong, C., Zhang, Y., & Fang, J. (2007). Dynamical stress characterization and energy evaluation of single cardiac myocyte actuating on flexible substrate. *Biochemical and Biophysical Research Communications*, *360*(2), 352–356.

Rajewsky, K. (1996). Clonal selection and learning in the antibody system. *Nature, 381*(6585), 751–758.

Rehfeldt, F., Engler, A. J., Eckhardt, A., Ahmed, F., & Discher, D. E. (2007). Cell responses to the mechanochemical microenvironment—Implications for regenerative medicine and drug delivery. *Advanced Drug Delivery Reviews, 59*(13), 1329–1339.

Rodriguez-Fernandez, J. L., Riol-Blanco, L., & Delgado-Martin, C. (2010). What is an immunological synapse? *Microbes and Infection, 12*(6), 438–445.

Rosenbluth, M. J., Lam, W. A., & Fletcher, D. A. (2006). Force microscopy of nonadherent cells: A comparison of leukemia cell deformability. *Biophysical Journal, 90*(8), 2994–3003.

Ross, T. D., Coon, B. G., Yun, S., Baeyens, N., Tanaka, K., Ouyang, M., et al. (2013). Integrins in mechanotransduction. *Current Opinion in Cell Biology, 25*(5), 613–618.

Saez, A., Buguin, A., Silberzan, P., & Ladoux, B. (2005). Is the mechanical activity of epithelial cells controlled by deformations or forces? *Biophysical Journal, 89*(6), L52–L54.

Saitakis, M., Dogniaux, S., Goudot, C., Bufi, N., Asnacios, S., Maurin, M., et al. (2017). Different TCR-induced T lymphocyte responses are potentiated by stiffness with variable sensitivity. *eLife, 6*, e23190.

Saito, T., & Yokosuka, T. (2006). Immunological synapse and microclusters: The site for recognition and activation of T cells. *Current Opinion in Immunology, 18*(3), 305–313.

Sarkar, R., & Rybenkov, V. V. (2016). A guide to magnetic tweezers and their applications. *Frontiers in Physics, 4*, 48.

Sawada, Y., & Sheetz, M. P. (2002). Force transduction by Triton cytoskeletons. *The Journal of Cell Biology, 156*(4), 609–615.

Sawada, Y., Tamada, M., Dubin-Thaler, B. J., Cherniavskaya, O., Sakai, R., Tanaka, S., et al. (2006). Force sensing by mechanical extension of the Src family kinase substrate p130Cas. *Cell, 127*(5), 1015–1026.

Schaefer, L. (2010). Extracellular matrix molecules: Endogenous danger signals as new drug targets in kidney diseases. *Current Opinion in Pharmacology, 10*(2), 185–190.

Schiller, H. B., Hermann, M. R., Polleux, J., Vignaud, T., Zanivan, S., Friedel, C. C., et al. (2013). Beta1- and alphav-class integrins cooperate to regulate myosin II during rigidity sensing of fibronectin-based microenvironments. *Nature Cell Biology, 15*(6), 625–636.

Schnyder, T., Castello, A., Feest, C., Harwood, N. E., Oellerich, T., Urlaub, H., et al. (2011). B cell receptor-mediated antigen gathering requires ubiquitin ligase Cbl and adaptors Grb2 and Dok-3 to recruit dynein to the signaling microcluster. *Immunity, 34*(6), 905–918.

Schwickert, T. A., Victora, G. D., Fooksman, D. R., Kamphorst, A. O., Mugnier, M. R., Gitlin, A. D., et al. (2011). A dynamic T cell-limited checkpoint regulates affinity-dependent B cell entry into the germinal center. *The Journal of Experimental Medicine, 208*(6), 1243–1252.

Shaheen, S., Wan, Z., Li, Z., Chau, A., Li, X., Zhang, S., et al. (2017). Substrate stiffness governs the initiation of B cell activation by the concerted signaling of PKCβ and focal adhesion kinase. *eLife, 6*, e23060.

Shen, B., Delaney, M. K., & Du, X. (2012). Inside-out, outside-in, and inside-outside-in: G protein signaling in integrin-mediated cell adhesion, spreading, and retraction. *Current Opinion in Cell Biology, 24*(5), 600–606.

Shinohara, H., Yasuda, T., Aiba, Y., Sanjo, H., Hamadate, M., Watarai, H., et al. (2005). PKC beta regulates BCR-mediated IKK activation by facilitating the interaction between TAK1 and CARMA1. *The Journal of Experimental Medicine, 202*(10), 1423–1431.

Shlomchik, M. J. (2009). Activating systemic autoimmunity: B's, T's, and tolls. *Current Opinion in Immunology, 21*(6), 626–633.

Slack-Davis, J. K., Martin, K. H., Tilghman, R. W., Iwanicki, M., Ung, E. J., Autry, C., et al. (2007). Cellular characterization of a novel focal adhesion kinase inhibitor. *The Journal of Biological Chemistry*, *282*(20), 14845–14852.

Spaargaren, M., Beuling, E. A., Rurup, M. L., Meijer, H. P., Klok, M. D., Middendorp, S., et al. (2003). The B cell antigen receptor controls integrin activity through Btk and PLCgamma2. *The Journal of Experimental Medicine*, *198*(10), 1539–1550.

Spillane, K. M., & Tolar, P. (2017). B cell antigen extraction is regulated by physical properties of antigen-presenting cells. *The Journal of Cell Biology*, *216*(1), 217–230.

Springer, T. A., & Dustin, M. L. (2012). Integrin inside-out signaling and the immunological synapse. *Current Opinion in Cell Biology*, *24*(1), 107–115.

Su, T. T., Guo, B., Kawakami, Y., Sommer, K., Chae, K., Humphries, L. A., et al. (2002). PKC-beta controls I kappa B kinase lipid raft recruitment and activation in response to BCR signaling. *Nature Immunology*, *3*(8), 780–786.

Sun, Y., Chen, C. S., & Fu, J. (2012). Forcing stem cells to behave: A biophysical perspective of the cellular microenvironment. *Annual Review of Biophysics*, *41*, 519–542.

Sun, Z., Guo, S. S., & Fässler, R. (2016). Integrin-mediated mechanotransduction. *The Journal of Cell Biology*, *215*(4), 445–456.

Tabdanov, E., Gondarenko, S., Kumari, S., Liapis, A., Dustin, M. L., Sheetz, M. P., et al. (2015). Micropatterning of TCR and LFA-1 ligands reveals complementary effects on cytoskeleton mechanics in T cells. *Integrative Biology*, 7(10), 1272–1284.

Tamzalit, F., Wang, M. S., Jin, W., Tello-Lafoz, M., Boyko, V., Heddleston, J. M., et al. (2019). Interfacial actin protrusions mechanically enhance killing by cytotoxic T cells. *Science Immunology*, *4*(33), eaav5445.

Tan, J. L., Tien, J., Pirone, D. M., Gray, D. S., Bhadriraju, K., & Chen, C. S. (2003). Cells lying on a bed of microneedles: An approach to isolate mechanical force. *Proceedings of the National Academy of Sciences of the United States of America*, *100*(4), 1484–1489.

Tang, S., Wan, Z., Gao, Y., Zheng, J.-S., Wang, J., Si, Y.-Y., et al. (2016). Total chemical synthesis of photoactivatable proteins for light-controlled manipulation of antigen–antibody interactions. *Chemical Science*, 7(3), 1891–1895.

Tesniere, A., Panaretakis, T., Kepp, O., Apetoh, L., Ghiringhelli, F., Zitvogel, L., et al. (2008). Molecular characteristics of immunogenic cancer cell death. *Cell Death and Differentiation*, *15*(1), 3.

Thauland, T. J., & Parker, D. C. (2010). Diversity in immunological synapse structure. *Immunology*, *131*(4), 466–472.

Tolar, P. (2017). Cytoskeletal control of B cell responses to antigens. *Nature Reviews. Immunology*, *17*(10), 621.

Tolar, P., Hanna, J., Krueger, P. D., & Pierce, S. K. (2009). The constant region of the membrane immunoglobulin mediates B cell-receptor clustering and signaling in response to membrane antigens. *Immunity*, *30*(1), 44–55.

Tolar, P., & Spillane, K. M. (2014). Force generation in B-cell synapses: Mechanisms coupling B-cell receptor binding to antigen internalization and affinity discrimination. *Advances in Immunology*, *123*, 69–100.

Trappmann, B., Gautrot, J. E., Connelly, J. T., Strange, D. G., Li, Y., Oyen, M. L., et al. (2012). Extracellular-matrix tethering regulates stem-cell fate. *Nature Materials*, *11*(7), 642–649.

Treanor, B., Depoil, D., Bruckbauer, A., & Batista, F. D. (2011). Dynamic cortical actin remodeling by ERM proteins controls BCR microcluster organization and integrity. *The Journal of Experimental Medicine*, *208*(5), 1055–1068.

Treanor, B., Depoil, D., Gonzalez-Granja, A., Barral, P., Weber, M., Dushek, O., et al. (2010). The membrane skeleton controls diffusion dynamics and signaling through the B cell receptor. *Immunity*, *32*(2), 187–199.

Tremblay, L., Hauck, W., Aprikian, A. G., Begin, L. R., Chapdelaine, A., & Chevalier, S. (1996). Focal adhesion kinase (pp125FAK) expression, activation and association with paxillin and p50CSK in human metastatic prostate carcinoma. *International Journal of Cancer, 68*(2), 164–171.

Trichet, L., Le Digabel, J., Hawkins, R. J., Vedula, S. R., Gupta, M., Ribrault, C., et al. (2012). Evidence of a large-scale mechanosensing mechanism for cellular adaptation to substrate stiffness. *Proceedings of the National Academy of Sciences of the United States of America, 109*(18), 6933–6938.

Tse, K. W., Lin, K. B., Dang-Lawson, M., Guzman-Perez, A., Aspnes, G. E., Buckbinder, L., et al. (2012). Small molecule inhibitors of the Pyk2 and FAK kinases modulate chemoattractant-induced migration, adhesion and Akt activation in follicular and marginal zone B cells. *Cellular Immunology, 275*(1–2), 47–54.

Tuson, H. H., Auer, G. K., Renner, L. D., Hasebe, M., Tropini, C., Salick, M., et al. (2012). Measuring the stiffness of bacterial cells from growth rates in hydrogels of tunable elasticity. *Molecular Microbiology, 84*(5), 874–891.

Tuson, H. H., Renner, L. D., & Weibel, D. B. (2012). Polyacrylamide hydrogels as substrates for studying bacteria. *Chemical Communications, 48*(10), 1595–1597.

Uffmann, K., Maderwald, S., Ajaj, W., Galban, C. G., Mateiescu, S., Quick, H. H., et al. (2004). In vivo elasticity measurements of extremity skeletal muscle with MR elastography. *NMR in Biomedicine, 17*(4), 181–190.

Upadhyaya, A. (2017). Mechanosensing in the immune response. *Seminars in Cell & Developmental Biology, 71*, 137–145.

van der Pluijm, Vloedgraven, H., Papapoulos, S., Lowick, C., Grzesik, W., Kerr, J., et al. (1997). Attachment characteristics and involvement of integrins in adhesion of breast cancer cell lines to extracellular bone matrix components. *Laboratory Investigation, 77*(6), 665–675.

Van Seventer, G. A., Shimizu, Y., Horgan, K. J., & Shaw, S. (1990). The LFA-1 ligand ICAM-1 provides an important costimulatory signal for T cell receptor-mediated activation of resting T cells. *Journal of Immunology, 144*(12), 4579–4586.

von Wichert, G., Jiang, G., Kostic, A., De Vos, K., Sap, J., & Sheetz, M. P. (2003). RPTP-alpha acts as a transducer of mechanical force on alphav/beta3-integrin-cytoskeleton linkages. *The Journal of Cell Biology, 161*(1), 143–153.

Walker, A. J., Lacchini, A. H., Sealey, K. L., Mackintosh, D., & Davies, A. J. (2010). Spreading by snail (*Lymnaea stagnalis*) defence cells is regulated through integrated PKC, FAK and Src signalling. *Cell and Tissue Research, 341*(1), 131–145.

Wan, Z., Chen, X., Chen, H., Ji, Q., Chen, Y., Wang, J., et al. (2015). The activation of IgM-or isotype-switched IgG-and IgE-BCR exhibits distinct mechanical force sensitivity and threshold. *eLife, 4*, e06925.

Wan, Z., & Liu, W. (2012). The growth of B cell receptor microcluster is a universal response of B cells encountering antigens with different motion features. *Protein & Cell, 3*(7), 545–558.

Wan, Z., Xu, C., Chen, X., Xie, H., Li, Z., Wang, J., et al. (2018). PI (4, 5) P2 determines the threshold of mechanical force-induced B cell activation. *The Journal of Cell Biology, 217*(7), 2565–2582.

Wan, Z., Zhang, S., Fan, Y., Liu, K., Du, F., Davey, A. M., et al. (2013). B cell activation is regulated by the stiffness properties of the substrate presenting the antigens. *The Journal of Immunology, 190*(9), 4661–4675.

Wang, H. B., Dembo, M., Hanks, S. K., & Wang, Y. (2001). Focal adhesion kinase is involved in mechanosensing during fibroblast migration. *Proceedings of the National Academy of Sciences of the United States of America, 98*(20), 11295–11300.

Wang, X., & Ha, T. (2013). Defining single molecular forces required to activate integrin and notch signaling. *Science, 340*(6135), 991–994.

Wang, J., Lin, F., Wan, Z., Sun, X., Lu, Y., Huang, J., et al. (2018). Profiling the origin, dynamics, and function of traction force in B cell activation. *Science Signaling*, *11*(542), eaai9192.

Wang, X., Rodda, L. B., Bannard, O., & Cyster, J. G. (2014). Integrin-mediated interactions between B cells and follicular dendritic cells influence germinal center B cell fitness. *Journal of Immunology*, *192*(10), 4601–4609.

Wang, J., Tang, S., Wan, Z., Gao, Y., Cao, Y., Yi, J., et al. (2016). Utilization of a photo-activatable antigen system to examine B-cell probing termination and the B-cell receptor sorting mechanisms during B-cell activation. *Proceedings of the National Academy of Sciences of the United States of America*, *113*(5), E558–E567.

Wang, J., Xu, L., Shaheen, S., Liu, S., Zheng, W., Sun, X., et al. (2017). Growth of B cell receptor microclusters is regulated by PIP2 and PIP3 equilibrium and Dock2 recruitment and activation. *Cell Reports*, *21*(9), 2541–2557.

Weber, M., Treanor, B., Depoil, D., Shinohara, H., Harwood, N. E., Hikida, M., et al. (2008). Phospholipase C-gamma2 and Vav cooperate within signaling microclusters to propagate B cell spreading in response to membrane-bound antigen. *The Journal of Experimental Medicine*, *205*(4), 853–868.

Wegener, K. L., & Campbell, I. D. (2008). Transmembrane and cytoplasmic domains in integrin activation and protein-protein interactions (review). *Molecular Membrane Biology*, *25*(5), 376–387.

Xia, T., Zhao, R., Liu, W., Huang, Q., Chen, P., Waju, Y. N., et al. (2018). Effect of substrate stiffness on hepatocyte migration and cellular Young's modulus. *Journal of Cellular Physiology*, *233*(9), 6996–7006.

Xie, C., Zhu, J., Chen, X., Mi, L., Nishida, N., & Springer, T. A. (2010). Structure of an integrin with an alphaI domain, complement receptor type 4. *The EMBO Journal*, *29*(3), 666–679.

Xing, R., Li, S., Liu, K., Yuan, Y., Li, Q., Deng, H., et al. (2014). HIP-55 negatively regulates myocardial contractility at the single-cell level. *Journal of Biomechanics*, *47*(11), 2715–2720.

Xu, C., Fang, Y., Yang, Z., Jing, Y., Zhang, Y., Liu, C., et al. (2019). MARCKS regulates tonic and chronic active B cell receptor signaling. *Leukemia*, *33*(3), 710.

Xu, L., Li, G., Wang, J., Fan, Y., Wan, Z., Zhang, S., et al. (2014). Through an ITIM-independent mechanism the FcgammaRIIB blocks B cell activation by disrupting the colocalized microclustering of the B cell receptor and CD19. *Journal of Immunology*, *192*(11), 5179–5191.

Xu, L., Xia, M., Guo, J., Sun, X., Li, H., Xu, C., et al. (2016). Impairment on the lateral mobility induced by structural changes underlies the functional deficiency of the lupus-associated polymorphism FcgammaRIIB-T232. *The Journal of Experimental Medicine*, *213*(12), 2707–2727.

Xu, C., Xie, H., Guo, X., Gong, H., Liu, L., Qi, H., et al. (2017). A PIP2-derived amplification loop fuels the sustained initiation of B cell activation. *Science Immunology*, *2*(17), eaan0787.

Yaffe, L. J., Mond, J. J., Ahmed, A., & Scher, I. (1983). Analysis of the B cell subpopulations influenced by allogeneic effect factor. I. MHC restricted enhancement of b cell responses to thymic-independent antigens, types 1 and 2, in normal and CBA/N mice. *Journal of Immunology*, *130*(2), 632–636.

Yanaba, K., Bouaziz, J. D., Matsushita, T., Magro, C. M., St Clair, E. W., & Tedder, T. F. (2008). B-lymphocyte contributions to human autoimmune disease. *Immunological Reviews*, *223*, 284–299.

Ye, F., Kim, C., & Ginsberg, M. H. (2011). Molecular mechanism of inside-out integrin regulation. *Journal of Thrombosis and Haemostasis*, *9*(Suppl. 1(0 1)), 20–25.

Yi, J., Wu, X. S., Crites, T., & Hammer, J. A., 3rd. (2012). Actin retrograde flow and actomyosin II arc contraction drive receptor cluster dynamics at the immunological synapse in Jurkat T cells. *Molecular Biology of the Cell*, *23*(5), 834–852.

Yu, Y., Fay, N. C., Smoligovets, A. A., Wu, H. J., & Groves, J. T. (2012). Myosin IIA modulates T cell receptor transport and CasL phosphorylation during early immunological synapse formation. *PLoS One*, 7(2), e30704.

Zeng, Y., Yi, J., Wan, Z., Liu, K., Song, P., Chau, A., et al. (2015). Substrate stiffness regulates B-cell activation, proliferation, class switch, and T-cell-independent antibody responses in vivo. *European Journal of Immunology*, *45*(6), 1621–1634.

Zhang, Y., Ge, C., Zhu, C., & Salaita, K. (2014). DNA-based digital tension probes reveal integrin forces during early cell adhesion. *Nature Communications*, *5*, 5167.

Zhao, D., Xue, C., Li, Q., Liu, M., Ma, W., Zhou, T., et al. (2018). Substrate stiffness regulated migration and angiogenesis potential of A549 cells and HUVECs. *Journal of Cellular Physiology*, *233*(4), 3407–3417.

Zhu, J., Luo, B. H., Xiao, T., Zhang, C., Nishida, N., & Springer, T. A. (2008). Structure of a complete integrin ectodomain in a physiologic resting state and activation and deactivation by applied forces. *Molecular Cell*, *32*(6), 849–861.

CHAPTER THREE

Ionic protein-lipid interactions at the plasma membrane regulate the structure and function of immunoreceptors

Hua Li[a,*], Chengsong Yan[a], Jun Guo[a], Chenqi Xu[a,b,c,*]
[a]State Key Laboratory of Molecular Biology, Shanghai Science Research Center, CAS Center for Excellence in Molecular Cell Science, Shanghai Institute of Biochemistry and Cell Biology, Chinese Academy of Sciences, University of Chinese Academy of Sciences, Shanghai, China
[b]School of Life Science and Technology, ShanghaiTech University, Shanghai, China
[c]Fountain-Valley Institute for Life Sciences, Guangzhou, China
*Corresponding authors: e-mail address: lihua@sibcb.ac.cn; cqxu@sibcb.ac.cn

Contents

Abstract

Adaptive lymphocytes express a panel of immunoreceptors on the cell surface. Phospholipids are the major components of cell membranes, but they have functional roles beyond forming lipid bilayers. In particular, acidic phospholipids forming microdomains in the plasma membrane can ionically interact with proteins via polybasic sequences, which can have functional consequences for the protein. We have shown

Advances in Immunology, Volume 144
ISSN 0065-2776
https://doi.org/10.1016/bs.ai.2019.08.007

that negatively charged acidic phospholipids can interact with positively charged juxtamembrane polybasic regions of immunoreceptors, such as TCR-CD3, CD28 and IgG-BCR, to regulate protein structure and function. Furthermore, we pay our attention to protein transmembrane domains. We show that a membrane-snorkeling Lys residue in integrin αLβ2 regulates transmembrane heterodimer formation and integrin adhesion through ionic interplay with acidic phospholipids and calcium ions (Ca^{2+}) in T cells, thus providing a new mechanism of integrin activation. Here, we review our recent progress showcasing the importance of both juxtamembrane and intramembrane ionic protein-lipid interactions.

1. Introduction

Adaptive lymphocytes express a plethora of transmembrane immunoreceptors on their surface orchestrating immune responses against invading pathogens and tumor cells. The transmembrane immunoreceptors are located at the plasma membrane that contains two distinct lipid bilayers, the outer leaflet being enriched of sphingolipid, cholesterol, and phosphatidylcholine, whereas the inner leaflet comprising of acidic phospholipids such as phosphatidylserine and phosphatidylinositides (Balla, 2013; Leventis & Grinstein, 2010; Sezgin, Levental, Mayor, & Eggeling, 2017). Lipids can regulate protein structure and function mainly through two types of protein-lipid interactions: protein domain-lipid interaction and ionic protein-lipid interaction (Li, Shi, Guo, Li, & Xu, 2014). The interactions between lipid head groups and protein domains have long been studied. Conserved protein domains, such as PH and C2 domains, can interact with specific lipid head groups (Lemmon, 2008). These globular domains interact with the negatively charged head groups of acidic glycero-phospholipids using their positively charged pockets or surfaces. In addition to this type of specific interaction, there is another type of relatively nonspecific interaction, termed ionic protein-lipid interaction that can occur between protein polybasic regions and acidic glycerophospho-lipids. The lipid-interacting polybasic regions are often unstructured and located adjacent to transmembrane domains or lipid-modification sites. It has been well demonstrated that acidic phospholipids are able to bind to juxtamembrane polybasic sequences of transmembrane proteins and membrane-anchored proteins to regulate protein signaling (Chen et al., 2015; Guo et al., 2017; Shi et al., 2013; Xu et al., 2008), clustering (van den Bogaart et al., 2011; Wang et al., 2014), and localization (Heo et al., 2006; Zhou et al., 2015). The list of proteins regulated by ionic protein-lipid interaction has been rapidly expanding and now includes several receptors, channels, kinases and GTPases (Arkhipov et al., 2013; Endres et al., 2013; Heo et al., 2006).

Intriguingly, recent evidences suggest that the intramembrane basic residue, so-called membrane-snorkeling basic residue, could also ionically interact with acidic phospholipids (Guo et al., 2018; Kim, Schmidt, et al., 2011). This intramembrane ionic protein-lipid interaction thus constitutes a third type of protein-lipid interaction.

Several key aspects of immunoreceptor signaling remain elusive. How is the immunoreceptor activity restrained in the resting T (or B) cells? How is the immunoreceptor signaling dependent on each other? How does the immunoreceptor signaling contribute to the antigen sensitivity and specificity? Given these transmembrane immunoreceptor are expressed on the surface of T and B cells, the ionic protein-lipid interaction has become an active player in the regulation of structure and function of immunoreceptors. In this review, we discuss how juxtamembrane and intramembrane ionic protein-lipid interactions address these key questions about immunoreceptor signaling, and discuss how these interactions are further regulated by Ca^{2+} ions.

2. General relevance of juxtamembrane polybasic regions and membrane-snorkeling basic residue in immunoreceptors

To explore whether ionic protein-lipid regulation occurs in a general manner, we first carried out a systematic bioinformatics analysis to calculate the isoelectric point (pI) value of the first 10-residue stretch in the cytoplasmic domain of single-pass plasma membrane proteins (Yang et al., 2017). The result shows that most proteins have pI values of >7, and more than 40% have pI values of >11 in immune cells. Many important membrane proteins in immune cells, such as CD3ε, CD28, IgG, Notch1 (NOTC1), and PD1L1, contain juxtamembrane polybasic regions (PBRs). Further analysis shows that there is no clear difference between membrane proteins in immune and total cells.

To investigate whether the presence of intramembrane basic residue is a general feature of transmembrane proteins, we analyzed the transmembrane domain (TMD) sequences of single-span transmembrane proteins from yeast and human (Guo et al., 2018). More than 40% of the TMDs from both yeast and human contain Lys or Arg. These basic residues mainly localize close to the border between TMD and the cytoplasmic domain (CD). More specifically, we analyzed the human single-span transmembrane proteins located at the plasma membrane and confirmed the high frequency of intramembrane basic residues and their membrane-snorkeling positions (Lomize, Lomize, Krolicki, & Pogozheva, 2017). Therefore, the presence of the membrane-snorkeling basic residue is a common feature of transmembrane proteins. Within the list, we found that all eight members of human integrin β subunits contain an intramembrane Lys/Arg residue at the position that is six residues away from the TMD/CD border.

3. Membrane insertion of immunoreceptor functional sites

3.1 CD3 cytoplasmic domain

T-cell receptor (TCR) on T cell surface interacts specifically with antigenic peptide presented by major histocompatibility complex (pMHC) on the surface of antigen presenting cell (APC). This interaction can trigger activating signaling pathways in T-cells that lead to cell proliferation and differentiation, cytokine production and other effector functions, therefore initiating the adaptive immune responses against invading pathogens (Chakraborty & Weiss, 2014; Smith-Garvin, Koretzky, & Jordan, 2009). TCR is a complicated membrane protein complex, composed of four subunits, an antigen-binding TCRαβ subunit and three signaling subunits, CD3εδ, CD3εγ and CD3ζζ (Fig. 1A) (Wucherpfennig, Gagnon, Call, Huseby, & Call, 2010). The TCRαβ subunit recognizes antigen on the extracellular side but cannot trigger intracellular signaling because its cytoplasmic domain do not contain signaling motif. TCR signaling depends on four CD3 chains that all contain a consensus sequence YxxL/Ix_{6-12}YxxL/I, named immunoreceptor tyrosine-based activating motif (ITAM), in their cytoplasmic domains (Reth, 1989). CD3ε, δ, γ chain each contains a single ITAM whereas CD3ζ chain contains three ITAMs. Besides ITAMs, CD3ε and CD3ζ chains also contain PBRs and the Nck-interacting proline-rich sequence (PRS) in CD3ε chain. The two tyrosines are phosphorylated by a Src kinase, Lck or Fyn, and a dually phosphorylated ITAM recruits the ZAP-70 protein tyrosine kinase, which in turn phosphorylates downstream components of the signaling pathway (Weiss & Littman, 1994). In resting T cells, how TCR activity is restrained in resting T cells is one of the key aspects of TCR signaling remain obscure.

Previous studies using in vitro assays with synthetic lipid vesicles showed that the PBR-containing cytoplasmic domains of CD3ε and CD3ζ chains bound to vesicles with net negative charges (Aivazian & Stern, 2000; Xu et al., 2008). Mutation of two clusters of basic residues in the amino-terminal

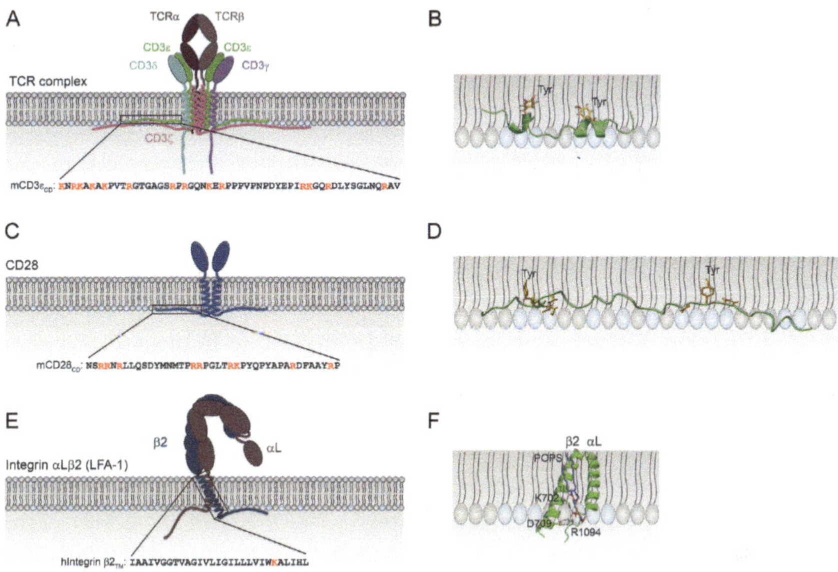

Fig. 1 Schematic presentation of immunoreceptors containing juxtamembrane polybasic regions and membrane-snorkeling basic residues. (A) T cell receptor (TCR) complex is composed of four subunits, an antigen-binding TCRαβ subunit and three signaling subunits, CD3εδ, CD3εγ and CD3ζζ. CD3ε and CD3ζ chains contains juxtamembrane PBRs. The amino acid sequence of the cytoplasmic domain of CD3ε from mouse is shown. (B) NMR structure of the immunoreceptor tyrosine-based activation motif (ITAM) of the cytoplasmic domain of CD3ε within a membrane bilayer (PDB entry 2K4F). Two key tyrosine residues inserted deeply into the membrane are indicated. (C) CD28 signaling relies on its conserved 41-residue cytoplasmic domain, which has multiple signaling motifs but lacks catalytic activity. The amino acid sequence of the cytoplasmic domain of CD28 from mouse is shown. (D) NMR structure of the cytoplasmic domain of CD28 within a membrane bilayer (PDB entry 2NAE). Two key tyrosine residues from YxxM and PYAP motifs are indicated. (E) Integrin αLβ2. A membrane-snorkeling lysine is positioned in the TMD of β2 subunit. The amino acid sequence of the TMD of β2 subunit from human is shown. (F) MD simulation structure of αLβ2 in lipid bilayer highlighting the trimeric interaction among αL, β2, and POPS. The lipid phosphate group simultaneously engages the β2-K702 amino group and the αL-R1094 guanidino group. β2-D709 and αL-R1094 form salt bridges. In (A), (C) and (E), the basic residues are shown in red. Acidic phospholipids are shown in blue, and zwitterionic phospholipids are shown in gray.

part of the CD3ε cytoplasmic domain abrogated lipid binding, confirming the importance of electrostatic interactions. Live-cell imaging studies showed a close interaction of the CD3ε cytoplasmic domain of TCR with the plasma membrane through fluorescence resonance energy transfer (FRET) between a C-terminal fluorescent protein and a membrane fluorophore (Xu et al., 2008). The same FRET-based method was extended to the study of CD3ζ cytoplasmic domain. In the native TCR-CD3 complex, the cytoplasmic domain of CD3ζ is associated closely with the plasma membrane and this association is dependent on PBR motifs (Zhang, Cordoba, Dushek, & van der Merwe, 2011). The high resolution structure of membrane-bound CD3ε cytoplasmic domain has been determined by nuclear magnetic resonance (NMR) spectroscopy, using a big lipid bicelle system to mimic membrane bilayer (Xu et al., 2008). The structure showed that the cytoplasmic domain was actually inserted into the bilayer, with the peptide backbone being located at the interface between the hydrophilic headgroup region and the hydrophobic acyl chain layer. Especially, the two tyrosines of the ITAM are all deeply inserted in the hydrophobic interior of the lipid bilayer (Fig. 1B). Functional studies showed that lipid binding of CD3ε or ζ prevented their phosphorylation by Lck (Aivazian & Stern, 2000; Xu et al., 2008). These data suggest that membrane sequestration of the key tyrosines of CD3ε cytoplasmic domain into the lipid bilayer functions as a safety control of receptor activation.

3.2 CD28 cytoplasmic domain

CD28 provides an essential costimulatory signal for T cell activation (Chen & Flies, 2013). CD28 signaling relies on its conserved 41-residue cytoplasmic domain, which has multiple signaling motifs but lacks catalytic activity (Fig. 1C) (Boomer & Green, 2010; Esensten, Helou, Chopra, Weiss, & Bluestone, 2016; Kong et al., 2011; Rudd, Taylor, & Schneider, 2009). YxxM and PYAP are dominant motifs localized at the N- and C-terminal regions of the cytoplasmic domain of CD28 ($CD28_{CD}$). The YxxM motif recruits the p85 subunit of PI3K, GRB2 and GADS through phosphor-Tyr-dependent interaction with SH2 domains. The PYAP motif interacts with signaling proteins, such as Lck and GRB2, through phosphorylation-independent interaction with their SH3 domains. The phosphorylated PYAP motif can interact with the Lck SH2 domain and in turn recruit PKC-θ (Kong et al., 2011). These molecular interactions eventually lead to the activation of transcription factors NFAT1, NF-κB, and AP-1 to regulate T cell activation and function. Besides the YxxM and PYAP motifs, CD28 also contains the highly conserved juxtamembrane PBR in the cytoplasmic domain.

We studied the lipid binding of $CD28_{CD}$ using biochemical and live cell imaging methods (Yang et al., 2017). Aromatic fluorescence emission (AFE) and live-cell FRET experiment showed that $CD28_{CD}$ PBRs can bind to acidic phospholipids via ionic interactions. A high resolution structure of membrane-bound $CD28_{CD}$ determined by NMR spectroscopy showed its backbone was mainly localized at the interface between the hydrophilic head-group region and the hydrophobic core of the membrane. This position of $CD28_{CD}$ can facilitate ionic interactions of basic residue side chains with phosphate groups in lipid head groups, as well as insertions of hydrophobic residue side chains into the membrane hydrophobic interior. Furthermore, the N terminus tended to be inserted deeper into the lipid bilayer than the C terminus. The key tyrosines in both YxxM and PYAP motifs were inserted into the membrane's hydrophobic core, which rendered them inaccessible to cytosolic tyrosine kinases. Furthermore, the basic residues in PBRs were oriented toward the membrane head groups, which facilitated their ionic interactions. These data also suggest that membrane sequestration of the key tyrosines of CD28 cytoplasmic domain into the lipid bilayer functions as a gatekeeper of receptor activation.

3.3 IgG cytoplasmic domain

The B cell receptor (BCR) molecule is a complex composed of a membrane-bound immunoglobulin (mIg) and a heterodimer of Igα and Igβ (Schamel & Reth, 2000). It is generally accepted that the function of the mIg is to recognize antigens, while the Igα and Igβ heterodimer initiates signaling through the immunoreceptor tyrosine activation motifs (ITAMs) in the cytoplasmic domains (Reth, 1992). Upon the first encounter with an antigen, the IgM- and IgD-BCR expressing naive B cells generate slow and low-titerd primary antibody responses. Memory B cell that expresses class switched IgG-BCR is one of the driving forces responsible for IgG antibody memory. The cytoplasmic domains of mIgM and mIgD contain only three amino acid (aa) residues, KVK, and thus cannot trigger signaling. In contrast, all mIgG subtypes harbor 28 aa cytoplasmic tails, which are highly conserved across species and contain an immunoglobulin tail tyrosine (ITT) motif.

The acidic phospholipid binding of the cytoplasmic domain of the mIgG (mIgG-tail) was demonstrated using fluorescence polarization (FP) and tryptophan fluorescence emission spectrum (TFES) assay (Chen et al., 2015). Furthermore, we used multidimensional NMR to test whether the key signaling tyrosine (Y21) located in the ITT motif was sequestered within the membrane hydrophobic core. Two-dimensional (2D) aromatic-filter nuclear Overhauser effect (NOE) experiments showed that Y21 had substantial NOE signals to lipid acyl chains, indicating that the tyrosine side chain was inserted into the membrane hydrophobic core. Moreover, W5 and F7 at the N-terminus of the mIgG-tail also had NOE signals to lipid acyl chains, implying that the entire mIgG-tail was bound to the plasma membrane (PM) with Y21 buried in the membrane hydrophobic core. A live cell FRET imaging assay in A20 B cells demonstrated that the mIgG-tail associates with the PM in quiescent B cells, and this interaction performed using the mIgG-tail construct was confirmed in the context of IgG-BCR complex.

To evaluate the function of IgG-BCR with a solvent-exposed cytoplasmic tail, we designed a linker mutant in which a 25 aa flexible linker is inserted between the transmembrane domain of the mIgG and N-terminus of the mIgG-tail (mIgG-Linker25-tail), as the basic-residue mutant of mIgG-tail (mIgG-tail-K/2A) shows impaired cell surface expression (Chen et al., 2015). Upon the antigen engagement, Igα and Igβ-ITAMs are phosphorylated by Lyn, and then recruit downstream signaling molecules to induce Ca^{2+} mobilization. Ca^{2+} mobilization analysis showed that the solvent-exposed mIgG-Linker25-tail exhibited dramatic hyperactivation with faster and stronger Ca^{2+} mobilization than the mIgG-tail upon IgG-BCR crosslinking. Furthermore, mIgG-Linker25-tail expressing primary B cells exhibited significantly faster proliferation than the mIgG-tail expressing primary B cells. Using high-resolution total internal reflection fluorescence microscopy (TIRFM) imaging technique, we found that, upon antigen recognition, the mIgG-Linker25-tail induced the recruitment of a significantly greater amount of BCR microclusters into the center of the contact zone to form a larger B cell immunological synapse than the mIgG-tail.

3.4 Membrane-snorkeling lysine of integrin αLβ2

Integrin αLβ2, also known as lymphocyte function-associated antigen 1 (LFA-1), is the major integrin in T cells that regulates T cell activation, effector function and differentiation (Fig. 1E) (Arnaout, 2016; Capece et al., 2017; Meli et al., 2016; Perez et al., 2003; Springer & Dustin, 2012; Varga et al., 2010). There is a highly conserved lysine in the TMD of β2. We applied solution NMR to study the role of the membrane-snorkeling Lys in αLβ2 transmembrane interaction. We first determined the monomer structure of the TMD of β2, and confirmed the position of the membrane-snorkeling

K702 using the hydrophobic paramagnetic probe 16-DSA (Guo et al., 2018). The structure of β2 monomer showed that the TMD ranging from I679 to L707 formed a nearly straight α-helix that extended till E712 in the CD. Upon addition of 16-DSA, V683-L704 showed significant signal broadening, suggesting that K702 should snorkel in the lipid environment instead of locating in the cytoplasmic domain. NMR measurements employing three lipid bicelle systems with different charge properties, i.e., zwitterionic phospholipid bicelles (100% POPC), mixture phospholipid bicelles (33% POPG, 67% POPC) and acidic phospholipid bicelles (100% POPG), showed that higher percentage of acidic phospholipids caused higher dimerization level, consistent with the previous study on αIIbβ3 (Lau, Kim, Ginsberg, & Ulmer, 2009). These data implicate that the membrane-snorkeling K702 stabilizes αLβ2 transmembrane interaction in the context of acidic phospholipids, likely through the ionic protein-lipid interaction.

Since the αLβ2 transmembrane dimer structure is too dynamic to be directly solved by solution NMR, we applied all-atom MD simulation to study the dynamic association between αL and β2 transmembrane domains (Guo et al., 2018). The MD simulated αLβ2 dimer structure showed that the N-terminal interactions were mainly stabilized through the hydrophobic stacking, while the C-terminal stabilizations were contributed by both hydrophobic stacking and salt-bridge interactions (β2-D709 and αL-R1094). Intriguingly, the lipid phosphate group of POPS simultaneously engages the β2-K702 amino group and the αL-R1094 guanidino group to mediate local contacts and thus stabilizes αLβ2 transmembrane dimer (Fig. 1F). Further functional assays using two types of FRET experiments (i.e., Head FRET and Tail FRET) and a flow chamber assay showed that the membrane-snorkeling Lys on β2 chain can stabilize αLβ2 transmembrane dimer and thus plays a gatekeeper function to maintain αLβ2 at basal activity in T cells.

Taken together, the functional sites of immunoreceptors in the immune system are lipid-bound in quiescent cells via ionic protein-lipid interactions. The sequestration of the key tyrosines into the hydrophobic core of the lipid bilayer visualized by the NMR structures of $CD3\varepsilon_{CD}$ and $CD28_{CD}$ provide the structural basis for regulation of receptor activation. Furthermore, the simultaneous engagement of the lipid phosphate group of POPS with the β2-K702 amino group and the αL-R1094 guanidino group reported in αLβ2 MD simulation study plays a critical role in αLβ2 transmembrane dimerization. These findings may be generally applicable for many other transmembrane receptors that contain juxtamembrane PBR and transmembrane snorkeling basic residues.

4. Dissociation of immunoreceptor functional sites from the membrane

In resting immune cells, ionic protein-lipid binding in immunoreceptors provides a safety control for immunoreceptor functional sites, which can prevent spontaneous phosphorylation of the signature tyrosine of ITAM or ITT. Upon antigen engagement, dissociation of the signaling motifs from the membrane is thus required to render the signature tyrosine accessible to kinases. This section mainly discusses our current understanding of the dissociation process of signaling motifs. Given the fact that protein-lipid interactions are dominated by ionic force, any factor that can change the local charge environment could essentially affect the binding of functional sites with the plasma membrane. Studies from different groups have suggested that the increase of Ca^{2+} concentration, the decrease of lipid concentration and tyrosine phosphorylation could lead to the disruption of ionic protein-lipid interactions. The effects of the decrease of lipid concentration and tyrosine phosphorylation have been extensively discussed in recent reviews (Li et al., 2014; Wu et al., 2015). Here we discuss the effect of the increase of Ca^{2+} concentration. The consequence of ionic protein-lipid binding is illustrated along the scenario of T or B cell activity from basal signaling to activation and signaling amplification. The potential role of immunoreceptor conformational change and dynamics in the dissociation process is also depicted.

4.1 Transient release of the IgG-BCR signaling motif provides insights into lymphocyte basal signaling

Membrane sequestration of tyrosine-based signaling motifs of antigen receptors effectively restricts the signaling activities in resting lymphocytes. However, low level of TCR/BCR basal signaling in resting cells is required for lymphocyte survival and antigen responsiveness (Chakraborty & Weiss, 2014; Monroe, 2004, 2006). However, the molecular mechanism of the basal signaling remains obscure. Using NMR spectroscopy, the hydrogen exchange rates of amide protons were measured to detect the transient release of the cytoplasmic domain of the membrane-bound IgG heavy chain (mIgG-tail) (Wang et al., 2017). The hydrogen exchange rates are sensitive probes reporting on the solvent accessibility of individual residues of proteins (Hwang, van Zijl, & Mori, 1998; Long, Bouvignies, & Kay, 2014). Distinct signals originated from the water magnetization were detected from the C-terminal region including the critical ITT motif, attesting to the transient release of the C-terminal region. Further analysis based on the hydrogen exchange values of lipid-free and lipid-bound mIgG-tail showed that the population of the transiently solvent-exposed state of ITT motif is estimated to be ~10%. The intrinsic dissociation propensity of the ITT motif thus provides a mechanistic explanation of the basal level signaling of mIgG-tail observed in the quiescent B cells in the absence of antigen stimulation.

4.2 Lipid-dependent conformational dynamics underlie the functional versatility of TCR

T cell signaling can be divided into three stages: initial triggering by antigen, signaling amplification and signaling sustainment. In resting T cells, no basal phosphorylation of CD3ε is detected and only a small fraction of CD3ζ is partially phosphorylated (van Oers et al., 1993), which strongly suggests that CD3ε/ζ cytoplasmic domains adopt a closed conformation at quiescent stage. Membrane binding of CD3ε/ζ cytoplasmic domains has been in previous studies. The NMR structure of the lipid-bound CD3 cytoplasmic domain ($CD3\varepsilon_{CD}$) shows that $CD3\varepsilon_{CD}$ protein backbone is localized at the interface of the lipid hydrophobic acyl-chain region and hydrophilic headgroup region (Xu et al., 2008). The ITAM tyrosine side-chains insert deeply into the membrane hydrophobic core, rendering them inaccessible to Lck in resting T cells. The PBR and PRS regions are also protected by the membrane from being recognized by downstream signaling molecules. This conformation is referred as a "closed" state. Upon antigen stimulation, the lipid-bound CD3ε/ζ cytoplasmic domains need to be dissociated from the membrane and become "open" to allow biochemical modification or binding with downstream molecules. Until now, it is still unknown how CD3 becomes open at the initial antigen triggering stage. Nevertheless, the binary "closed" and "open" CD3 conformations cannot explain the functional versatility of TCR. We hypothesized that there might be multiple intermediate conformations of CD3 cytoplasmic domains with different openness of the three functional motifs. Antigens with different TCR binding kinetics might stabilize different conformations of CD3 cytoplasmic domains to trigger distinct downstream signaling.

We have studied the functional relevance of this hypothesis in TCR signaling, using CD3ε as an example because it has all three types of functional motifs, including ITAM, PBR and PRS. We first developed an atomic force microscopy (AFM) system to study the closed-to-open conformational transition of CD3ε cytoplasmic domain at the single-molecule level (Guo et al., 2017). In AFM experiments, in addition to one-peak events, we also observed a substantial amount of two-peak events, indicating the detection of a secondary lipid-binding site of CD3ε_{CD}. Since the major binding site is located at the N-terminal PBR, the secondary lipid-binding site should be located in the middle of CD3ε_{CD}. NMR spectroscopy experiments, mainly solvent paramagnetic resonance enhancement (sPRE), were performed to probe the conformational dynamics of CD3ε cytoplasmic domain at the atomic resolution (Guo et al., 2017). Different regions of CD3ε cytoplasmic domain showed heterogeneous lipid-dependent dynamics, which provided the basis for the multiple conformations. Furthermore, sPRE data agreed well with AFM finding showing that the secondary lipid-binding site should be located in the middle of CD3ε_{CD}, including the first Tyr of ITAM. Live-cell imaging experiment confirmed the physiological relevance of heterogeneous CD3ε conformations induced by different antigen stimulations. Our study thus presents a new concept that lipid-dependent CD3 conformation dynamics directly regulates antigen-specific signaling of TCR (Fig. 2).

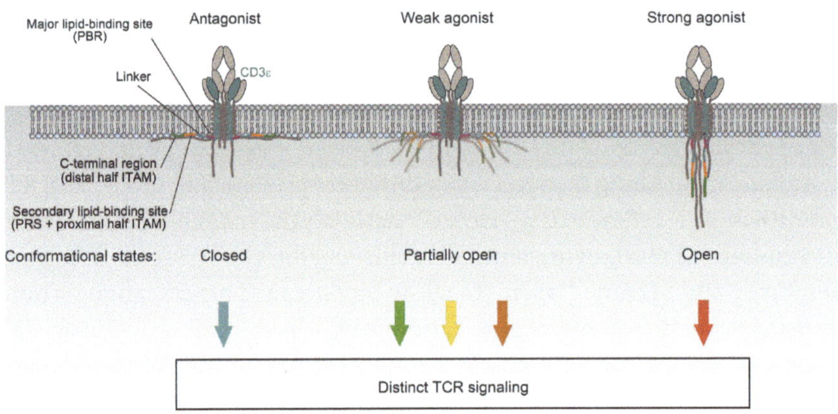

Fig. 2 Lipid-dependent conformational dynamics underlie the functional versatility of TCR. The lipid-dependent conformational dynamics of CD3 cytoplasmic domain play a key role in regulating the conformational change from closed to open (or partially open) state in activated T cells. Different TCR stimulations can stabilize CD3 cytoplasmic domains at different open conformations with different openness of the three functional motifs (PBR, PRS and ITAM), which therefore result in distinct activated states of TCR to trigger distinct immune responses. Four regions of CD3ε cytoplasmic domain are indicated to show the feature of CD3ε-lipid binding kinetics: major lipid-binding site (PBR), secondary lipid-binding site (PRS and proximal half ITAM), the linker between major and secondary lipid-binding site, and C-terminal region (distal half ITAM). Acidic phospholipids are shown in blue, and zwitterionic phospholipids are shown in gray.

4.3 Neutralization of the negative charge of lipids by Ca^{2+}

4.3.1 TCR signaling amplification regulated by Ca^{2+}

At the quiescent stage of T cells, the cytoplasmic domains of CD3ε/ζ insert deeply into the plasma membrane (Fig. 3A). After ligation with pMHC, TCR can trigger a comprehensive downstream signaling network to activate T-cell. Ca^{2+} influx is an early hallmark of TCR signaling, which happens in 6.4 s after antigen engagement (Feske, 2007; Huse et al., 2007). Recent studies reported that the major Ca^{2+} channel in T-cell, Ca^{2+}-release-activated Ca^{2+} channel (CRAC), co-localized with TCR in the immunological synapse (Lioudyno et al., 2008). The TCR proximal Ca^{2+} concentration was much higher than the global Ca^{2+} concentration (Lioudyno et al., 2008; Shi et al., 2013). When PM Ca^{2+} channels open, Ca^{2+} ions quickly influx into cells, raising the global cytoplasmic Ca^{2+} concentration and generating Ca^{2+} microdomains with high micromolar concentrations surrounding the open channels (Fig. 3B). These membrane-proximal Ca^{2+} microdomains should be in close vicinity to acidic phospholipids in the PM. Use of NMR to monitor the chemical environment of phosphorus in phospholipids revealed that Ca^{2+} at physiological micromolar concentrations can directly bind to the phosphate of an acidic phospholipid and perturb the phosphorus signal, but cannot bind to the phosphate of a zwitterionic phospholipid. Ca^{2+}-phosphate binding should thus neutralize the phospholipid negative charge and lead to the disruption of ionic CD3-lipid interaction. Cellular experiments showed that Ca^{2+} influx indeed could significantly enhance CD3 phosphorylation in activated T-cells (Fig. 3C). But since Ca^{2+} is a powerful molecule that can trigger multiple signaling pathways, it is possible that Ca^{2+} signaling may also contribute to Ca^{2+}-mediated enhancement of CD3 phosphorylation. To rule out this possibility, we replaced Ca^{2+} by a nonsignaling divalent cation Sr^{2+} that could influx into T-cell via the same CRAC channel (Yeromin et al., 2006). Sr^{2+} can also trigger the membrane dissociation of CD3 cytoplasmic domain and facilitate CD3 phosphorylation, thus indicating that it is the positive charge but not Ca^{2+} signaling to the enhancement of CD3 phosphorylation. It should be noticed that CRAC channel only opens after initial TCR triggering. Therefore, CRAC-mediated Ca^{2+} influx should facilitate TCR phosphorylation mainly at the signal amplification stage following the initial step. But this is critical for T-cell function because the physiological levels of foreign antigens are often very low so the initial TCR triggering is generally very weak. The positive feedback regulation of TCR phosphorylation by Ca^{2+} thus is critical for T-cell to acquire full effector function at physiological conditions.

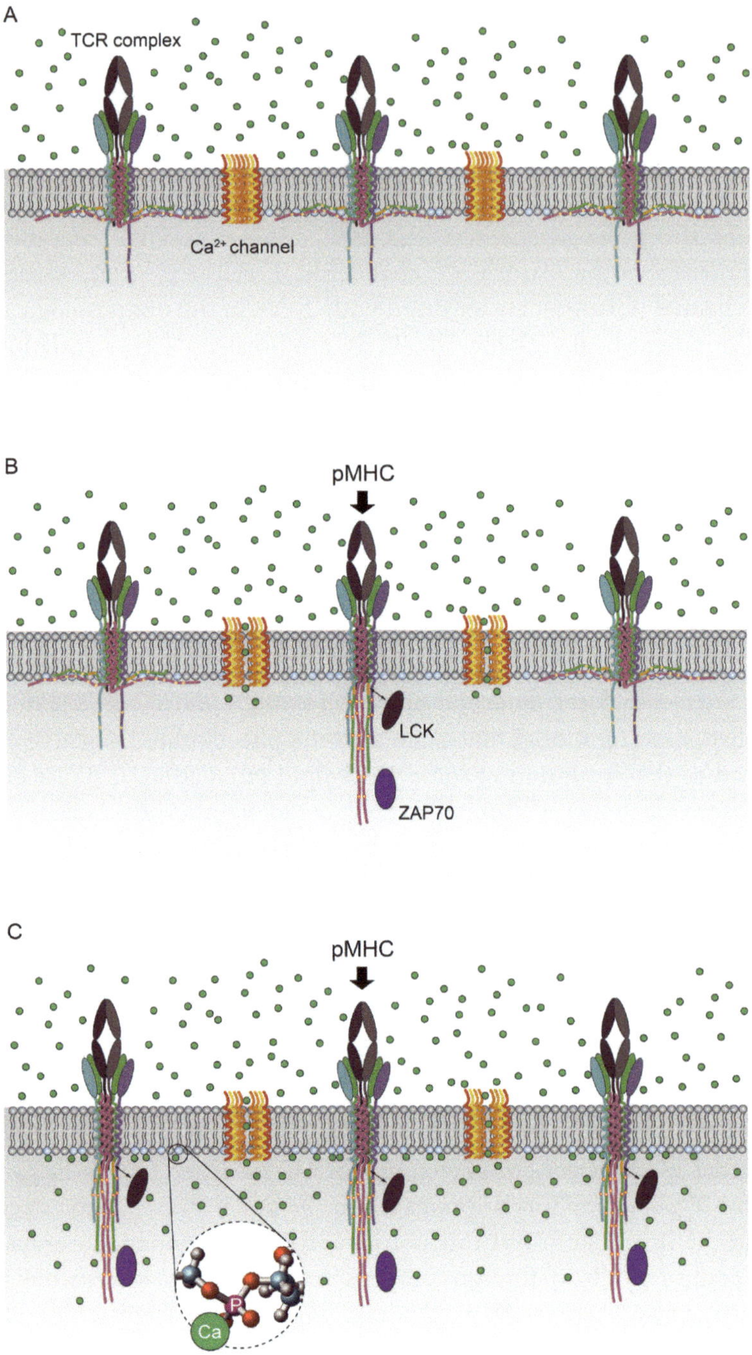

Fig. 3 See legend on opposite page.

4.3.2 TCR-Ca^{2+}-CD28 positive feedback circuit increases T cell sensitivity

At the resting T cells, the activity of both TCR and CD28 is restricted by membrane binding. After T cell activation, Ca^{2+} influx happens and CD28 is initially colocalized with TCR in peripheral microclusters that move toward the center of the immune synapse. Ca^{2+} imaging experiments showed that TCR signaling induced local Ca^{2+} ion enrichment around CD28 (Yang et al., 2017). NMR and FRET measurements showed that the ionic CD28-lipid interaction is disrupted in response to the increase of Ca^{2+} concentration, and the tyrosine side chains in the signaling motifs were no longer fully inserted into the membrane interior but dissociated from the membrane. Enhanced phosphorylation of CD28 and recruitment of downstream signaling proteins such as p85, Lck and GRB2 in the presence of TCR ligation were demonstrated in the functional experiments in primary T cells. These results together show that Ca^{2+} can use its charge to enhance the opening and signaling of CD28. TCR-induced Ca^{2+} influx removes this safety control and leads to the opening and signaling of CD28, which explains the dependence of CD28 signaling on TCR signaling. As we have shown that TCR-Ca^{2+} forms positive feedback in previous study, we integrated the TCR-Ca^{2+} and CD28-Ca^{2+} feedback through Ca^{2+} to form a dual-feedback circuit. The underlying positive-feedback circuit of TCR-Ca^{2+}-CD28 provides a signaling basis for

---

Fig. 3 A schematic illustration of the Ca^{2+}-induced TCR signaling amplification and hypersensitivity model. (A) In the resting state, the positively charged TCR CD3ε/ζ cytoplasmic domains interact with acidic phospholipids in the inner leaflet of the plasma membrane and key tyrosine residues are sequestered in the membrane bilayer, which provides a "safety" control on TCR triggering. (B) After ligation with pMHC, TCR can trigger a comprehensive downstream signaling network to activate T cells. Key tyrosines are phosphorylated by a Src kinase, e.g., Lck, and a dually phosphorylated ITAM recruits the ZAP-70 protein tyrosine kinase, which in turn phosphorylates downstream components of the signaling pathway. Ca^{2+} influx is an early hallmark of TCR signaling. TCR signaling induces local Ca^{2+} ion enrichment around TCR. Unphosphorylated and phosphorylated tyrosine residues are shown by yellow dots and yellow dots with red rims. (C) Membrane-proximal Ca^{2+} ions can then bind to the phosphate group in acidic phospholipids and neutralize their negative charges, which results in the dissociation of CD3ε/ζ cytoplasmic domains from the membrane and increases the accessibility of ITAM for Lck. Ca^{2+} can thus facilitate the phosphorylation of TCR-CD3 complexes, especially those contacting with low-affinity self-antigens or even bystanders. This TCR-Ca^{2+} feedback regulation can amplify the initial antigen-stimulated signal to a greater magnitude, which helps explain the unique nature of the hypersensitivity of T cells to even a single antigen. Acidic phospholipids are shown in blue, and zwitterionic phospholipids are shown in gray.

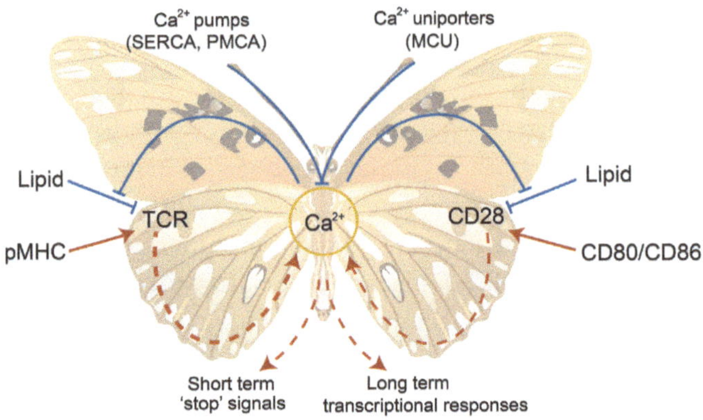

Fig. 4 TCR-Ca^{2+}-CD28 positive feedback circuit provides a signaling basis for the high antigen sensitivity of T cells. In resting T cells, membrane sequestration of tyrosine-based signaling motifs of TCR and CD28 effectively restricts their signaling activities. After ligation with pMHC, TCR can trigger a comprehensive downstream signaling network to activate T-cell. Ca^{2+} influx is an early hallmark of TCR signaling. Ca^{2+} influx induces the dissociation of $CD3_{CD}$ and $CD28_{CD}$ from the membrane and the solvent exposure of tyrosine residues through competitive binding to the phosphate groups of acidic phospholipids, thus facilitating CD3 and CD28 signaling in activated T cells. The signal transduction of TCR and CD28 can further induce Ca^{2+} influx. The underlying positive-feedback circuit of TCR-Ca^{2+}-CD28 amplifies the initial antigen-stimulated signal to a greater magnitude and provides a signaling basis for the high antigen sensitivity of T cells. Intracellular Ca^{2+} concentrations are also negatively regulated by Ca^{2+} pumps (e.g., SERCA and PMCA) and Ca^{2+} uniporters (e.g., MCU), keeping the intracellular Ca^{2+} level to be maintained in a reasonable range. The physiological roles of Ca^{2+} signaling in T cells mainly include short-term integrin-mediated "stop" signals and long-term transcriptional responses.

the high antigen sensitivity of T cells (Fig. 4). This work thus reports a new regulatory mechanism for CD28 signaling that addresses several key questions of costimulation in T cell activation.

4.3.3 Integrin activation regulated by Ca^{2+}

The major Ca^{2+} channel of T cells (CRAC) colocalizes with integrin αLβ2 in the immunological synapse to trigger high local Ca^{2+} concentration (Lioudyno et al., 2008). Ca^{2+} has been recognized as a master regulator of T-cell adhesion for long time. Increase of intracellular Ca^{2+} concentration is both necessary and sufficient to induce the stop-signal of T cells (Feske, 2007). The NMR system showed in vitro that Ca^{2+} can specifically disrupt the ionic interaction between the membrane-snorkeling K702 and lipids to destabilize αLβ2 transmembrane heterodimer (Guo et al., 2018).

Cellular functional experiments showed that Ca^{2+} influx induced by Thapsigargin (TG) could induce the high affinity conformation of αLβ2 and upregulate its activity, thus confirming that intracellular [Ca^{2+}] elevation alone is sufficient to activate αLβ2. Inside-out signaling of integrin depends on the recruitment of adaptor proteins such as Talins and kindlins to the β subunit tail (Kim, Ye, & Ginsberg, 2011; Luo, Carman, & Springer, 2007; Tadokoro et al., 2003). In the system using a cytoplasmic domain truncation of β2 (β2-ΔCT) to abolish integrin inside-out signaling, Ca^{2+}-induced αLβ2 activation was still observed. Therefore, the mechanism of Ca^{2+}-induced αLβ2 activation is through the modulation of the ionic Lys-lipid interaction but not through the canonical Ca^{2+} signaling or integrin inside-out signaling.

5. Concluding remarks

It has been generally accepted that ionic protein-lipid interactions play essential roles in regulation on the structure and function of membrane. We found that the immunoreceptor activity is regulated by negatively charged acidic phospholipids and positively charged Ca^{2+} ions. Acidic phospholipids sequester immunoreceptor signaling motifs within the membrane via ionic protein-lipid interaction, which provides a safety control for immunoreceptor activation in resting T or B cells. Ca^{2+} influx is an early hallmark of T cell activation. Influxed Ca^{2+} can bind to the phosphate groups of acidic phospholipids, thus neutralizing the negative charges of phospholipids and leading to the disruption of ionic protein-lipid interaction. Ca^{2+} can thus facilitate the phosphorylation of signaling motifs in immunoreceptors. This Ca^{2+}-mediated positive feedback regulation of TCR-CD3 can amplify the initial antigen-stimulated signal to a greater magnitude, which helps explain the unique nature of the hypersensitivity of T cells to even a single antigen. Furthermore, the Ca^{2+}-mediated positive feedback regulation of CD28 can be integrated with TCR-Ca^{2+} to form a dual-feedback circuit. The underlying positive-feedback TCR-Ca^{2+}-CD28 circuit thus provides a signaling basis for the high antigen sensitivity of T cells, reporting a new regulatory mechanism for CD28 signaling that addresses several key questions of costimulation in T cell activation. The Ca^{2+} can further activate the major integrin molecule in T cells by interfering with intramembrane protein-lipid interaction. The T cell signaling amplification mechanism mediated by Ca^{2+} can also be applied to B cells where Ca^{2+} influx amplify the antigen-initiated signaling to a greater magnitude and thus contribute to the enhanced activation of IgG-BCR expressing memory B cells in comparison with the case of IgM-BCR expressing mature naive B cells. Furthermore, Ca^{2+} can similarly interfere with intramembrane protein-ipid interaction thus activating the major integrin molecule in T cells. It is also worth noting that the cytoplasmic domains of immunoreceptors exhibit heterogeneous lipid-dependent conformational dynamics, which is comprehensively illustrated in the study on CD3ε cytoplasmic domains. Lipid-dependent conformational dynamics thus provides structural basis for the versatile signaling property of TCR. The NMR study on IgG-BCR reveals transient solvent exposure of the ITT signaling motif that can be further enhanced by calcium ion, and provides insight into the mechanism of lymphocyte basal signaling.

The finding reported here about how ionic protein-lipid interactions at the plasma membrane regulate the structure and function of immunoreceptors might have general relevance, as bioinformatics analysis shows the presence of juxtamembrane polybasic regions and membrane-snorkeling basic residue is a common feature of transmembrane proteins. Despite major recent progress, many questions still remain to be answered. How is the immunoreceptor signaling regulated among the immunoreceptor pool on the surface of lymphocytes? How is the signaling controlled spatiotemporally when one immunoreceptor contains multiple signaling motifs? In the future, new tools and technologies will need to be developed to fully understand the specific roles of ionic protein-lipid interactions in diverse biological systems.

Acknowledgments

The work is supported equally by the following grants: CAS grants (Strategic Priority Research Program XDB29030203; Facility-based Open Research Program; QYZDB-SSW-SMC048), NSFC grants (31530022, 31425009, 31830026, 31621003, 31861133009), STSMC 16JC1404800, Fountain-Valley Life Sciences Fund of University of Chinese Academy of Sciences Education Foundation to C.X.; NSFC grant 31670751 to H.L.

References

Aivazian, D., & Stern, L. J. (2000). Phosphorylation of T cell receptor zeta is regulated by a lipid dependent folding transition. *Nature Structural Biology*, 7(11), 1023–1026. https://doi.org/10.1038/80930.

Arkhipov, A., Shan, Y., Das, R., Endres, N. F., Eastwood, M. P., Wemmer, D. E., et al. (2013). Architecture and membrane interactions of the EGF receptor. *Cell*, *152*(3), 557–569. https://doi.org/10.1016/j.cell.2012.12.030.

Arnaout, M. A. (2016). Biology and structure of leukocyte beta 2 integrins and their role in inflammation. *F1000Research*, *5*, 2433. https://doi.org/10.12688/f1000research.9415.1.

Balla, T. (2013). Phosphoinositides: Tiny lipids with giant impact on cell regulation. *Physiological Reviews*, *93*(3), 1019–1137. https://doi.org/10.1152/physrev.00028.2012.

Boomer, J. S., & Green, J. M. (2010). An enigmatic tail of CD28 signaling. *Cold Spring Harbor Perspectives in Biology*, *2*(8), a002436. https://doi.org/10.1101/cshperspect.a002436.

Capece, T., Walling, B. L., Lim, K., Kim, K. D., Bae, S., Chung, H. L., et al. (2017). A novel intracellular pool of LFA-1 is critical for asymmetric CD8(+) T cell activation and differentiation. *The Journal of Cell Biology*, *216*(11), 3817–3829. https://doi.org/10.1083/jcb.201609072.

Chakraborty, A. K., & Weiss, A. (2014). Insights into the initiation of TCR signaling. *Nature Immunology*, *15*(9), 798–807. https://doi.org/10.1038/ni.2940.

Chen, L., & Flies, D. B. (2013). Molecular mechanisms of T cell co-stimulation and co-inhibition. *Nature Reviews. Immunology*, *13*(4), 227–242. https://doi.org/10.1038/nri3405.

Chen, X., Pan, W., Sui, Y., Li, H., Shi, X., Guo, X., et al. (2015). Acidic phospholipids govern the enhanced activation of IgG-B cell receptor. *Nature Communications*, *6*, 8552. https://doi.org/10.1038/ncomms9552.

Endres, N. F., Das, R., Smith, A. W., Arkhipov, A., Kovacs, E., Huang, Y., et al. (2013). Conformational coupling across the plasma membrane in activation of the EGF receptor. *Cell*, *152*(3), 543–556. https://doi.org/10.1016/j.cell.2012.12.032.

Esensten, J. H., Helou, Y. A., Chopra, G., Weiss, A., & Bluestone, J. A. (2016). CD28 costimulation: From mechanism to therapy. *Immunity*, *44*(5), 973–988. https://doi.org/10.1016/j.immuni.2016.04.020.

Feske, S. (2007). Calcium signalling in lymphocyte activation and disease. *Nature Reviews. Immunology*, 7(9), 690–702. https://doi.org/10.1038/nri2152.

Guo, X., Yan, C., Li, H., Huang, W., Shi, X., Huang, M., et al. (2017). Lipid-dependent conformational dynamics underlie the functional versatility of T-cell receptor. *Cell Research*, *27*(4), 505–525. https://doi.org/10.1038/cr.2017.42.

Guo, J., Zhang, Y., Li, H., Chu, H., Wang, Q., Jiang, S., et al. (2018). Intramembrane ionic protein-lipid interaction regulates integrin structure and function. *PLoS Biology*, *16*(11). e2006525https://doi.org/10.1371/journal.pbio.2006525.

Heo, W. D., Inoue, T., Park, W. S., Kim, M. L., Park, B. O., Wandless, T. J., et al. (2006). PI(3,4,5)P3 and PI(4,5)P2 lipids target proteins with polybasic clusters to the plasma membrane. *Science*, *314*(5804), 1458–1461. https://doi.org/10.1126/science.1134389.

Huse, M., Klein, L. O., Girvin, A. T., Faraj, J. M., Li, Q. J., Kuhns, M. S., et al. (2007). Spatial and temporal dynamics of T cell receptor signaling with a photoactivatable agonist. *Immunity*, *27*(1), 76–88. https://doi.org/10.1016/j.immuni.2007.05.017.

Hwang, T. L., van Zijl, P. C., & Mori, S. (1998). Accurate quantitation of water-amide proton exchange rates using the phase-modulated CLEAN chemical EXchange (CLEANEX-PM) approach with a fast-HSQC (FHSQC) detection scheme. *Journal of Biomolecular NMR*, *11*(2), 221–226.

Kim, C., Schmidt, T., Cho, E. G., Ye, F., Ulmer, T. S., & Ginsberg, M. H. (2011). Basic amino-acid side chains regulate transmembrane integrin signalling. *Nature*, *481*(7380), 209–213. https://doi.org/10.1038/nature10697.

Kim, C., Ye, F., & Ginsberg, M. H. (2011). Regulation of integrin activation. *Annual Review of Cell and Developmental Biology*, *27*, 321–345. https://doi.org/10.1146/annurev-cellbio-100109-104104.

Kong, K. F., Yokosuka, T., Canonigo-Balancio, A. J., Isakov, N., Saito, T., & Altman, A. (2011). A motif in the V3 domain of the kinase PKC-theta determines its localization in the immunological synapse and functions in T cells via association with CD28. *Nature Immunology*, *12*(11), 1105–1112. https://doi.org/10.1038/ni.2120.

Lau, T. L., Kim, C., Ginsberg, M. H., & Ulmer, T. S. (2009). The structure of the integrin alphaIIbbeta3 transmembrane complex explains integrin transmembrane signalling. *The EMBO Journal*, *28*(9), 1351–1361. https://doi.org/10.1038/emboj.2009.63.

Lemmon, M. A. (2008). Membrane recognition by phospholipid-binding domains. *Nature Reviews. Molecular Cell Biology*, *9*(2), 99–111. https://doi.org/10.1038/nrm2328.
Leventis, P. A., & Grinstein, S. (2010). The distribution and function of phosphatidylserine in cellular membranes. *Annual Review of Biophysics*, *39*, 407–427. https://doi.org/10.1146/annurev.biophys.093008.131234.
Li, L., Shi, X., Guo, X., Li, H., & Xu, C. (2014). Ionic protein-lipid interaction at the plasma membrane: What can the charge do? *Trends in Biochemical Sciences*, *39*(3), 130–140. https://doi.org/10.1016/j.tibs.2014.01.002.
Lioudyno, M. I., Kozak, J. A., Penna, A., Safrina, O., Zhang, S. L., Sen, D., et al. (2008). Orai1 and STIM1 move to the immunological synapse and are up-regulated during T cell activation. *Proceedings of the National Academy of Sciences of the United States of America*, *105*(6), 2011–2016. https://doi.org/10.1073/pnas.0706122105.
Lomize, A. L., Lomize, M. A., Krolicki, S. R., & Pogozheva, I. D. (2017). Membranome: A database for proteome-wide analysis of single-pass membrane proteins. *Nucleic Acids Research*, *45*(D1), D250–D255. https://doi.org/10.1093/nar/gkw712.
Long, D., Bouvignies, G., & Kay, L. E. (2014). Measuring hydrogen exchange rates in invisible protein excited states. *Proceedings of the National Academy of Sciences of the United States of America*, *111*(24), 8820–8825. https://doi.org/10.1073/pnas.1405011111.
Luo, B. H., Carman, C. V., & Springer, T. A. (2007). Structural basis of integrin regulation and signaling. *Annual Review of Immunology*, *25*, 619–647. https://doi.org/10.1146/annurev.immunol.25.022106.141618.
Meli, A. P., Fontes, G., Avery, D. T., Leddon, S. A., Tam, M., Elliot, M., et al. (2016). The integrin LFA-1 controls T follicular helper cell generation and maintenance. *Immunity*, *45*(4), 831–846. https://doi.org/10.1016/j.immuni.2016.09.018.
Monroe, J. G. (2004). Ligand-independent tonic signaling in B-cell receptor function. *Current Opinion in Immunology*, *16*(3), 288–295. https://doi.org/10.1016/j.coi.2004.03.010.
Monroe, J. G. (2006). ITAM-mediated tonic signalling through pre-BCR and BCR complexes. *Nature Reviews. Immunology*, *6*(4), 283–294. https://doi.org/10.1038/nri1808.
Perez, O. D., Mitchell, D., Jager, G. C., South, S., Murriel, C., McBride, J., et al. (2003). Leukocyte functional antigen 1 lowers T cell activation thresholds and signaling through cytohesin-1 and Jun-activating binding protein 1. *Nature Immunology*, *4*(11), 1083–1092. https://doi.org/10.1038/ni984.
Reth, M. (1989). Antigen receptor tail clue. *Nature*, *338*(6214), 383–384. https://doi.org/10.1038/338383b0.
Reth, M. (1992). Antigen receptors on B lymphocytes. *Annual Review of Immunology*, *10*, 97–121. https://doi.org/10.1146/annurev.iy.10.040192.000525.
Rudd, C. E., Taylor, A., & Schneider, H. (2009). CD28 and CTLA-4 coreceptor expression and signal transduction. *Immunological Reviews*, *229*(1), 12–26. https://doi.org/10.1111/j.1600-065X.2009.00770.x.
Schamel, W. W., & Reth, M. (2000). Monomeric and oligomeric complexes of the B cell antigen receptor. *Immunity*, *13*(1), 5–14.
Sezgin, E., Levental, I., Mayor, S., & Eggeling, C. (2017). The mystery of membrane organization: Composition, regulation and roles of lipid rafts. *Nature Reviews. Molecular Cell Biology*, *18*(6), 361–374. https://doi.org/10.1038/nrm.2017.16.
Shi, X., Bi, Y., Yang, W., Guo, X., Jiang, Y., Wan, C., et al. (2013). Ca2+ regulates T-cell receptor activation by modulating the charge property of lipids. *Nature*, *493*(7430), 111–115. https://doi.org/10.1038/nature11699.
Smith-Garvin, J. E., Koretzky, G. A., & Jordan, M. S. (2009). T cell activation. *Annual Review of Immunology*, *27*, 591–619. https://doi.org/10.1146/annurev.immunol.021908.132706.

Springer, T. A., & Dustin, M. L. (2012). Integrin inside-out signaling and the immunological synapse. *Current Opinion in Cell Biology*, *24*(1), 107–115. https://doi.org/10.1016/j.ceb.2011.10.004.
Tadokoro, S., Shattil, S. J., Eto, K., Tai, V., Liddington, R. C., de Pereda, J. M., et al. (2003). Talin binding to integrin beta tails: A final common step in integrin activation. *Science*, *302*(5642), 103–106. https://doi.org/10.1126/science.1086652.
van den Bogaart, G., Meyenberg, K., Risselada, H. J., Amin, H., Willig, K. I., Hubrich, B. E., et al. (2011). Membrane protein sequestering by ionic protein-lipid interactions. *Nature*, *479*(7374), 552–555. https://doi.org/10.1038/nature10545.
van Oers, N. S., Tao, W., Watts, J. D., Johnson, P., Aebersold, R., & Teh, H. S. (1993). Constitutive tyrosine phosphorylation of the T-cell receptor (TCR) zeta subunit: Regulation of TCR-associated protein tyrosine kinase activity by TCR zeta. *Molecular and Cellular Biology*, *13*(9), 5771–5780. https://doi.org/10.1128/mcb.13.9.5771.
Varga, G., Nippe, N., Balkow, S., Peters, T., Wild, M. K., Seeliger, S., et al. (2010). LFA-1 contributes to signal I of T-cell activation and to the production of T(h)1 cytokines. *The Journal of Investigative Dermatology*, *130*(4), 1005–1012. https://doi.org/10.1038/jid.2009.398.
Wang, Y., Gao, J., Guo, X., Tong, T., Shi, X., Li, L., et al. (2014). Regulation of EGFR nanocluster formation by ionic protein-lipid interaction. *Cell Research*, *24*(8), 959–976. https://doi.org/10.1038/cr.2014.89.
Wang, H., Wang, S., Li, C., Li, H., Mao, Y., Liu, W., et al. (2017). Probing transient release of membrane-sequestered tyrosine-based signaling motif by solution NMR spectroscopy. *Journal of Physical Chemistry Letters*, *8*(16), 3765–3769. https://doi.org/10.1021/acs.jpclett.7b01662.
Weiss, A., & Littman, D. R. (1994). Signal transduction by lymphocyte antigen receptors. *Cell*, *76*(2), 263–274.
Wu, W., Yan, C., Shi, X., Li, L., Liu, W., & Xu, C. (2015). Lipid in T-cell receptor transmembrane signaling. *Progress in Biophysics and Molecular Biology*, *118*(3), 130–138. https://doi.org/10.1016/j.pbiomolbio.2015.04.004.
Wucherpfennig, K. W., Gagnon, E., Call, M. J., Huseby, E. S., & Call, M. E. (2010). Structural biology of the T-cell receptor: Insights into receptor assembly, ligand recognition, and initiation of signaling. *Cold Spring Harbor Perspectives in Biology*, *2*(4), a005140. https://doi.org/10.1101/cshperspect.a005140.
Xu, C., Gagnon, E., Call, M. E., Schnell, J. R., Schwieters, C. D., Carman, C. V., et al. (2008). Regulation of T cell receptor activation by dynamic membrane binding of the CD3epsilon cytoplasmic tyrosine-based motif. *Cell*, *135*(4), 702–713. https://doi.org/10.1016/j.cell.2008.09.044.
Yang, W., Pan, W., Chen, S., Trendel, N., Jiang, S., Xiao, F., et al. (2017). Dynamic regulation of CD28 conformation and signaling by charged lipids and ions. *Nature Structural & Molecular Biology*, *24*(12), 1081–1092. https://doi.org/10.1038/nsmb.3489.
Yeromin, A. V., Zhang, S. L., Jiang, W., Yu, Y., Safrina, O., & Cahalan, M. D. (2006). Molecular identification of the CRAC channel by altered ion selectivity in a mutant of Orai. *Nature*, *443*(7108), 226–229. https://doi.org/10.1038/nature05108.
Zhang, H., Cordoba, S. P., Dushek, O., & van der Merwe, P. A. (2011). Basic residues in the T-cell receptor zeta cytoplasmic domain mediate membrane association and modulate signaling. *Proceedings of the National Academy of Sciences of the United States of America*, *108*(48), 19323–19328. https://doi.org/10.1073/pnas.1108052108.
Zhou, Y., Wong, C. O., Cho, K. J., van der Hoeven, D., Liang, H., Thakur, D. P., et al. (2015). Signal transduction. Membrane potential modulates plasma membrane phospholipid dynamics and K-Ras signaling. *Science*, *349*(6250), 873–876. https://doi.org/10.1126/science.aaa5619.

CHAPTER FOUR

Non-canonical Hippo signaling regulates immune responses

Lanfen Chen*
State Key Laboratory of Cellular Stress Biology, Innovation Center for Cell Signaling Network, School of Life Sciences, Xiamen University, Xiamen, Fujian, China.
*Corresponding author: e-mail address: chenlanfen@xmu.edu.cn

Contents

Abstract

The Hippo signaling pathway has been shown to play a pivotal role in controlling organ size and maintaining tissue homeostasis in multiple organisms ranging from *Drosophila* to mammals. Recently, we and others have demonstrated that Hippo signaling is also essential for maintaining the immune system homeostasis. Unlike the canonical Mst-Lats-Yap signal pathway, which controls tissue growth during development and regeneration, most studies regarding Hippo signaling in immune regulation is focusing in Mst1/2, the core kinases of Hippo signaling, cross-talking with other signaling pathways in various immune cells. In particular, patients bearing a loss-of-function mutation of Mst1 develop a complex immunodeficiency syndrome. Regarding the Hippo signaling in innate immunity, we have reported that Mst1/2 kinases are required for phagocytosis and efficient clearance of bacteria in phagocytes by regulating reactive oxygen species (ROS) production; and at the same time, by sensing the excessive ROS, Mst1/2 kinases maintain cellular redox homeostasis and prevent phagocytes aging and death through modulating the stability of the key antioxidant transcription factor Nrf2. In addition, we have revealed that the Mst1/2 kinases are critical in regulating T cells activation and Mst1/2-TAZ axis regulates the reciprocal differentiation of Treg cells and Th17 cells to modulate autoimmune inflammation by altering interactions between the transcription factors Foxp3 and RORγt. These results indicate that Hippo signaling maintains the balance between tolerance and inflammation of adaptive immunity.

Advances in Immunology, Volume 144
ISSN 0065-2776
https://doi.org/10.1016/bs.ai.2019.07.001

1. Hippo signaling and immune homeostasis

Homeostasis, referred to internal balance, keeps fairly stable conditions for a system to operate properly. A living organism needs to maintain homeostasis constantly in order to properly grow, function, and survive. The Hippo signaling pathway, first identified in *Drosophila*, is an evolution conserve signaling pathway for controlling organ size and maintaining tissue homeostasis (Avruch et al., 2012; Chen, Qin, Deng, Avruch, & Zhou, 2012; Du et al., 2014; Yu, Zhao, & Guan, 2015). The core members of the Hippo pathway in mammals have been identified, including mammalian Ste20-like kinases 1 and 2 (Mst1/2, orthologs of the *Drosophila* Hippo) and its scaffold protein WW domain containing protein 1 (WW45), the nuclear dbf2-related (NDR) family kinases large tumor suppressor 1 and 2 (Lats1/2) and its scaffold protein Mps one binder 1A and B (Mob1A/B), and two transcriptional co-activators Yes-associated protein (YAP) and WW domain containing transcription regulator 1 (WWTR1 or TAZ). The canonical Hippo signaling is mainly through phosphorylation of Mst1/2-WW45 complex and activation of their downstream Lats1/2-Mob1A/B complex, which then phosphorylates YAP or its paralogue TAZ. Phosphorylated YAP/TAZ is either targeted for proteosomal degradation or sequestered in the cytoplasm by the 14-3-3 protein, thus YAP/TAZ cannot bind to TEA domain (TEAD) family transcription factors and turn on the expression of the downstream genes (Fig. 1). Numerous studies have shown that Hippo signaling is critical for maintaining tissues homeostasis (Dong et al., 2007; Fan et al., 2016; Harvey, Zhang, & Thomas, 2013; Ji et al., 2019; Wu et al., 2013; Zhang, Chen, et al., 2017; Zhou et al., 2009, 2011). For examples, loss of the core kinase components Mst1/2 or overexpression of the downstream effector YAP in liver will result in a YAP-dependent accelerated liver cell proliferation, resistance to apoptosis and massive organ overgrowth (Dong et al., 2007; Lee et al., 2010; Lu et al., 2010; Zhou et al., 2009); in contrast, knockout of YAP in liver will lead to enhanced liver cell death and eventually liver failure (Wu et al., 2013). In brief, the function of the canonical Hippo signaling pathway is to inhibit the activation of YAP, and ultimately inhibit cell proliferation and promote cell apoptosis for maintaining the tissues homeostasis.

The immune system is a well-organized and tightly regulated network that is able to maintain immune homeostasis under normal physiological conditions. This network consists of the innate and adaptive immune cells

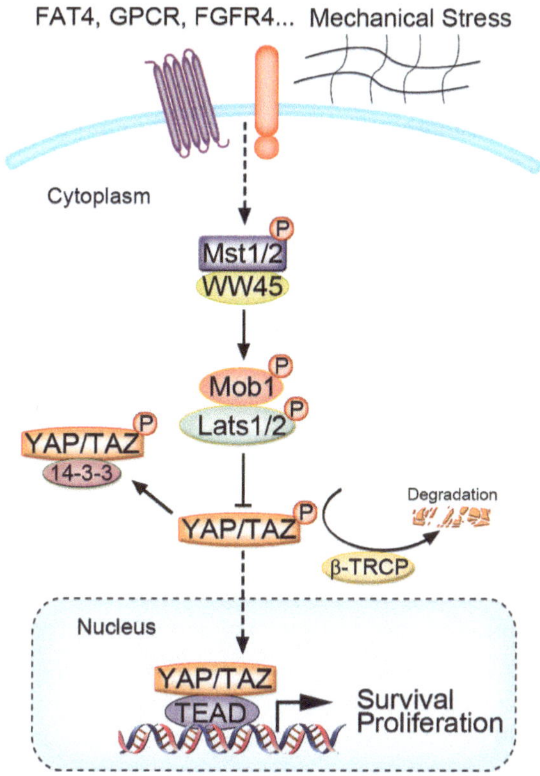

Fig. 1 Schematic representation of the canonical Hippo pathway in mammals. The canonical Hippo signaling pathway consists of a core kinase cascade formed by kinases Mst1 and Mst2 (Mst1/2), scaffolding protein WW45, downstream NDR family kinases Lats1 and Lats2 (Lats1/2), and adaptor protein Mob1, the transcription co-activators YAP and its paralog TAZ and the TEAD family of transcription factors. Mst1/2 phosphorylates and activates Lats1/2-Mob1, which then phosphorylates YAP/TAZ. Phospho-YAP/TAZ is either degraded or sequestered in the cytoplasm by the 14-3-3 protein. When the Hippo pathway is off, YAP/TAZ accumulates in the nucleus and forms a functional hybrid transcriptional factor with TEADs to turn on targeted genes expression.

that continually monitor their environment, actively distinguishing between self and none-self, establishing cell-cell communication to protect the organism from pathogen infections, autoimmunity or cancer development. When challenged with foreign antigen, specific appropriate immune responses are initiated that are aimed at restoring normal homeostasis. However, under particular circumstances, this balance is not maintained and the immune responses either under or over react. For examples, when the immune response is inefficient or unresponsive, the host might develop cancers resulted from mutated cells escaped from immune surveillance and the uncontrolled growth of the cancer cells, or encounter severe infections due to the insufficient host defense; Conversely, when the immune response over-reacts, the host might encounter some immunopathology conditions such as autoimmunity or the inflammatory cytokine storm following infections. So far, many studies have revealed that the outcome of an immune response can be modulated through receptors, sequential signaling pathways and/or the feedback loop in a context-dependent manner to maintain the immune homeostasis. Exploring the molecular mechanism for maintaining the immune homeostasis will allow us to understand the pathogenesis of autoimmune diseases, infections and cancers, and provide us new targets for the design of novel therapies for these diseases.

Recently, more and more studies uncovered that Hippo signaling is also essential for maintaining immune system homeostasis. Unlike the canonical Mst1/2-Lats1/2-Yap Hippo signaling cassette, which controls tissue growth during development and regeneration, most studies regarding Hippo signaling in immune regulation have focused on its core kinases, Mst1/2, which initial multiple non-canonical Hippo signaling pathways. Mst1 and Mst2 kinases, as well as its binding partner Nore1b (also called RAPL) and substrate Mob1, are most abundant in tissues of the lymphoid system (Zhou, Medoff, et al., 2008). The first few studies that demonstrated the indispensable role of Hippo signaling in the immune system were in vitro studies showing that, the Mst1/RAPL complex is required for lymphocyte function associated antigen-1 (LFA-1)-mediated T-cell adhesion and migration upon T-cell receptor (TCR) or chemokine stimulation (Katagiri et al., 2004; Katagiri, Maeda, Shimonaka, & Kinashi, 2003). Later on, studies of Mst1-deficient mice revealed that, unexpectedly and in contrast to the *Drosophila* loss-of-function (LOF) phenotypes, loss of Mst1 results in a mixed immunodeficiency phenotype in affected mice (Dong et al., 2009; Mou et al., 2012; Zhou, Medoff, et al., 2008). Consistently, biallelic LOF mutations in human *MST1* also lead to an autosomal recessive primary immunodeficiency syndrome (Abdollahpour et al., 2012; Nehme et al., 2012). MST1-deficient patients showed recurrent infections and autoimmune manifestations, as well as clinical signs of T- and B-cell lymphopenia and a progressive loss of naive T cells, which were also observed in Mst1-deficient mice. However, mice lacking Mst2 alone have normal lymphoid function and no obvious phenotype, but global deficiency of both Mst1 and Mst2 gives embryonic lethality (Mou et al., 2012; Zhou et al., 2009). All evidences obtained from genetic mutated mice and human patients suggested that Hippo signaling has important roles in regulating both innate and adaptive immune responses.

In general, Mst1/2 kinases act through the non-canonical Hippo signaling to regulate the immune responses by cross-talking with other essential pathways in specific immune cell types, such as integrin signaling (Katagiri et al., 2003, 2004, 2009; Katagiri, Imamura, & Kinashi, 2006), B cell receptor (BCR) or TCR signaling (Bagherzadeh Yazdchi et al., 2019; Mou et al., 2012; Park et al., 2017; Zhou, Medoff, et al., 2008) Toll-like receptors (TLRs) signaling (Alsufyani et al., 2018; Geng et al., 2015; Li, Xiao, et al., 2015), cytokine receptors signaling (Lee et al., 2019; Shi et al., 2018), MAPK signaling (Li et al., 2017; Novakova, Talacko, Novak, & Valis, 2019) and antiviral signaling (Meng et al., 2016; Wang et al., 2017; Zhang, Meng, et al., 2017) (Fig. 2). Our previous work demonstrated that Mst1/2 kinases is an intrinsic negative regulator of the proliferative response of naïve T cells in response to TCR stimulation and is important for maintaining the proper lymphocytes pool as loss of Mst1 resulted in lymphopenia (Mou et al., 2012; Zhou, Medoff, et al., 2008. Recently, we found that Mst1/2-TAZ signaling inhibits

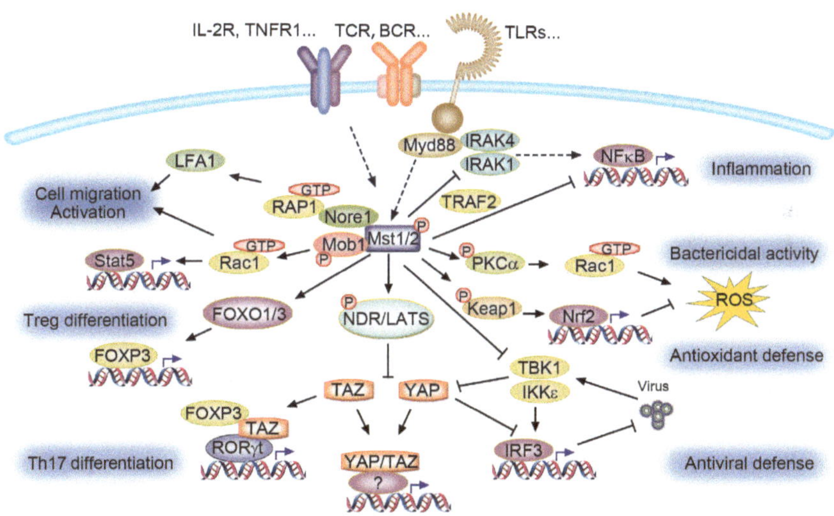

Fig. 2 Schematic illustration of immune responses regulated by Hippo signaling. Upon the stimulation of the specific upstream receptors, Mst1/2 kinases act through the non-canonical Hippo signaling to regulate the immune responses by cross-talking with other essential pathways in specific immune cell types. Collectively, the non-canonical Hippo signaling plays important roles in both innate and adaptive immunity by regulating immune cell migration and activation, inflammation, Th17 cell and Treg cell differentiation, bactericidal activity, antiviral responses, and antioxidant defense.

the development of inflammatory Th17 cells, but enhances the differentiation of immune suppressive Treg cells, supporting that properly regulation of Hippo signing in T cell is critical for preventing the development of autoimmune diseases and maintaining the immune homeostasis (Geng et al., 2017). In addition, our studies also revealed that Mst1/2 may be key coordinators of ROS generation and scavenging in phagocytes. TLR-Mst1/2-Rac1 signaling is essential for ROS induction and bactericidal activity in innate immune cells (Geng et al., 2015); while the Mst1/2-Nrf2 axis plays an important role in ROS-sensing and antioxidant defense for maintaining the redox homeostasis in macrophages during an antimicrobial response (Wang et al., 2019).

2. Hippo signaling in T lymphocytes

Emerging results showed that Mst1/2 kinases are critical for T-lymphocyte development, migration, homing, and differentiation (Dong et al., 2009; Du et al., 2014; Geng et al., 2017; Katagiri et al., 2006, 2009, 2003, 2004; Mou et al., 2012; Shi et al., 2018; Zhou, Medoff, et al., 2008). T lymphocytes are crucial players in the immune system. T lymphoid precursors migrate from the bone marrow to the thymus, where they encounter a series of selective processes for proper development and maturation. Once T cells have completed their development in the thymus, they enter the venous circulation and traffic to secondary lymphoid organs, awaiting an antigenic stimulus. Naïve T cells, which have not yet encountered their specific antigens, circulate through lymphatic vessels, peripheral blood and tissue fluid to play a role in cellular immunity and immune regulation. T cells recirculation facilitates extensive exposure to antigens in the body, strengthens immune response and maintains immune memory for a long period.

2.1 Expression of the Hippo pathway components in T cells

To explore the role of Hippo signaling in T cells, the expression levels of the core kinases and regulators of the Hippo pathway were analyzed in different stages of T cell maturation, activation and differentiation. During the T cell development process in thymus, the protein levels of Mst1 and Mst2, as well as Nore1b, are progressively increased from detectable low levels in $CD4^+CD8^+$ double positive (DP) thymocytes to higher levels in $CD4^+$ and $CD8^+$ single positive (SP) thymocytes with a similar extent (Mou et al., 2012). The protein levels of Mob1, a physiological substrate of Mst1/2 kinases, are comparable in DP and SP thymocytes, but the phosphorylated Mob1 can only be detected in SP thymocytes. The low expression and activity of Mst1 and Mst2 in DP as compared with SP thymocytes suggests that Mst1/2 kinases might have little or no role in thymocytes development till the DP stage. In periphery, the abundance of Mst1 and Mst2 remains high in mature naïve T cells freshly out of thymus. In contrast, the mRNA and protein levels of Mst1 and Mst2 in $CD4^{+}CD62L^{low}$ effector/memory T cells are reduced approximately 10-fold compared with that in the $CD4^{+}CD62L^{hi}$ naïve T cells (Zhou, Medoff, et al., 2008). In combination with the observation that Mst1-null mice exhibit the greatly enhanced T cell activation and increased the percentage of $CD4^{+}CD62L^{low}$ effector/memory T cells, these results suggested that down-regulation of Mst1/2 expression is a normal part of the program for the transition of T cells from a naïve to an activated effector or memory phenotype and Mst1 might act as determinant of the threshold for activation of naïve T cells (Zhou, Medoff, et al., 2008) (Fig. 3A).

In the canonical Hippo signaling pathway, Mst1/2 directly phosphorylates Lats1, which, combined with Lats1 autophosphorylation, is activated, and in turn phosphorylates and inhibits YAP by promoting its nuclear exit. Binding of Mob1A or Mob1B promotes the autophosphorylation of Lats1/2 or NDR1/2 kinases on their activation loop contributing to their catalytic activation (Dong et al., 2007; Hao, Chun, Cheung, Rashidi, & Yang, 2008; Zhao et al., 2007). Mst1 and/or Mst2-mediated Mob1A/B phosphorylation at Thr12 and Thr35 promotes the binding of Mob1 with Lats1/2 (Praskova, Xia, & Avruch, 2008). In the context of T cells, although the expression of Lats1/2 and YAP can be detected in $CD3^{+}$ T cells, TCR signaling can only slightly increase Lats1/2 and YAP phosphorylation, and their activities are relative insensitivity to Mst1 elimination, suggesting that Lats1/2 and YAP might be not involved in T cell activation and function. However, Mob1 is abundant in T cells. TCR signaling mediated activation of Mob1, which in turn binds and activates the DOCK8 rac1 guanyl nucleotide exchange factor (GEF) to control Rho GTPase activation for migratory responses of SP thymocytes, indicating that the Mst1/2-Mob1 axis plays a crucial role in T cell migration and activation (Mou et al., 2012). These results may also explain the similarity of immunological defects found in Mst1 or DOCK8 deficiencies in humans and mice (Abdollahpour et al., 2012; Nehme et al., 2012; Purcell, Cant, & Irvine, 2015).

Upon antigen recognition and environmental cytokines stimulation, naive $CD4^{+}$ T cells differentiate into several functional classes of effector T cells, such as helper T cell 1 (Th1), Th2, Th17, T follicular helper

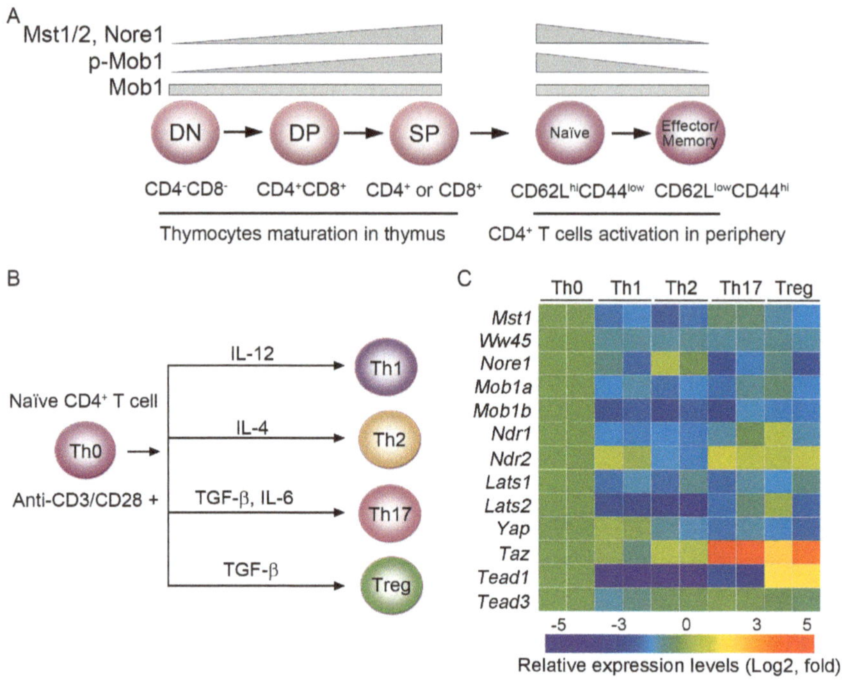

Fig. 3 Schematic illustration of the Hippo pathway components expression in T cells. (A) The protein levels of Mst1, Mst2, Nore1, Mob1 and phosphorylated (p-) Mob1 in thymocytes at different stages of development and in mature periphery T cells at naïve or activated stages. (B) Naïve CD4$^+$ T Cells were activated by anti-CD3 and anti-CD28 in the presence of IL-12 for Th1 polarization; IL-4 for Th2 polarization; TGF-β and IL-6 for Th17 polarization; or TGF-b for Treg cell polarization. (C) Expression of mRNA encoding components of the Hippo pathway in various T cell subsets (two culture replicates per subset (one per column)) differentiated from naive CD4$^+$ T cells in vitro as shown at B. Results were normalized (key) and are presented relative to those of Th0 cells, set as 1. *Adapted from Geng, J., Yu, S., Zhao, H., Sun, X., Li, X., Wang, P., et al. (2017). The transcriptional coactivator TAZ regulates reciprocal differentiation of TH17 cells and Treg cells.* Nature Immunology, 18*(7), 800–812. doi: 10.1038/ni.3748.*

(Tfh) and regulatory T cell (Treg), that are specialized for different immunological functions (Saravia, Chapman, & Chi, 2019). To study the role of Hippo signaling in different effecter T cell subsets, the expression levels of the major components in above mentioned effector T cell subsets, which were generated in vitro with standard polarization conditions respectively, were compared by using real-time PCR analysis (Geng et al., 2017) (Fig. 3B and C). The mRNA levels of *Mst1*, *Ww45*, *Nore1b*, *Mob1a*, *Mob1b*, *Lats1*, *Lats2*, *Yap* were lower or no different in these T cell subsets, when compared with that in Th0 cells (unstimulated CD4$^+$ naïve T cells). Unlike *Lats1* and

Last2, the mRNA levels of *Ndr2*, the gene of another NDR family kinase, were slightly higher in Th1, Th17 and Treg subsets. *Tead1* mRNA was much more abundant in Treg cells than in Th0 cells, but was undetectable in other subsets analyzed. Notably, *Taz* mRNA, but not *Yap1* mRNA, was robustly induced in both Treg cells and Th17 cells but underwent the greatest induction in Th17 cells (Geng et al., 2017).

The increased protein levels of TAZ in mouse Th17 cells and Treg cells were confirmed by the immunoblot analysis. Higher TAZ expression was also observed in human Th17 and Treg cells, but not in Th1 cells or Th2 cells, relative to its expression in Th0. TGF-β is needed for the differentiation of both Treg and Th17 cells cell subsets, whereas IL-6 promotes Th17, but suppresses regulatory T cell differentiation (Saravia et al., 2019). The abundance *Taz* mRNA was significantly increased by TGF-β alone but not by IL-6 alone and that this increase was further enhanced by stimulation with a combination of TGF-β and IL-6. We identified that, Smad3 and STAT3, the main transcription factor downstream of signaling of TGF-β or IL-6, respectively, are the major transcription factors for *Taz* expression. Knockdown of Smad3 or knockout of STAT3 significantly decreased TAZ expression in naïve $CD4^+$ T cells cultured under Th17-skewing conditions, while overexpression of Smad3 resulted in the induction of TAZ expression, and co-expression Smad3 with STAT3 further enhanced the TAZ expression. Consistent with that, Smad3 increased the transcriptional activity of the *Taz* promoter, but STAT3 did not, while Smad3 together with STAT3 synergistically enhanced this activity. There are 10 known Smad-binding sequences (GAG(A/C)C) and 10 STAT-binding sequences (TT(N5)AA) in the 2-kb region of the *Taz* promoter (Geng et al., 2017). Further analysis revealed that a Smad-binding site in the region −225 bp to −192 bp and a STAT3-binding site in the region of −282 bp to −240 bp (all positions relative to the transcription start site) are essential for inducing the transcription of *Taz* gene (Geng et al., 2017).

2.2 Kinases Mst1 and Mst2 regulate T cell migration and activation

Initially, by analyzing Mst1 knockout mice (*Mst1*$^{-/-}$) generated from an ES cell line bearing a gene trap inserted between the first and second exons of Mst1 gene, we found that loss of Mst1 resulted in a variety of T cell abnormalities (Zhou, Medoff, et al., 2008). There is a reduction in white pulp, decreased numbers of total $CD4^+$ T cells, $CD8^+$ T cells and $B220^+$ B cells and absence of marginal zone B cells in the spleen of *Mst1*$^{-/-}$ mouse.

Further analysis revealed that loss of Mst1 results in fewer peripheral mature naïve T cells ($CD62L^{hi}CD44^{lo}$) and relatively normal numbers of effector/memory ($CD62L^{lo}CD44^{hi}$) T cells in blood, lymph nodes and spleen. In contrast, unlike Mst1, a global deletion of murine Mst2, which shares 76% identical and an identical activation loop sequence, caused no changes in lymphocyte numbers in any compartment (Zhou, Medoff, et al., 2008). However, additional elimination of Mst2 in the entire hematopoietic lineage on $Mst1^{-/-}$ mice ($Mst1^{-/-}$ $Mst2^{fl/fl}$ *Vav*-Cre) causes a more severe reduction in the number of mature T cell in the circulation and the secondary lymphoid organs suggesting that Mst2 might play a redundant role in lymphoid tissues during the absence of Mst1 (Mou et al., 2012). The kinase activity of Mst1 is essential for T cell homeostasis, since the defective phenotype of Mst1 deficiency in the lymphoid compartments can only be restored by the transgenic expression of wild type but not catalytically inactive Mst1 (Mou et al., 2012).

Inactivation of Mst1, or both Mst1 and Mst2 does not have obvious effect on the thymocytes development, which might due to the very low abundance and activity of Mst1/2 kinases in the developmentally earlier thymocytes (Mou et al., 2012). However, the total numbers of $CD4^+$ and $CD8^+$ SP thymocytes are increased in $Mst1^{-/-}$ $Mst2^{fl/fl}$ *Vav*-Cre mice compared with that of their wild-type counterparts. These SP thymocytes of $Mst1^{-/-}$ $Mst2^{fl/fl}$ *Vav*-Cre mice resemble mature T cells of wild-type mice, undergo excessive apoptosis and their egress from the thymus is severely reduced. Qa-2 and CD24 are two markers for indicating the mature thymocytes and periphery T cells. Qa-2, a nonpolymorphic MHC class 1 type molecule, is expressed in late stage of the thymocyte development and its expression increases further on recent thymic emigrants and periphery mature T cells, whereas CD24 is highly expressed throughout thymocyte development but its abundance greatly decreases on recent thymic emigrants and diminishes further in the periphery. $CD4^+$ and $CD8^+$ SP thymocytes from $Mst1^{-/-}$ $Mst2^{fl/fl}$ *Vav*-Cre mouse exhibits a $Qa\text{-}2^{hi}CD24^{lo}$ phenotype (Boursalian, Golob, Soper, Cooper, & Fink, 2004; Mou et al., 2012). In additions, the fraction of $Qa\text{-}2^{hi}CD24^{lo}$ $CD4^+$ or $CD8^+$ SP cells in the $Mst1^{-/-}$ $Mst2^{fl/fl}$ *Vav*-Cre thymus also expresses higher levels of S1PR1, the sphingosine-1 phosphate (S1P) receptor, which expresses very late in thymocyte development (Carlson et al., 2006). Compared with wild-type SP thymocytes, the Mst1/2-deficient SP thymocytes expressed comparable levels of the chemokine receptors CCR7, CXCR3, CXCR4 and CCR5, as well as the integrins CD11b and LFA-1. However, these Mst1/2 deficient

SP thymocytes failed to enter secondly lymphoid tissues, even when they are placed directly in the circulation (Mou et al., 2012). All these evidence suggested that Mst1/2-deficient thymocytes have uninterrupted maturation toward the mature naive peripheral T cells, but are defective on thymic egress. Further studies revealed that loss of Mst1/2 kinases disables S1P and chemokine-induced chemotaxis, actin polarization, and activation of rho family GTPases in SP thymocytes. Mechanically, in mature thymocytes, the chemokine (CCL19) or S1P, stimulates the Mst1/2-dependent phosphorylation of Mob1, promotes the interaction of Mob1 with DOCK8 and stimulates the DOCK8 GEF activity toward the activation of rho family GTPases, such as Rac1, which promote the thymic egress and migration of mature thymocytes (Mou et al., 2012).

$Mst1^{-/-}$ $Mst2^{fl/fl}$ *Vav*-Cre mice or $Mst1^{-/-}$ $Mst2^{fl/fl}$ *Lck*-Cre mice, in which Mst2 was deleted in entire hematopoietic lineage or a later stage of T cell development in thymus of $Mst1^{-/-}$ mice, respectively, exhibit the defective thymic egress and decreased number of, but more activated, peripheral T cells (Mou et al., 2012). To explore the role of Mst1/2 in the activation of peripheral T cells, we also generated the $Mst1^{fl/fl}Mst2^{fl/fl}$ *Ox40*-Cre mice, in which Mst1 and Mst2 are eliminated only in mature and activated T cells. $Mst1^{fl/fl}Mst2^{fl/fl}$ *Ox40*-Cre mice exhibits normal T cell development in the thymus and normal numbers of T cells in peripheral lymphoid tissues, but slightly more effector/memory T cells in the spleen than those of their wild-type littermates (Geng et al., 2017). Mst1 might act as a negative regulator of the commitment of naive T cells to a proliferative response upon TCR activation, as the enhanced proliferation rate and the increased production of the cytokines IL-2, IFN-γ and IL-4 was found in Mst1-deficient T cells in response to anti-CD3 or anti-CD3/anti-CD28 stimulation when compared with that of wild-type T cells. Upon the TCR stimulation, the increase in tyrosine phosphorylation of CD3ζ, ZAP70, Lck, and PLCγ is similar in splenic T cells from wild-type and Mst1-deficient mice, whereas the phosphorylation of Mob1A/B observed in the wild-type T cells is lost entirely in the Mst1-deficient T cells. Elimination of Mst1 has little effect on the Lats1 carboxyl-terminal phosphorylation, Lats1/2 autophosphorylation and YAP phosphorylation in T cells. Thus the activation of Mob1A/B might serve as the effector of Mst1's antiproliferative effect in naïve T cells (Zhou, Medoff, et al., 2008). In additions, freshly isolated Mst1-deficient T cells exhibit high levels of ongoing apoptosis. The Mst1-null effector/memory $CD4^+$ T cells continue to exhibit the higher rate of apoptosis in response to TCR stimulation in vitro, indicating that loss of Mst1 might enhance the activation induce cell death (AICD) and Mst1 exerts an appreciable anti-apoptotic effect in this T cell subset (Zhou, Medoff, et al., 2008).

2.3 Hippo signaling regulates Th17 cell and Treg cell subsets differentiation

Th17 cells play critical roles in autoimmunity and tissue damage, while Foxp3^{+} Treg cells are essential for mediating immune tolerance and immunosuppressive. The dysregulation of Th17 and Treg cells is often linked with several immune diseases (Saravia et al., 2019). It is interesting that there is plasticity between the Th17 cell lineage and Treg cell lineage and the developmental pathways for Th17 cells and Treg cells are reciprocally interconnected. Mice with the elimination of Mst1, or both Mst1 and Mst2 in the hematopoietic lineage, were prone to autoimmune diseases, such as Sjögren's syndrome and colitis (Du et al., 2014; Geng et al., 2017). Recent studies revealed that Mst1 kinases promote the differentiation of Treg cell or enhance its regulatory function by modulating the activity of Foxo1/3 (Du et al., 2014), Sirt1 (Li, Du, et al., 2015; Li, Xiao, et al., 2015), Akt (Du et al., 2014) or Rac1-DOCK8 (Shi et al., 2018). Our group reported that activated T cells specific knockout Mst1/2 mice ($Mst1^{fl/fl}Mst2^{fl/fl}$ *Ox40*-Cre) exhibits a substantial higher frequency of Th17 cells and a modest decreased frequency of Treg cells in the draining lymph nodes upon the immunization of keyhole limpet hemocyanin (KLH) in complete Freund's adjuvant (CFA). In T cell transfer model of colitis, $Rag1^{-/-}$ mice received adoptive transfer of $Mst1^{-/-}$ naïve T cells exhibited more severe intestinal inflammation than that of mice that received wild-type naïve T cells. As a downstream transcriptional cofactor of the Hippo signaling pathway, TAZ is highly enriched in Th17 cells. Interestingly, $Rag1^{-/-}$ mice received *Mst1* and *Taz* double-knockout naïve CD4^{+} T cells showed less severe intestinal inflammation than that of mice received $Mst1^{-/-}$ naïve CD4^{+} T cells suggesting that TAZ might serve as a critical downstream effector of Mst1/2 kinases to mediate autoimmunity. Mice with TAZ-deficiency in T cells were resistant to the induction of Th17 cell-dependent inflammatory diseases, such as EAE and colitis. In contrast, adoptive transfer of TAZ-overexpressing naïve T cells, which are isolated from T cell-specific expression of *Taz* transgenic mice, elicited more-severe colitis in $Rag1^{-/-}$ mice with a significantly higher frequency of Th17 cells in the colonic lamina propria (LP) than that elicited by the transfer of control wild-type naïve T cells. In additions, the expression levels of *RORC*, which encodes

RAR related orphan receptor gamma T (RORγt), the main transcription factor of Th17 cells, and *TAZ* were positively correlated and were significantly upregulated in memory $CD4^+$ T cells isolated from peripheral blood of patients with rheumatoid arthritis or Sjögren's syndrome when compared with these from healthy individuals (Geng et al., 2017).

Further studies revealed that the transcriptional co-activator TAZ acts as a molecular switch for reciprocal differentiation of Th17 and Treg regulation. Under Th17-inducing conditions, TAZ is highly induced by TGF-β and IL-6 stimulation and acts as a critical co-activator of RORγt for Th17 differentiation. The tryptophan-tryptophan (WW) domain of TAZ physically binds to RORγt on its DNA-binding domain (DBD) and ligand-binding domain (LBD) in vitro and in vivo. Moreover, the WW domain of TAZ interacted with the LBD of RORγt via the WW-domain-binding motif PPxY (Pro-Pro-x-Tyr) located in the carboxy-terminal activation-function region AF2, which is the main transcription-activation motif of RORγt. Luciferase assays showed that wild-type TAZ, but not the WW domain-truncated form of TAZ ($TAZ^{\Delta WW}$), which was unable to interact with RORγt, increased RORγt-mediated activity of the *Il17a* promoter in a dose-dependent manner. Consistent with that, overexpression of wild-type TAZ in naive $CD4^+$ T cells resulted in a significantly higher frequency of IL-17^+ cells under Th17-skewing conditions, but overexpression of the truncated form of $TAZ^{\Delta WW}$ did not. Moreover, overexpression of TAZ in RORγt-deficient naive $CD4^+$ T cells was unable to induce Th17 differentiation indicating that RORγt is required for the TAZ-mediated development of Th17 cells and TAZ is a critical co-activator of RORγt for Th17 differentiation (Geng et al., 2017).

TCR signaling and the treatment of TGF-β and IL-6 are essential for differentiation of Th17 cells from naïve $CD4^+$ T cells (Bettelli et al., 2006). TGF-β treatment is capable of inducing both Foxp3 and RORγt expression (Zhou, Lopes, et al., 2008). Foxp3 was found to be able to associate with RORγt and to inhibit its ability to act as a transcriptional activator. In the presence of IL-6, this inhibition was abrogated, and Th17 differentiation was initiated. Interestingly, we observed that, under both the Th17-skewing condition and the Treg-skewing condition, TAZ deficiency resulted in increased production of Foxp3 in T cells, but comparable *Foxp3* mRNA levels as that of wild-type T cells, indicating that TAZ might regulate the stability of Foxp3 protein. Indeed, we found under Th17-skewing conditions, TAZ attenuates the effect of the Tat interactive protein 60 kDa (Tip60) and p300 on the acetylation and stabilization of Foxp3 and then targeted Foxp3 for proteasomal degradation, thus blocked its inhibitory effect on RORγt. Tip60 and p300 mediated acetylation of Foxp3 is essential for inhibiting proteasomal degradation of Foxp3, as well as enhancing Foxp3 activity (van Loosdregt & Coffer, 2014). Notably, TAZ-deficient Treg cells exhibited greater acetylation but less ubiquitination of endogenous Foxp3 than that of wild-type cells, while overexpression of TAZ attenuated the effect of Tip60 and p300 on the acetylation and stabilization of Foxp3. The interaction assays with truncated protein revealed that the coiled-coil domain of TAZ (residues 158–249) interacts with the zinc domain of Tip60 (residues 113–283), while Foxp3 binds to the zinc-and-acetyltransferase-MYST domain of Tip60 (residues 113–513), which indicated that TAZ might compete with Foxp3 to bind to the same region between residues 113 and 283 of Tip60. Indeed, further analysis showed that TAZ has higher affinity for Tip60 and efficiently disrupts the interaction between Tip60 and Foxp3, thus sequesters Tip60 from Foxp3 and diminishing the Tip60-mediated acetylation of Foxp3 and targeting it for proteasomal degradation. In addition, we found that TAZ not only just negatively regulates the stability of Foxp3, but also blocks the inhibitory activity of Foxp3 on RORγt in the context of Th17 cells. Interestingly, TAZ and RORγt binds to distinct regions of Foxp3, while Foxp3 and RORγt binds to the same site of TAZ at the WW domain. However, Foxp3 does not compete with RORγt for binding to TAZ. In contrast, dimerized or polymerized TAZ functions as a scaffold to promote assembly of the Foxp3-TAZ-RORγt complex. Since Foxp3 can inhibit Th17 differentiation by antagonizing the function of RORγt (Zhou, Lopes, et al., 2008). The result that co-expression of TAZ with Foxp3 and RORγt efficiently blocks the inhibitory effect of Foxp3 on RORγt activity suggested that the inhibitory effect of Foxp3 on RORγ might be blocked by the hindrance created by TAZ in the complex of TAZ, RORγt and Foxp3 (Geng et al., 2017).

Paradoxically, TAZ is also expressed in TGF-β-activated Treg cells at a slightly lower level than that in Th17 cells, so how stabilization of Foxp3 is achieved in Treg cells. Interestingly, in addition to TAZ, TEAD1, a transcription factor downstream of canonical Hippo signaling, is also induced in Treg cells under the Treg-inducing condition. However, unlike TAZ, whose expression is highly induced in Th17 cells, the expression of TEAD1 is down-regulated in Th17 cells. In the canonical Hippo signaling pathway, TAZ binds to TEADs and enhances the expression of its downstream target genes encoding molecules that promote survival and proliferation, and eventually leads to organ growth and cancer development. It is interesting that we found that, under the Treg-inducing condition, highly induced TEAD1 has a higher affinity for TAZ than that of Foxp3 and is able to disrupt the interaction of TAZ with Foxp3. In addition, TEAD1 sequesters TAZ from Tip60, and thereby allow Tip60-mediated acetylation and stabilization of Foxp3 in Treg cells. The antagonistic sequestration of TEAD1-TAZ also favors inhibition of RORγt's activity by Foxp3 to further advance the development of Treg cells. Since TEAD1 is not induced in Th17 cells, our result suggested that IL-6/STAT3 signaling directly suppresses TEAD1-encoding genes as a mechanism for tipping the balance in favor of Th17 cells rather than Treg cells (Geng et al., 2017).

It has been previously shown that the transcriptional factor, Runx1 influences Th17 differentiation by inducing RORγt expression and by binding to and acting together with RORγt during IL-17 transcription (Lazarevic et al., 2011; Zhang, Meng, & Strober, 2008). Similar to TAZ, Runx1 also interacts with the transcription factor Foxp3, and this interaction is necessary for the negative effect of Foxp3 on Th17 differentiation. However, we found that either knockout or overexpression of TAZ has no effect on RORγt expression. Although TAZ could interact with Runx1, TAZ shows much higher affinity with RORγt than Runx1. TAZ/RORγt shows significantly higher *Il17a* promoter reporter activity than Runx1/RORγt. Importantly, knockdown of Runx1 has no significant effect on TAZ-mediated Th17 polarization indicating that TAZ-mediated Th17 development does not depend on Runx1. These data demonstrated that TAZ and Runx1 regulate Th17 differentiation through distinct mechanisms by which TAZ mediates Th17 polarization through directly activating RORγt while Runx1-induced Th17 polarization might mainly depend on the upregulation of RORγ, and it would be interesting to determine the role of TAZ in Runx1-mediated Th17 differentiation in the future.

Taken together, we concluded that inactivation of Hippo signaling promotes translocation of TAZ nucleus, which is able to attenuate the function of Foxp3 and enhance RORγt-mediated Th17 cells development. On the other hand, in the Treg cells differentiation context, high expression of TEAD1 sequesters TAZ from RORγt and Foxp3 to positively promote Treg cell differentiation (Fig. 4) (Geng et al., 2017).

3. Hippo signaling in innate immune cells

The innate immune system is the first critical line of host defense by discriminating self- from non-self- components, and it is referred to as innate

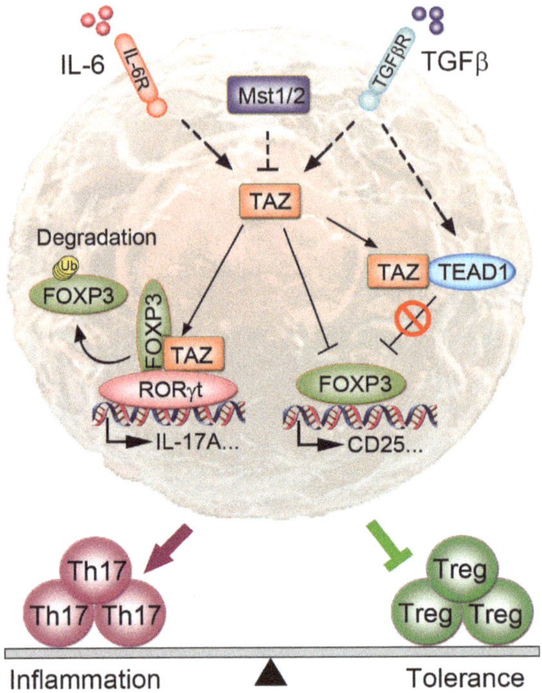

Fig. 4 A proposed working model for Mst1/2-TAZ signaling regulates reciprocal differentiation of Th17 or Treg cells. Differentiation. TAZ potentiates Th17 differentiation through direct transcriptional activation of RORγt and promoting Foxp3 degradation by reducing Tip60-mediated acetylation of Foxp3, while under Treg-skewing conditions, upregulated TEAD1 sequesters TAZ from RORγt, Tip60 and Foxp3, thereby negatively regulating TAZ mediated Th17 differentiation but promoting Treg differentiation. Thus, Hippo signaling is critical for preventing development of autoimmune diseases and maintaining the immune homeostasis.

due to its immediately response upon infection to defend against various pathogens, such as viruses, bacteria and parasites. Mononuclear phagocytes of the innate immune system are essential for the development of inflammation and, together with neutrophils, are the phagocytic cells involved in the clearance of microbial agents. When a pathogen enters the body, those innate myeloid immune cells recognize the specific pathogen-associated molecular patterns (PAMPs), such as carbohydrate, polypeptide, and nucleic acid that expressed on the pathogen's surface, via complementary pattern recognition receptors (PRRs), such as the Toll-like receptor (TLR) family, the C-type lectin-like family, scavenger receptors, and complement receptors (Brubaker, Bonham, Zanoni, & Kagan, 2015).

As primary sentinels for the detection of pathogens by binding microbe PAMPs, TLRs serve to initiate pro-inflammatory responses (Liu & Cao, 2016). When wild-type bone marrow–derived macrophages (BMDMs) were stimulated with an array of TLR ligands, we observed that the stimulation of cell-surface TLRs (TLR1, TLR2 and TLR4) substantially enhances the phosphorylation of Mob1, a physiological substrate of Mst1 and Mst2, whereas the ligands of endosomal TLRs (TLR7, TLR8 and TLR9) do not change the phosphorylation of Mob1, except for a moderate increase in its phosphorylation induced by poly(I:C) (an agonist of TLR3) (Geng et al., 2015). By using MyD88-deficient RAW264.7 cell line, we further demonstrated that LPS (an agonist of TLR4), Pam3CSK4 (an agonist of TLR1 and TLR2) and LTA (an agonist of TLR2) activate Mst1 and Mst2 via a MyD88-dependent pathway. The deletion of Mst1 and Mst2 does not alter the TLR-induced activation of the mitogen-activated protein kinases (MAPKs) p38, Jnk or Erk. However, in response to LPS stimulation, the phosphorylation levels of IκB kinase (IKKα/β), as well as the phosphorylation levels of IκBα, are higher in Mst1/2-deficient BMDMs compared to that of wild-type control cells. This result suggested that the loss of Hippo signaling might enhance the LPS/TLR4-mediated activation of NF-κB, which could be responsible for increased induction of pro-inflammatory cytokines, such as IL-6 and TNFα, in Mst1/2-deficient BMDMs upon stimulation with LPS (Geng et al., 2015). Interestingly, Liu et al. reported that in the absence of Hippo function, Gram-positive bacteria and fungi, but not Gram-negative bacteria, infections resulted in increased lethality in flies (Liu et al., 2016). This immune phenotype is very similar to that observed in Toll signaling-deficient *Drosophila* indicating that the canonical Hippo pathway in fly fat bodies functions as a regulator of innate immunity. They further demonstrated that Hippo signaling enhances NF-κB signaling and promotes anti-microbial peptide expression in *Drosophila*. Without the inhibiting effect of Hippo signaling, Yorkie directly increases the transcription of the *Drosophila* IκB factor, Cactus, which prevents the nuclear translocation of the NFκB transcription factor(s) dorsal and the dorsal-related immunity factor (Dif), as well as the expression of anti-microbial peptides. Upon activation by Gram-positive bacteria, the Toll-Myd88-Pelle cascade leads to phosphorylation and degradation of the Cka subunit of the Hippo inhibitory complex, releasing Hippo to achieve Yorkie blockage and induction of anti-microbial effects (Liu et al., 2016). Thus, with regard to the regulation of NF-κB signaling by Hippo signaling, results are inconsistent between mammalian macrophages and *Drosophila* fat cells. Whether downstream effectors, such as YAP or TAZ, regulate the transcription of IκBα in mammalian macrophages remains to be investigated.

3.1 Regulation of phagocytosis and bactericide in phagocytes

Human patients bearing LOF mutation of MST1 have recurrent bacterial or viral infections. We observed that the hematopoietic cell-specific knockout of Mst1 and Mst2 ($Mst1^{-/-}$ $Mst2^{fl/fl}$ *Vav*-Cre) mice exhibited multiple or recurrent infections, such as pneumonia and lung abscesses. In contrast to $Mst1^{-/-}$ $Mst2^{fl/fl}$ *Vav*-Cre mice, the mice with the myeloid cell-specific knockout of Mst1 and Mst2 ($Mst1^{fl/fl}Mst2^{fl/fl}$ *Lyz2*-Cre) did not show spontaneous inflammation or infections over the first 7 months of life. However, compared to wild-type ($Mst1^{fl/fl}Mst2^{fl/fl}$) mice, much more $Mst1^{fl/fl}Mst2^{fl/fl}$ *Lyz2*-Cre mice died from the bacterial peritonitis in the cecal-ligation-and puncture (CLP) model of septic peritonitis. $Mst1^{fl/fl}Mst2^{fl/fl}$ *Lyz2*-Cre mice showed significantly higher levels of bacterial invasion of the lungs, liver, spleen, kidneys and peritoneal fluid after CLP than that in their wild-type littermates. In additions, $Mst1^{fl/fl}Mst2^{fl/fl}$ *Lyz2*-Cre mice exhibited more severe inflammation in lung and kidney tissues and significantly higher serum concentrations of the inflammatory cytokines IL-6, TNF and IL-1β than their wild-type littermates after CLP induction, suggesting that the greater susceptibility of $Mst1^{fl/fl}Mst2^{fl/fl}$ *Lyz2*-Cre mice to CLP-induced bacterial sepsis was not due to a lack of a pro-inflammatory response to bacterial infection (Geng et al., 2015). Our further studies revealed that TLR/MyD88-mediated activation of Mst1/2 in phagocytes was required for phagocytosis and efficient clearance of bacteria. Flow cytometry and immunofluorescence micrographs showed that Mst1/2-deficient phagocytes exhibited less phagocytosis of both *E. coli* and *L. monocytogenes*, but higher number of live intracellular bacteria at late time points (more than 30 min) after bacterial infection, than did wild-type cells, which indicated that in addition to showing a modest uptake of bacteria, Mst1/2-deficient phagocytes were significantly defective in the intracellular killing of bacteria (Geng et al., 2015).

ROS play a critical role in bacterial killing by phagocytes, in which both phagosomal NADPH-oxidase and mitochondrial ROS (mROS) are major sources of ROS for killing bacteria inside phagosomes. Interestingly, the induction of both phagosomal ROS and mROS is considerably impaired in Mst1/2 deficient phagocytes after bacterial infection, which might be responsible to their defective in bactericide activity. Consistent with its ability to activate Mst1/2 by different TLRs, engagement of the cell-surface TLRs (TLR1, TLR2 and TLR4) augments mROS and total cellular ROS in BMDMs and neutrophils, but engagement of the endosomal TLRs (TLR3, TLR7, TLR8 and TLR9) does not. Notably, Mst1/2-deficient BMDMs or neutrophils show little or no increase in mROS and cellular ROS in response to the stimulation of TLR1, TLR2 or TLR4 (Geng et al., 2015). Previously study showed that recruitment of mitochondria and releasing mROS to phagosomes containing intracellular pathogens are required to kill the pathogens (West et al., 2011). Mst1/2-deficient BMDMs display much less mitochondrial cupping around phagocytosed Pam3CSK4- or LPS-coated beads, or fewer co-localization of mitochondria and bacteria during infection with GFP-*E. coli*, than did wild-type BMDMs, suggesting that Mst1/2 kinases might control the mitochondrion-phagosome juxtaposition during the infections. Mechanically, we found that TLR-mediated Mst1/2 kinases activate the small GTPase Rac via the kinase PKC-α and the GDP-dissociation inhibitor LyGDI, and induce the TRAF6-ECSIT complex assembly for recruitment of mitochondria to phagosomes and generation of ROS to kill engulfed bacteria (Geng et al., 2015).

Mst1/2 kinases regulate chemokine-stimulated reorganization of F-actin in thymocytes by promoting activation of the small GTPase Rac1 (Mou et al., 2012). Interestingly, upon the Rac inhibitor NSC23766 treatment, the co-localization of mitochondria with GFP-*E. coli* or LPS-induced mROS and total cellular ROS is decreased or blocked in both in BMDMs and neutrophils. Consistently, the levels of activated form of Rac1, GTP charged Rac1 (Rac1-GTP), are much lower in Mst1/2-deficient phagocytes, and the reintroducing of constitutively active form of Rac1 ($Rac1^{G12V}$) restores the normal organization of F-actin, mitochondrion-phagosome juxtaposition and production of mROS and cellular ROS in Mst1/2 deficient phagocytes upon stimulation with LPS (Geng et al., 2015). We then identified and confirmed that PKCα protein and LyGDI can form complex in macrophages by mass spectrometry and co-immunoprecipitation assays respectively. LyGDI belongs to a family of three Rho-GDP-dissociation inhibitors that bind Rac-GDP in a cytosolic complex, and PKC-α-mediated phosphorylation of LyGDI at Ser31 disrupts the interaction between LyGDI and Rac, which releases Rac-GDP and promotes its translocation to the membrane for undergoing guanyl nucleotide exchange (Mehta, Rahman, & Malik, 2001). We found that Mst1/2 can bind and directly phosphorylate PKC-α at Ser226 and Thr228. The Mst1/2-mediated phosphorylation of

PKC-α at Ser226 and Thr228 is required for the optimal activation of PKC-α, as the phosphorylation of PKC-α at Thr638, an autophosphorylation site reflective of PKC-α activation, is much lower in Mst1/2 deficient BMDMs than that in wild-type BMDMs upon the stimulation of LPS. In addition, co-expression of PKC-α with Mst2 enhances the interaction between PKC-α and LyGDI, and this in turn promotes the PKC-α-mediated phosphorylation of LyGDI, which leads to LyGDI dissociation from the LyGDI-Rac1 complex and enhances the activation of Rac-GTP. Consistently, the ability of LPS to diminish the interaction between LyGDI and Rac1 is much lower in Mst1/2-deficient BMDMs than in wild-type BMDMs (Geng et al., 2015).

The co-localization of Rac1 with phagosomes is enhanced in wild-type BMDMs upon infection of *E. coli*, and this response is much lower in Mst1/2-deficient BMDMs. In our study, the E3 ubiquitin ligase TRAF6, a key intermediate in TLR signaling, is identified to specifically interact with the inactive form of Rac1 ($Rac1^{T17N}$), but not with a constitutively active form of Rac ($Rac1^{G12V}$). Furthermore, TRAF6 catalyzes the K63-linked ubiquitination of Rac1 at Lys16 and enhances the activation state of Rac1. Knockdown of endogenous TRAF6 is accompanied by a marked reduction in total and K63-linked ubiquitination of Rac1 and the activation of Rac1 in resting or LPS-stimulated BMDMs. On the other hand, the GTP charging of activated Rac1 is required for undergoing the TRAF6-catalyzed ubiquitination on Rac1, i.e. TRAF6 preferentially ubiquitinates the GTP-charged active form of Rac1. Thus, upon infection, TLRs initiate GTP charging of Rac1 by releasing LyGDI from Rac-GDP, which enables the TRAF6-mediated K63-linked polyubiquitination of Rac-GTP, followed by the dissociation of TRAF6 from Rac-GTP. Thus, the ubiquitination of Rac, although it is catalyzed subsequent to charging of Rac1 with GTP, further enhances and stabilizes the activation of GTP-charged Rac1 (Geng et al., 2015).

Previous study has shown that the recruitment of mitochondria to phagosomes and increased mROS production to kill the intracellular bacteria are mediated by the assembly of a complex of TRAF6 with ECSIT in the mitochondria (West et al., 2011). We found that the co-localization of TRAF6 and ECSIT with the bacteria is occurred in wild-type BMDMs, but not in Mst1/2-deficient BMDMs after infection with *E. coli*, and this defect is "rescued" in Mst1/2-deficient BMDMs expressing the constituted activated $Rac1^{G12V}$. Interestingly, the immunoprecipitation assays revealed that both ECSIT and Rac1 interacted with the carboxy-terminal MATH domain (amino acids 351–522) of TRAF6. Co-expression of TRAF6 and ECSIT with Rac1 variants shows that wild-type Rac1 only modestly displaces ECSIT from TRAF6, but inactive $Rac1^{T17N}$ does so substantially. In contrast, $Rac1^{G12V}$ had little or no effect on the TRAF6-ECSIT complex. Immunofluorescence staining further confirmed that active Rac1 greatly enhances the co-localization of ECSIT and TRAF6 in HeLa cells, but inactive Rac1 does not (Geng et al., 2015). These data indicated that, in Mst1/2-deficient phagocytes, inactive Rac has a dominant-negative effect to block the association of TRAF6-ECSIT through the competitive binding of ECIST and inactive Rac to TRAF6. These results also explained that the inactivating $Rac2^{D57N}$ substitution causes a human immunodeficiency syndrome characterized by a substantial reduction in ROS production in phagocytes (Ambruso et al., 2000; Gu et al., 2001; Williams et al., 2000). Taken together, upon the bacterial infection, the process of Mst1/2 kinases-mediated phosphorylation of PKCα/LyGDI, followed by GTP-charging and ubiquitination of Rac in BMDMs is critical for the dissociation of Rac from the TRAF6 to enable assembly of the TRAF6-ECSIT complex, and that in turn mediates mitochondrion phagosome juxtaposition and an increase in mROS production for killing intracellular pathogens (Geng et al., 2015).

In summary, our work demonstrated that kinases Mst1 and Mst2 are key regulators of microbe-elicited ROS production and that they act through a previously unrecognized signaling cascade: TLR-Mst1/2-PKC-Rac-TRAF6-ECIST (Geng et al., 2015) (Fig. 5). These results demonstrated that the signaling downstream of TLRs is not simply directed to transcriptional regulation of genes for the innate immune responses, but is also able to rapidly reorganize organelles and sculpt their subcellular composition to augment host defense through post-translational modification. However, the downstream effectors of the TLR-MyD88 complex for the activation of Mst1 and Mst2 remain to be identified. Recently, Li et al. showed that Mst1 binds and phosphorylates IL-1 receptor–associated kinase 1 (IRAK1), which results in IRAK1 degradation, to dampened TLR4/9-induced proinflammatory cytokine secretion but enhanced TLR3/4-triggered IFN-β production (Li, Xiao, et al., 2015). Mst1 differentially regulates TLR3/4/9-mediated inflammatory responses in macrophages and thereby is protective against chronic inflammation–associated HCC (Li, Xiao, et al., 2015). In additions, the kinase Mst4 has also been shown to limit inflammatory responses through direct phosphorylation of TRAF6 (Jiao et al., 2015). It will be interesting to determine whether Mst1 and Mst2

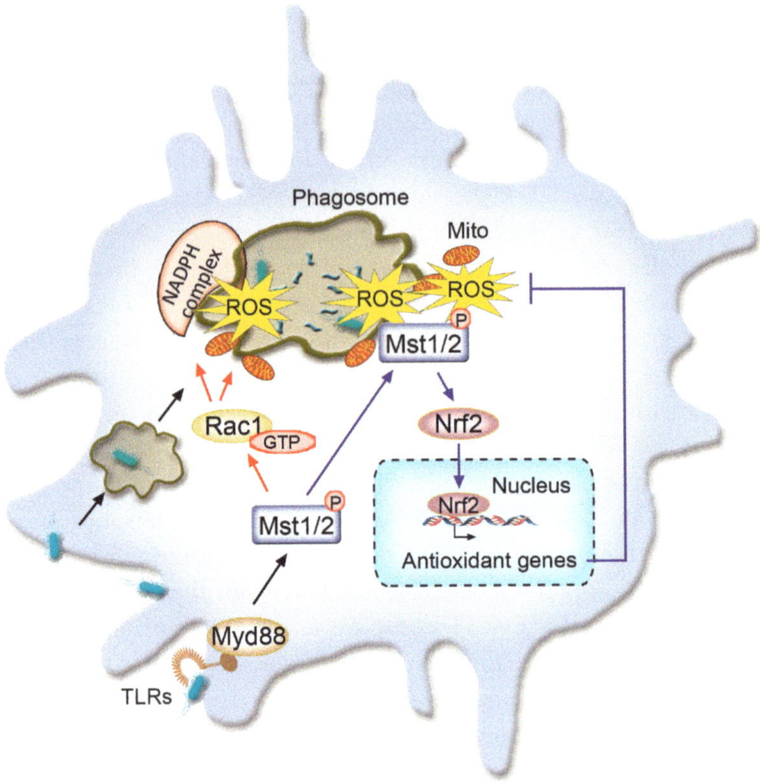

Fig. 5 A proposed working model of kinases Mst1/2 acting as molecular switches to maintaining redox homeostasis by coordinating induction of ROS to kill microbes and clearance excess ROS to attenuate ROS-induced damage in macrophages. During an antimicrobial response, Toll-like receptor (TLR) signaling triggers the activation of Mst1 and Mst2 kinases, enhances the GTP charging of Rac1. Activated Rac1 then promotes mitochondrion phagosome juxtaposition and thereby augmenting mitochondrial, as well as phagosomal, ROS production for killing bacteria inside the phagosome. On the other hand, phagosomal or mitochondrial ROS attract Mst1/2 to cap around phagosome or mitochondrion from the cytosol and activate Mst1/2; activated Mst1/2 kinases stabilize Nrf2 and induce the expression of antioxidant enzymes to protect macrophages from oxidative damage.

can also phosphorylate TRAF6 and, if so, whether this affects the TRAF6-mediated regulation of Rac activation. Thus, how the TLR signaling pathway interplays with the Hippo signaling pathway will be an interesting field to be studied.

3.2 Macrophage redox homeostasis and aging

ROS are a double-edged sword: they are critical for maintaining the normal physiological function of cells and are also toxic species that cause cellular injury. Ample ROS production in phagocytes is a major defense mechanism against pathogen infection; on the other hand, ROS lead to impaired physiological function through cumulative cellular damage of DNA, proteins, lipids, and other macromolecules, which results in oxidative stress, aging and antioxidant defense decreases with age (Balaban, Nemoto, & Finkel, 2005; Holmstrom & Finkel, 2014). In additions, oxidative damage affects mitochondrial DNA replication and transcription and results in decreased mitochondrial function, which in turn leads to enhanced ROS production and further oxidative damage to cells (Balaban et al., 2005). A previous study showed that knockdown of *C. elegans* CST-1, the orthologue of the Hippo kinase, accelerates aging and shortens life span (Lehtinen et al., 2006). Hydrogen peroxide is commonly used to activate Mst1/2 in vitro and several mechanisms of ROS-mediated Mst1/2 activation have been proposed (Avruch et al., 2012; Creasy, Ambrose, & Chernoff, 1996; Rawat & Chernoff, 2015; Rawat, Creasy, Peterson, & Chernoff, 2013). However, it is not clear whether model systems exposed to exogenous hydrogen peroxide have relevance to systems in which the oxidant is generated endogenously. As above mentioned, macrophages engulf harmful microorganisms and destroy them in phagosomes, and these processes depend mainly on the production of large amounts of phagosomal and mitochondrial ROS (Geng et al., 2015). Thus the dedicated balance between the generation and elimination of ROS is essential to suppress excess ROS and thus attenuate ROS induced damage and the aging process in macrophages. Our recent studies demonstrated that oxidants generated endogenously by phagosomes or mitochondria during the infection recruited Mst1/2 to phagosomes or mitochondria and markedly activated these kinases (Wang et al., 2019). The activation of Mst1/2 and the association of Mst1/2 with phagosomes containing engulfed bacteria or the mitochondrial compartments can be abolished or disrupted by the antioxidant *N*-acetylcysteine (NAC) treatment. Thus, Mst1/2 kinases are able to sense and then are activated by the phagosomal and mitochondrial ROS produced in macrophages during the respiration or upon infections (Wang et al., 2019).

3.2.1 Increased oxidative stress and premature aging in Mst1/2-deficient macrophages

Although the induction of phagosomal and mitochondrial ROS is defect in Mst1/2-deficient phagocytes upon the infection of pathogens, we surprisingly observed that Mst1/2-deficient BMDMs exhibit higher basal levels of ROS than that of wild-type BMDMs (Wang et al., 2019). Further analysis revealed that loss of Mst1/2 results in oxidative stress in phagocytes, as shown by increased levels of protein carbonylation (a biomarker of oxidative stress) and phosphorylated (p)-H2A.X (an DNA damage indicator), as well as increased apoptotic events associated with enhanced cleavage of PARPγ and caspase 3, and more importantly NAC, a ROS scavenger, can significantly downregulate these oxidative stress phenomena, indicating that Mst1/2 kinases are critical in protecting macrophages from oxidative stress (Wang et al., 2019). Notably, we observed that the mRNA and protein levels of Mst1 and Mst2, as well as the p-Mob levels were dramatically reduced in aged macrophages (20 months) suggesting that Mst1/2 kinases might also involve in preventing macrophages aging process (Wang et al., 2019). Recently, Meng et al. reported that the disintegration of redox-stress response capacity (RRC) is a substantive characteristic of aging (Meng et al., 2017). RRC refers to the ability of cells to respond to oxidative stress, specifically three major activities: the ability to generate ROS or RNS, the ability to regulate antioxidants, and the ability to degrade damaged proteins for maintaining cellular redox and protein homeostasis (Meng et al., 2017). As mentioned above, loss of Mst1/2 kinases results in the defective clearance of bacteria in phagocytes, as well as the increased proinflammtory cytokines production during the infection, which resembles the features of aged phagocytes (Geng et al., 2015; Plowden, Renshaw-Hoelscher, Engleman, Katz, & Sambhara, 2004). Previous study showed that the expression levels of TLRs(1–9) downregulated in activated aged peritoneal macrophages (Renshaw et al., 2002). In comparison of the TLRs in wild-type and Mst1/2-deficient macrophages, we observed that the expression levels of TLR1, 2, 5, 8, and 9 are comparable in 2-month old macrophages, but are significantly decreased in Mst1/2-deficient macrophages from the 12- and 20-month old mice. While the expression levels TLR3, 4, 6, and 7 are all much lower in Mst1/2-deficient macrophages compared with that of WT macrophages at any given ages. In additions, we found that the ability of macrophages to activate OVA-specific OT-II $CD4^+$ T cells as measured by the proliferation assay is gradually decreased with increasing age. Mst1/2-deficient macrophages (12- and 20-month) exhibit much lower capacity to activated $CD4^+$ T cells when compared with that of the same ages wild-type macrophages. In addition, lipofuscin granules, a recognized hallmark of aging, are also observed in Mst1/2-deficient Mst1/2 macrophages at younger ages, and are more abundance when compared with wild-type cells at the same age (Wang et al., 2019). Numerous data have shown that ROS-mediated accumulation of cellular damage results in increased telomere shortening and dysfunction, which are associated with aging, mortality and aging-related diseases (von Zglinicki, 2002). We observed that Mst1/2-deficient macrophages have shorter telomeres than that of wild-type cells at 8 months and 12 months of age, although the difference in telomere length is not significant at 2 months of age, suggesting that loss of Mst1/2 promotes telomeric loss (Wang et al., 2019). Taken together, these data indicate that loss of Mst1/2 resulted in premature aging in macrophages due to oxidative stress.

3.2.2 Kinases Mst1 and Mst2 regulate Nrf2 function for defensing oxidative stress in macrophages

Interestingly, we observed that the enzymatic antioxidant system is defective in Mst1/2-deficient macrophages. Upon LPS, antimycin A, rotenone, or H_2O_2 treatments, or *E. coli* infection, the mRNA and protein levels of various antioxidant genes such as, *Nqo1*, *Ho-1*, *Gclc*, and *Gclm*, which are critical for protecting cells against toxic free radical, are dramatically lower in Mst1/2-deficient BMDMs than that of wild-type BMDMs (Wang et al., 2019). Oxidative stress is involved in the activation of several major transcription factors, such as those in the Nrf2 and FoxO1/3 families, which induce the expression of the antioxidant genes to promote cellular adaptation to oxidative stress (Gorrini, Harris, & Mak, 2013; Huang, Nguyen, & Pickett, 2000). Previous studies have shown that, in the nervous system, oxidative stress induces the Mst1-mediated phosphorylation of FoxO3 at Ser207, leading to the release of FoxO3 from 14 to 3-3 proteins and the consequent accumulation of FoxO3 in the nucleus, where FoxO3 induces the expression of antioxidant or apoptotic genes and thereby leads to either cell recovery or cell death in response to oxidative stress (Lee et al., 2013; Lee, Seo, Choi, & Koh, 2014; Lehtinen et al., 2006; Yuan et al., 2009). In T cell immunity, it has been demonstrated that Mst1 modulates FoxO1 and FoxO3 (FoxO1/3) stability to regulate Foxp3 expression and Treg development/function and inhibits autoimmunity (Choi et al., 2009; Du et al., 2014). By analyzing the expression prolife of Nrf2 and FoxO1/3, we surprisingly found that FoxO1/3 and Nrf2 are differentially expressed in various immune cell types (Wang et al., 2019). FoxO1 and FoxO3 are highly expressed in T lymphocytes and B lymphocytes, but are barely detectable in macrophages, whereas Nrf2 is preferentially expressed in macrophages. Consistently, loss of Nrf2, but not FoxO1 or FoxO3, results in elevated basal levels of ROS in macrophages without any stimulation (Wang et al., 2019). These results indicate that Nrf2 is the key transcriptional activator of the antioxidant response in macrophages.

Interestingly, although the increased Nrf2 mRNA level is not affected, the accumulation of Nrf2 protein is impaired in Mst1/2-deficient BMDMs in response to the oxidative stress caused by the treatment of antimycin A or rotenone, two drugs that block the mitochondrial respiratory chain and lead to the generation of mitochondrial ROS, mimicking the mitochondrial oxidative burst. This result suggested that Mst1/2 kinases might regulate the protein stability of Nrf2. Previous studies have shown that Nrf2 is predominantly degraded through the ubiquitination mediated proteasome pathway. Under unstressed conditions, Keap1, a substrate adapter subunit of a Cullin 3 (Cul3)-based ubiquitin E3 ligase, interacts with Nrf2 and promotes the ubiquitination and proteasomal degradation of Nrf2 (Kobayashi et al., 2004; Motohashi & Yamamoto, 2004; Zipper & Mulcahy, 2002). We observed that the ubiquitination level of Nrf2 is higher in Mst1/2-deficient BMDMs compared with that in wild-type cells, while under the oxidative stress conditions, the ubiquitination level Nrf2 is decreased in wild-type BMDMs, but not in Mst1/2-deficient BMDMs. Our further study showed that Mst1/2 kinases are able to bind to and phosphorylate Keap1 and their interaction is enhanced upon *E.coli* infection or antimycin A treatment, but disrupted by NAC treatment. Mass spectrometry and site-directed mutagenesis further revealed that Keap1 is phosphorylated by Mst1/2 at four amino acid residues (T51, S53, T55, and T80), located next to or within the BTB domain (amino acids 77–149), which are essential for binding the E3 ubiquitin ligase Cul3 or for Keap1 dimerization or polymerization. Mst1/2-mediated Keap1 phosphorylation does not affect the interaction between Keap1 and Cul3, but prevents the Keap1 dimerization or polymerization. Overexpression of nonphosphorylatable mutant Keap1^{4A} (T51A, S53A, T55A, and T80A), which mimics no Mst1/2-mediated phosphorylation and is able to form Keap1 dimers/polymers, dramatically enhances the ubiquitination level of Nrf2 and decreased Nrf2 protein levels, while overexpression of nonpolymerizable Keap1^{4D} (T51D, S53D, T55D, and T80D) leads to the lower Nrf2 ubiquitination level and no or little effect on the Nrf2 protein levels in BMDMs or Raw264.7 cells. In additions, nonphosphorylatable mutant Keap1^{4A} also has a higher binding affinity for Nrf2 suggesting that dimerization or polymerization of keap1 might cause a conformation change for better binding Nrf2 (Wang et al., 2019). Therefore, our study demonstrated that ROS triggered the activation of Mst1/2 to phosphorylate its substrate the adapter protein Keap1 in the Keap1-Cul3-Rbx1 E3 ubiquitin ligase complex, and prevent its polymerization and association with Nrf2, thereby block the targeting of Nrf2 for degradation.

These results revealed that the accumulation of Nrf2 is critical for Mst1/2-mediated antioxidative response (Wang et al., 2019). Indeed, reintroduction of adenovirus expressing Nrf2 (Ad-Nrf2), but not of control adenovirus expressing GFP (Ad-GFP), significantly downregulates basal ROS, increases the transcription of the *Ho-1* and *Nqo1* genes, decreases p-H2A.X levels, as well as decreases the percentage of apoptotic events in Mst1/2-deficient BMDM under unstressed or stressed conditions (Wang et al., 2019). Taken together, we identified the Mst-Nrf2 axis as an important ROS sensing, antioxidant, and anti-aging mechanism in phagocytes during an antimicrobial response (Fig. 5).

4. Conclusion

The Hippo signaling pathway regulates cellular proliferation and survival to maintain the tissue homeostasis during the development. Our recently work demonstrated that Hippo signaling also play pivotal roles in regulating immune homeostasis. Mst1/2, the core kinases of the Hippo signaling pathway, function as molecular switches to maintaining redox homeostasis by coordinating induction of ROS to kill microbes and clearance excess ROS to attenuate ROS-induced damage and the aging process in macrophages. These results reveal the importance of the subcellular localization and spatial coordination of innate immunological effectors and show how defects in this can result in impaired phagosome function, defective killing of microbes and oxidative stress induced cell death and aging, and eventually leading to immunodeficiency. Mst1/2-Nrf2 signaling as an oxidative stress response mechanism in macrophages suggests that this pathway may provide a mechanistic basis for how oxidative stress contributes to the pathogenesis of aging-associated inflammation and infection. In addition, Hippo signaling prevents the development of inflammatory Th17 cells but enhances the differentiation of immune suppressive Treg cells, supporting the likely physiopathologic relevance of the loss of Hippo signaling that engages. These findings highlight non-canonical activation of the Hippo pathway as a potential target in infection diseases, autoimmune diseases and immune cells aging, as well as raise new considerations for the current thinking on Hippo signaling as a cancer target. Targeting Hippo signaling in cancer patients raises a note of caution due to the potential for enhancing Treg cells, which might suppress tumor clearance. However, our findings suggest that the cancer therapy targeting Hippo might be useful for treating autoimmune diseases by blocking Th17 cells differentiation and increasing the abundance of Treg cells to provide long-term anti-inflammatory effects. Interestingly, recent work from Guan's group revealed a surprising role of the Hippo pathway kinases Lats1/2 in suppressing anti-tumor immunity (Moroishi et al., 2016). Anyhow, as a tumor suppressor pathway, as well as an immune function modulating pathway, the Hippo signaling pathway is a promising therapeutic target for the treatment of these diseases, however, its effects on either one need to be considered for safety reasons and more regulatory details remain to be explored.

Reference

Abdollahpour, H., Appaswamy, G., Kotlarz, D., Diestelhorst, J., Beier, R., Schaffer, A. A., et al. (2012). The phenotype of human STK4 deficiency. *Blood*, *119*(15), 3450–3457. https://doi.org/10.1182/blood-2011-09-378158.

Alsufyani, F., Mattoo, H., Zhou, D., Cariappa, A., Van Buren, D., Hock, H., et al. (2018). The Mst1 kinase is required for follicular B cell homing and B-1 B cell development. *Frontiers in Immunology*, *9*, 2393. https://doi.org/10.3389/fimmu.2018.02393.

Ambruso, D. R., Knall, C., Abell, A. N., Panepinto, J., Kurkchubasche, A., Thurman, G., et al. (2000). Human neutrophil immunodeficiency syndrome is associated with an inhibitory Rac2 mutation. *Proceedings of the National Academy of Sciences of the United States of America*, *97*(9), 4654–4659. https://doi.org/10.1073/pnas.080074897.

Avruch, J., Zhou, D., Fitamant, J., Bardeesy, N., Mou, F., & Barrufet, L. R. (2012). Protein kinases of the hippo pathway: Regulation and substrates. *Seminars in Cell & Developmental Biology*, *23*(7), 770–784. https://doi.org/10.1016/j.semcdb.2012.07.002.

Bagherzadeh Yazdchi, S., Witalis, M., Meli, A. P., Leung, J., Li, X., Panneton, V., et al. (2019). Hippo pathway kinase Mst1 is required for long-lived humoral immunity. *Journal of Immunology*, *202*(1), 69–78. https://doi.org/10.4049/jimmunol.1701407.

Balaban, R. S., Nemoto, S., & Finkel, T. (2005). Mitochondria, oxidants, and aging. *Cell*, *120*(4), 483–495. https://doi.org/10.1016/j.cell.2005.02.001.

Bettelli, E., Carrier, Y., Gao, W., Korn, T., Strom, T. B., Oukka, M., et al. (2006). Reciprocal developmental pathways for the generation of pathogenic effector TH17 and regulatory T cells. *Nature*, *441*(7090), 235–238. https://doi.org/10.1038/nature04753.

Boursalian, T. E., Golob, J., Soper, D. M., Cooper, C. J., & Fink, P. J. (2004). Continued maturation of thymic emigrants in the periphery. *Nature Immunology*, *5*(4), 418–425. https://doi.org/10.1038/ni1049.

Brubaker, S. W., Bonham, K. S., Zanoni, I., & Kagan, J. C. (2015). Innate immune pattern recognition: A cell biological perspective. *Annual Review of Immunology*, *33*, 257–290. https://doi.org/10.1146/annurev-immunol-032414-112240.

Carlson, C. M., Endrizzi, B. T., Wu, J., Ding, X., Weinreich, M. A., Walsh, E. R., et al. (2006). Kruppel-like factor 2 regulates thymocyte and T-cell migration. *Nature*, *442*(7100), 299–302. https://doi.org/10.1038/nature04882.

Chen, L., Qin, F., Deng, X., Avruch, J., & Zhou, D. (2012). Hippo pathway in intestinal homeostasis and tumorigenesis. *Protein & Cell*, *3*(4), 305–310. https://doi.org/10.1007/s13238-012-2913-9.

Choi, J., Oh, S., Lee, D., Oh, H. J., Park, J. Y., Lee, S. B., et al. (2009). Mst1-FoxO signaling protects naive T lymphocytes from cellular oxidative stress in mice. *PLoS One*, *4*(11). e8011https://doi.org/10.1371/journal.pone.0008011.

Creasy, C. L., Ambrose, D. M., & Chernoff, J. (1996). The Ste20-like protein kinase, Mst1, dimerizes and contains an inhibitory domain. *The Journal of Biological Chemistry*, *271*(35), 21049–21053. https://doi.org/10.1074/jbc.271.35.21049.

Dong, Y., Du, X., Ye, J., Han, M., Xu, T., Zhuang, Y., et al. (2009). A cell-intrinsic role for Mst1 in regulating thymocyte egress. *Journal of Immunology, 183*(6), 3865–3872. https://doi.org/10.4049/jimmunol.0900678.

Dong, J., Feldmann, G., Huang, J., Wu, S., Zhang, N., Comerford, S. A., et al. (2007). Elucidation of a universal size-control mechanism in Drosophila and mammals. *Cell, 130*(6), 1120–1133.

Du, X., Shi, H., Li, J., Dong, Y., Liang, J., Ye, J., et al. (2014). Mst1/Mst2 regulate development and function of regulatory T cells through modulation of Foxo1/Foxo3 stability in autoimmune disease. *Journal of Immunology, 192*(4), 1525–1535. https://doi.org/10.4049/jimmunol.1301060.

Fan, F., He, Z., Kong, L. L., Chen, Q., Yuan, Q., Zhang, S., et al. (2016). Pharmacological targeting of kinases MST1 and MST2 augments tissue repair and regeneration. *Science Translational Medicine, 8*(352). 352ra108https://doi.org/10.1126/scitranslmed.aaf2304.

Geng, J., Sun, X., Wang, P., Zhang, S., Wang, X., Wu, H., et al. (2015). Kinases Mst1 and Mst2 positively regulate phagocytic induction of reactive oxygen species and bactericidal activity. *Nature Immunology, 16*(11), 1142–1152. https://doi.org/10.1038/ni.3268.

Geng, J., Yu, S., Zhao, H., Sun, X., Li, X., Wang, P., et al. (2017). The transcriptional coactivator TAZ regulates reciprocal differentiation of TH17 cells and Treg cells. *Nature Immunology, 18*(7), 800–812. https://doi.org/10.1038/ni.3748.

Gorrini, C., Harris, I. S., & Mak, T. W. (2013). Modulation of oxidative stress as an anticancer strategy. *Nature Reviews. Drug Discovery, 12*(12), 931–947. https://doi.org/10.1038/nrd4002.

Gu, Y., Jia, B., Yang, F. C., D'Souza, M., Harris, C. E., Derrow, C. W., et al. (2001). Biochemical and biological characterization of a human Rac2 GTPase mutant associated with phagocytic immunodeficiency. *The Journal of Biological Chemistry, 276*(19), 15929–15938. https://doi.org/10.1074/jbc.M010445200.

Hao, Y., Chun, A., Cheung, K., Rashidi, B., & Yang, X. (2008). Tumor suppressor LATS1 is a negative regulator of oncogene YAP. *The Journal of Biological Chemistry, 283*(9), 5496–5509. https://doi.org/10.1074/jbc.M709037200.

Harvey, K. F., Zhang, X., & Thomas, D. M. (2013). The Hippo pathway and human cancer. *Nature Reviews. Cancer, 13*(4), 246–257. https://doi.org/10.1038/nrc3458.

Holmstrom, K. M., & Finkel, T. (2014). Cellular mechanisms and physiological consequences of redox-dependent signalling. *Nature Reviews. Molecular Cell Biology, 15*(6), 411–421. https://doi.org/10.1038/nrm3801.

Huang, H. C., Nguyen, T., & Pickett, C. B. (2000). Regulation of the antioxidant response element by protein kinase C-mediated phosphorylation of NF-E2-related factor 2. *Proceedings of the National Academy of Sciences of the United States of America, 97*(23), 12475–12480. https://doi.org/10.1073/pnas.220418997.

Ji, S., Liu, Q., Zhang, S., Chen, Q., Wang, C., Zhang, W., et al. (2019). FGF15 activates hippo signaling to suppress bile acid metabolism and liver tumorigenesis. *Developmental Cell, 48*(4), 460–474, e469. https://doi.org/10.1016/j.devcel.2018.12.021.

Jiao, S., Zhang, Z., Li, C., Huang, M., Shi, Z., Wang, Y., et al. (2015). The kinase MST4 limits inflammatory responses through direct phosphorylation of the adaptor TRAF6. *Nature Immunology, 16*(3), 246–257. https://doi.org/10.1038/ni.3097.

Katagiri, K., Imamura, M., & Kinashi, T. (2006). Spatiotemporal regulation of the kinase Mst1 by binding protein RAPL is critical for lymphocyte polarity and adhesion. *Nature Immunology, 7*(9), 919–928. https://doi.org/10.1038/ni1374.

Katagiri, K., Katakai, T., Ebisuno, Y., Ueda, Y., Okada, T., & Kinashi, T. (2009). Mst1 controls lymphocyte trafficking and interstitial motility within lymph nodes. *The EMBO Journal, 28*(9), 1319–1331. https://doi.org/10.1038/emboj.2009.82.

Katagiri, K., Maeda, A., Shimonaka, M., & Kinashi, T. (2003). RAPL, a Rap1-binding molecule that mediates Rap1-induced adhesion through spatial regulation of LFA-1. *Nature Immunology*, *4*(8), 741–748. https://doi.org/10.1038/ni950.

Katagiri, K., Ohnishi, N., Kabashima, K., Iyoda, T., Takeda, N., Shinkai, Y., et al. (2004). Crucial functions of the Rap1 effector molecule RAPL in lymphocyte and dendritic cell trafficking. *Nature Immunology*, *5*(10), 1045–1051. https://doi.org/10.1038/ni1111.

Kobayashi, A., Kang, M. I., Okawa, H., Ohtsuji, M., Zenke, Y., Chiba, T., et al. (2004). Oxidative stress sensor Keap1 functions as an adaptor for Cul3-based E3 ligase to regulate proteasomal degradation of Nrf2. *Molecular and Cellular Biology*, *24*(16), 7130–7139. https://doi.org/10.1128/MCB.24.16.7130-7139.2004.

Lazarevic, V., Chen, X., Shim, J. H., Hwang, E. S., Jang, E., Bolm, A. N., et al. (2011). T-bet represses T(H)17 differentiation by preventing Runx1-mediated activation of the gene encoding RORgammat. *Nature Immunology*, *12*(1), 96–104. https://doi.org/10.1038/ni.1969.

Lee, K. P., Lee, J. H., Kim, T. S., Kim, T. H., Park, H. D., Byun, J. S., et al. (2010). The hippo-Salvador pathway restrains hepatic oval cell proliferation, liver size, and liver tumorigenesis. *Proceedings of the National Academy of Sciences of the United States of America*, *107*(18), 8248–8253. https://doi.org/10.1073/pnas.0912203107.

Lee, I. Y., Lim, J. M., Cho, H., Kim, E., Kim, Y., Oh, H. K., et al. (2019). MST1 negatively regulates TNFalpha-induced NF-kappaB signaling through modulating LUBAC activity. *Molecular Cell*, *73*(6), 1138–1149, e1136. https://doi.org/10.1016/j.molcel.2019.01.022.

Lee, S. J., Seo, B. R., Choi, E. J., & Koh, J. Y. (2014). The role of reciprocal activation of cAbl and Mst1 in the oxidative death of cultured astrocytes. *Glia*, *62*(4), 639–648. https://doi.org/10.1002/glia.22631.

Lee, J. K., Shin, J. H., Hwang, S. G., Gwag, B. J., McKee, A. C., Lee, J., et al. (2013). MST1 functions as a key modulator of neurodegeneration in a mouse model of ALS. *Proceedings of the National Academy of Sciences of the United States of America*, *110*(29), 12066–12071. https://doi.org/10.1073/pnas.1300894110.

Lehtinen, M. K., Yuan, Z., Boag, P. R., Yang, Y., Villen, J., Becker, E. B., et al. (2006). A conserved MST-FOXO signaling pathway mediates oxidative-stress responses and extends life span. *Cell*, *125*(5), 987–1001. https://doi.org/10.1016/j.cell.2006.03.046.

Li, C., Bi, Y., Li, Y., Yang, H., Yu, Q., Wang, J., et al. (2017). Dendritic cell MST1 inhibits Th17 differentiation. *Nature Communications*, *8*, 14275. https://doi.org/10.1038/ncomms14275.

Li, J., Du, X., Shi, H., Deng, K., Chi, H., & Tao, W. (2015). Mammalian sterile 20-like kinase 1 (Mst1) enhances the stability of forkhead box P3 (Foxp3) and the function of regulatory T cells by modulating Foxp3 acetylation. *The Journal of Biological Chemistry*, *290*(52), 30762–30770. https://doi.org/10.1074/jbc.M115.668442.

Li, W., Xiao, J., Zhou, X., Xu, M., Hu, C., Xu, X., et al. (2015). STK4 regulates TLR pathways and protects against chronic inflammation-related hepatocellular carcinoma. *The Journal of Clinical Investigation*, *125*(11), 4239–4254. https://doi.org/10.1172/JCI81203.

Liu, J., & Cao, X. (2016). Cellular and molecular regulation of innate inflammatory responses. *Cellular & Molecular Immunology*, *13*(6), 711–721. https://doi.org/10.1038/cmi.2016.58.

Liu, B., Zheng, Y., Yin, F., Yu, J., Silverman, N., & Pan, D. (2016). Toll receptor-mediated hippo signaling controls innate immunity in Drosophila. *Cell*, *164*(3), 406–419. https://doi.org/10.1016/j.cell.2015.12.029.

Lu, L., Li, Y., Kim, S. M., Bossuyt, W., Liu, P., Qiu, Q., et al. (2010). Hippo signaling is a potent in vivo growth and tumor suppressor pathway in the mammalian liver. *Proceedings of the National Academy of Sciences of the United States of America*, *107*(4), 1437–1442. https://doi.org/10.1073/pnas.0911427107.

Mehta, D., Rahman, A., & Malik, A. B. (2001). Protein kinase C-alpha signals rho-guanine nucleotide dissociation inhibitor phosphorylation and rho activation and regulates the endothelial cell barrier function. *The Journal of Biological Chemistry*, *276*(25), 22614–22620. https://doi.org/10.1074/jbc.M101927200.

Meng, J., Lv, Z., Qiao, X., Li, X., Li, Y., Zhang, Y., et al. (2017). The decay of redox-stress response capacity is a substantive characteristic of aging: Revising the redox theory of aging. *Redox Biology*, *11*, 365–374. https://doi.org/10.1016/j.redox.2016.12.026.

Meng, F., Zhou, R., Wu, S., Zhang, Q., Jin, Q., Zhou, Y., et al. (2016). Mst1 shuts off cytosolic antiviral defense through IRF3 phosphorylation. *Genes & Development*, *30*(9), 1086–1100. https://doi.org/10.1101/gad.277533.116.

Moroishi, T., Hayashi, T., Pan, W. W., Fujita, Y., Holt, M. V., Qin, J., et al. (2016). The Hippo pathway kinases LATS1/2 suppress cancer immunity. *Cell*, *167*(6), 1525–1539. e1517. https://doi.org/10.1016/j.cell.2016.11.005.

Motohashi, H., & Yamamoto, M. (2004). Nrf2-Keap1 defines a physiologically important stress response mechanism. *Trends in Molecular Medicine*, *10*(11), 549–557. https://doi.org/10.1016/j.molmed.2004.09.003.

Mou, F., Praskova, M., Xia, F., Van Buren, D., Hock, H., Avruch, J., et al. (2012). The Mst1 and Mst2 kinases control activation of rho family GTPases and thymic egress of mature thymocytes. *The Journal of Experimental Medicine*, *209*(4), 741–759. https://doi.org/10.1084/jem.20111692.

Nehme, N. T., Pachlopnik Schmid, J., Debeurme, F., Andre-Schmutz, I., Lim, A., Nitschke, P., et al. (2012). MST1 mutations in autosomal recessive primary immunodeficiency characterized by defective naive T-cell survival. *Blood*, *119*(15), 3458–3468. https://doi.org/10.1182/blood-2011-09-378364.

Novakova, J., Talacko, P., Novak, P., & Valis, K. (2019). The MEK-ERK-MST1 axis potentiates the activation of the extrinsic apoptotic pathway during GDC-0941 treatment in jurkat T cells. *Cells*, *8*(2). E191https://doi.org/10.3390/cells8020191.

Park, E., Kim, M. S., Song, J. H., Roh, K. H., Lee, R., & Kim, T. S. (2017). MST1 deficiency promotes B cell responses by CD4(+) T cell-derived IL-4, resulting in hypergammaglobulinemia. *Biochemical and Biophysical Research Communications*, *489*(1), 56–62. https://doi.org/10.1016/j.bbrc.2017.05.094.

Plowden, J., Renshaw-Hoelscher, M., Engleman, C., Katz, J., & Sambhara, S. (2004). Innate immunity in aging: Impact on macrophage function. *Aging Cell*, *3*(4), 161–167. https://doi.org/10.1111/j.1474-9728.2004.00102.x.

Praskova, M., Xia, F., & Avruch, J. (2008). MOBKL1A/MOBKL1B phosphorylation by MST1 and MST2 inhibits cell proliferation. *Current Biology*, *18*(5), 311–321. https://doi.org/10.1016/j.cub.2008.02.006.

Purcell, C., Cant, A., & Irvine, A. D. (2015). DOCK8 primary immunodeficiency syndrome. *Lancet*, *386*(9997), 982. https://doi.org/10.1016/S0140-6736(14)62039-0.

Rawat, S. J., & Chernoff, J. (2015). Regulation of mammalian Ste20 (Mst) kinases. *Trends in Biochemical Sciences*, *40*(3), 149–156. https://doi.org/10.1016/j.tibs.2015.01.001.

Rawat, S. J., Creasy, C. L., Peterson, J. R., & Chernoff, J. (2013). The tumor suppressor Mst1 promotes changes in the cellular redox state by phosphorylation and inactivation of peroxiredoxin-1 protein. *The Journal of Biological Chemistry*, *288*(12), 8762–8771. https://doi.org/10.1074/jbc.M112.414524.

Renshaw, M., Rockwell, J., Engleman, C., Gewirtz, A., Katz, J., & Sambhara, S. (2002). Cutting edge: Impaired toll-like receptor expression and function in aging. *Journal of Immunology*, *169*(9), 4697–4701.

Saravia, J., Chapman, N. M., & Chi, H. (2019). Helper T cell differentiation. *Cellular & Molecular Immunology*, *16*, 634–643. https://doi.org/10.1038/s41423-019-0220-6.

Shi, H., Liu, C., Tan, H., Li, Y., Nguyen, T. M., Dhungana, Y., et al. (2018). Hippo kinases Mst1 and Mst2 sense and amplify IL-2R-STAT5 signaling in regulatory T cells to

establish stable regulatory activity. *Immunity*, *49*(5), 899–914. e896. https://doi.org/10.1016/j.immuni.2018.10.010.
van Loosdregt, J., & Coffer, P. J. (2014). Post-translational modification networks regulating FOXP3 function. *Trends in Immunology*, *35*(8), 368–378. https://doi.org/10.1016/j.it.2014.06.005.
von Zglinicki, T. (2002). Oxidative stress shortens telomeres. *Trends in Biochemical Sciences*, *27*(7), 339–344.
Wang, P., Geng, J., Gao, J., Zhao, H., Li, J., Shi, Y., et al. (2019). Macrophage achieves self-protection against oxidative stress-induced ageing through the Mst-Nrf2 axis. *Nature Communications*, *10*(1), 755. https://doi.org/10.1038/s41467-019-08680-6.
Wang, S., Xie, F., Chu, F., Zhang, Z., Yang, B., Dai, T., et al. (2017). YAP antagonizes innate antiviral immunity and is targeted for lysosomal degradation through IKKvarepsilon-mediated phosphorylation. *Nature Immunology*, *18*(7), 733–743. https://doi.org/10.1038/ni.3744.
West, A. P., Brodsky, I. E., Rahner, C., Woo, D. K., Erdjument-Bromage, H., Tempst, P., et al. (2011). TLR signalling augments macrophage bactericidal activity through mitochondrial ROS. *Nature*, *472*(7344), 476–480. https://doi.org/10.1038/nature09973.
Williams, D. A., Tao, W., Yang, F., Kim, C., Gu, Y., Mansfield, P., et al. (2000). Dominant negative mutation of the hematopoietic-specific Rho GTPase, Rac2, is associated with a human phagocyte immunodeficiency. *Blood*, *96*(5), 1646–1654.
Wu, H., Xiao, Y., Zhang, S., Ji, S., Wei, L., Fan, F., et al. (2013). The Ets transcription factor GABP is a component of the hippo pathway essential for growth and antioxidant defense. *Cell Reports*, *3*(5), 1663–1677. https://doi.org/10.1016/j.celrep.2013.04.020.
Yu, F. X., Zhao, B., & Guan, K. L. (2015). Hippo pathway in organ size control, tissue homeostasis, and cancer. *Cell*, *163*(4), 811–828. https://doi.org/10.1016/j.cell.2015.10.044.
Yuan, Z., Lehtinen, M. K., Merlo, P., Villen, J., Gygi, S., & Bonni, A. (2009). Regulation of neuronal cell death by MST1-FOXO1 signaling. *The Journal of Biological Chemistry*, *284*(17), 11285–11292. https://doi.org/10.1074/jbc.M900461200.
Zhang, S., Chen, Q., Liu, Q., Li, Y., Sun, X., Hong, L., et al. (2017). Hippo signaling suppresses cell ploidy and tumorigenesis through Skp2. *Cancer Cell*, *31*(5), 669–684. e667. https://doi.org/10.1016/j.ccell.2017.04.004.
Zhang, Q., Meng, F., Chen, S., Plouffe, S. W., Wu, S., Liu, S., et al. (2017). Hippo signalling governs cytosolic nucleic acid sensing through YAP/TAZ-mediated TBK1 blockade. *Nature Cell Biology*, *19*(4), 362–374. https://doi.org/10.1038/ncb3496.
Zhang, F., Meng, G., & Strober, W. (2008). Interactions among the transcription factors Runx1, RORgammat and Foxp3 regulate the differentiation of interleukin 17-producing T cells. *Nature Immunology*, *9*(11), 1297–1306. https://doi.org/10.1038/ni.1663.
Zhao, B., Wei, X., Li, W., Udan, R. S., Yang, Q., Kim, J., et al. (2007). Inactivation of YAP oncoprotein by the Hippo pathway is involved in cell contact inhibition and tissue growth control. *Genes & Development*, *21*(21), 2747–2761.
Zhou, D., Conrad, C., Xia, F., Park, J. S., Payer, B., Yin, Y., et al. (2009). Mst1 and Mst2 maintain hepatocyte quiescence and suppress hepatocellular carcinoma development through inactivation of the Yap1 oncogene. *Cancer Cell*, *16*(5), 425–438. https://doi.org/10.1016/j.ccr.2009.09.026.
Zhou, L., Lopes, J. E., Chong, M. M., Ivanov, I. I., Min, R., Victora, G. D., et al. (2008). TGF-beta-induced Foxp3 inhibits T(H)17 cell differentiation by antagonizing RORgammat function. *Nature*, *453*(7192), 236–240. https://doi.org/10.1038/nature06878.

Zhou, D., Medoff, B. D., Chen, L., Li, L., Zhang, X. F., Praskova, M., et al. (2008). The Nore1B/Mst1 complex restrains antigen receptor-induced proliferation of naive T cells. *Proceedings of the National Academy of Sciences of the United States of America*, *105*(51), 20321–20326. https://doi.org/10.1073/pnas.0810773105.

Zhou, D., Zhang, Y., Wu, H., Barry, E., Yin, Y., Lawrence, E., et al. (2011). Mst1 and Mst2 protein kinases restrain intestinal stem cell proliferation and colonic tumorigenesis by inhibition of yes-associated protein (Yap) overabundance. *Proceedings of the National Academy of Sciences of the United States of America*, *108*(49), E1312–E1320. https://doi.org/10.1073/pnas.1110428108.

Zipper, L. M., & Mulcahy, R. T. (2002). The Keap1 BTB/POZ dimerization function is required to sequester Nrf2 in cytoplasm. *The Journal of Biological Chemistry*, *277*(39), 36544–36552. https://doi.org/10.1074/jbc.M206530200.

CHAPTER FIVE

Molecular mechanisms of T helper 17 cell differentiation: Emerging roles for transcription cofactors

Yu Jiang[a], Xiaohu Wang[a], Chen Dong[a,b,*]
[a]Institute for Immunology and School of Medicine, Tsinghua University, Beijing, China
[b]Beijing Key Lab for Immunological Research on Chronic Diseases, Beijing, China
*Corresponding author: e-mail address: chendong@tsinghua.edu.cn

Contents

Abstract

T helper 17 (Th17) cells, characterized by secretion of IL-17 and IL-17F, are a specialized $CD4^+$ effector T cell lineage that not only facilitates host defense against pathogen infection and maintenance of mucosal barrier, but also potently induces tissue inflammation and autoimmune diseases. Since its discovery in 2005, the developmental program of Th17 cells has been characterized, which involves a number of key cytokines,

Advances in Immunology, Volume 144
ISSN 0065-2776
https://doi.org/10.1016/bs.ai.2019.09.003

transcription factors and multiple layers of epigenetic modifications. However, how these mechanisms integrate into the complex regulatory network in Th17 cells has not been well defined. Emerging evidences have revealed essential roles of cofactors in controlling chromosome accessibilities and activities of Th17-specific transcription factors. Moreover, cofactors also act as critical signaling integrators to coordinate multiple signaling pathways and transcriptional programs. Deficiency or dysregulation of these cofactors results in defects in Th17 responses and induction of associated autoimmune diseases. Our lab has recently reported several important cofactors in Th17 cells. Here we summarize our findings regarding this new scenario of developmental regulation of Th17 cells. These findings may benefit the development of innovative strategies to treat autoimmune diseases.

1. Introduction

1.1 Th17 cells: Effector cytokines and biological functions

$CD4^+$ T cells are key players in regulating immune responses toward diverse environmental threats. Upon activation, they can differentiate into different functional subsets, including T helper (Th) 1, Th2, Th17, T follicular helper (Tfh) and regulatory T (Treg) cells, characterized by expression of distinct transcription factors and effect cytokines (Zhu, Yamane, & Paul, 2010). Among them, Th17 cells mainly express the master transcription factor RORγt and effect cytokines IL-17, IL-17F and IL-22, and have been best known for their pathogenic role in various autoimmune diseases, despite their essential protective role in clearance of extracellular bacterial and fungal infections and maintenance of mucosal barrier functions (Dong, 2008; Korn, Bettelli, Oukka, & Kuchroo, 2009).

Th17 cells were initially characterized by our and other groups in 2005 (Harrington et al., 2005; Langrish et al., 2005; Park et al., 2005). Over the past years, we have witnessed a rapid expansion of our knowledge regarding the molecular mechanisms controlling the differentiation and function of Th17 cells under various experimental or physiological settings. Due to the broad distribution of receptors for Th17 cell produced cytokines, Th17 cells have a profound effect on various tissues and organs in diverse immune responses. For example, IL-17 and IL-17F are essential in protecting host against extracellular bacterial and fungi infections, such as *Staphylococcus aureus, Citrobacter rodentium* and *Candida albicans,* through inducing proinflammatory cytokines and anti-microbial peptides and by acting on both hematopoietic cells and non-hematopoietic cells including neutrophils, macrophages, epithelial cells, fibroblasts and so on (Jin & Dong, 2013), whereas IL-17 and IL-22 are critical for maintaining the integrity and function of mucosal barriers or surface through their direct effect on epithelial cells from various tissues (Aujla & Kolls, 2009; Kolls & Khader, 2010; Ouyang & Valdez, 2008). Dysregulated IL-17 and IL-17F production are often linked to persistent tissue inflammations and various autoimmune diseases, such as multiple sclerosis, rheumatoid arthritis, ankylosing spondylitis, psoriasis and inflammatory bowel disease (Dong, 2008; Korn et al., 2009). Since 2015, several humanized monoclonal antibodies against IL-17 or its receptor IL-17RA, including secukinumab, ixekizumab and brodalumab, have been approved in US, Europe and Japan for treatment of moderate to severe psoriasis, psoriatic arthritis and ankylosing spondylitis (Thomas, Lee, & Wu, 2019). Due to the essential functions of both beneficial and detrimental effects of Th17 cells, it is crucial to understand how the Th17 cell program is initiated, amplified, controlled and resolved in various immune responses.

1.2 Th17 cell differentiation regulation

1.2.1 Cytokines involved in Th17 cell differentiation and functions

Unlike Th1 and Th2 cells, the initiation of Th17 cell differentiation requires two cytokines with opposite functions, the proinflammatory cytokine IL-6 and the immune suppressive cytokine TGF-β (Bettelli et al., 2006; Mangan et al., 2006; Veldhoen, Hocking, Atkins, et al., 2006). Moreover, the differentiation, expansion, maturation or proinflammatory activities can also be reinforced or modulated by the combination of additional cytokines, including IL-1β, IL-21, IL-23 and TGF-β3 (Chung et al., 2009; Cua et al., 2003; Korn et al., 2007; Langrish et al., 2005; Lee et al., 2012; McGeachy et al., 2009; Nurieva et al., 2007; Zhou et al., 2007), further complicating the regulation of Th17 cell commitment.

1.2.1.1 IL-6 and TGF-β initiate Th17 cell differentiation

TGF-β is a pleiotropic cytokine belonging to the transforming growth factor superfamily and has three mammalian isoforms (TGF-β1, 2, 3). TGF-β probably represents the most extensively studied cytokine so far due to its diverse physiological functions in regulating cell proliferation, differentiation, survival, migration and so on, in both hematopoietic and non-hematopoietic systems (Massague, 2012). Shortly after the discovery of Th17 cells, TGF-β was found to be necessary for induction of Th17 cell differentiation *in vitro* cultures, in combination with IL-6 (Bettelli et al., 2006; Mangan et al., 2006; Veldhoen, Hocking, Atkins, et al., 2006).

Transgenic overexpression of TGF-β in T cells led to increased Th17 response and more severe experimental autoimmune encephalomyelitis (EAE) (Bettelli et al., 2006), an Th17 cell-dependent autoimmune disease model, whereas T-cell specific deficiency of TGF-β receptor caused defective Th17 cell differentiation and resistant to EAE (Veldhoen, Hocking, Flavell, & Stockinger, 2006). Though TGF-β is known to be produced by a variety of cell types and is abundantly present in the circulation, T cell-derived TGF-β appears to have an important role in supporting Th17 cell development, because T cell-specific ablation of TGF-β significantly dampened Th17 cell generation *in vivo*, and resulted in resistance to EAE induction (Li, Wan, & Flavell, 2007), suggesting TGF-β regulates *in vivo* Th17 cell differentiation through an autocrine manner, at least partly.

Similar to TGF-β, IL-6 is also an important pleiotropic cytokine with many physiological activities. In the immune system, IL-6 is produced by multiple cell types, including dendritic cells, monocytes, macrophages, B cells and certain T cell subsets, particularly during acute phase of infection, and is also a key mediator of fever response (Kishimoto, 2005). The combination of IL-6 and TGF-β potently induces Th17 cell differentiation in *in vitro* cultures (Bettelli et al., 2006; Veldhoen, Hocking, Atkins, et al., 2006). Blocking IL-6 in *in vitro* culture system completely inhibited naive T cell polarization into Th17 cells, and T cell specific deficiency of STAT3, the downstream signaling molecule of IL-6, impaired Th17 cell differentiation *in vitro* and *in vivo*, and caused resistance to EAE (Harris et al., 2007; Yang et al., 2007), suggesting an indispensable role of IL-6/STAT3 axis in regulating the differentiation and function of Th17 cells.

TGF-β is also required for induction of regulatory T cells (Chen et al., 2003; Kretschmer et al., 2005), the major suppressive T cell subset in the immune system. TGF-β alone is able to induce the expression of both RORγt and FOXP3, the master transcription factors for Th17 and Treg cells (Fontenot, Gavin, & Rudensky, 2003; Hori, Nomura, & Sakaguchi, 2003; Ivanov et al., 2006), respectively. It has been shown that FOXP3 can directly interact with RORγt and inhibit its transcriptional activity, and thus Th17 cell differentiation (Zhou et al., 2008). In the presence of IL-2, TGF-β potently drives T cells polarized into Treg cells (Fontenot, Rasmussen, Gavin, & Rudensky, 2005), whereas in the presence of IL-6, TGF-β robustly induces Th17 cell program (Bettelli et al., 2006; Veldhoen, Hocking, Atkins, et al., 2006). It appears that the balance of IL-2 and IL-6 signals is critical to dictate the fate between Th17 and Treg program. IL-6 regulates Th17 cell differentiation mainly through activating STAT3 (Harris et al., 2007; Yang et al., 2007). ChIP-seq studies reveal that STAT3 can bind to both the *Rorc* and *Il17-17f* gene loci, and STAT3-deficiency in T cells not only diminishes *Rorc* expression and Th17 cell differentiation, but also lead to increased *Foxp3* expression (Durant et al., 2010), suggesting STAT3 has multiple functions in Th17 cells. In contrast, IL-2 mainly activates STAT5, which binds the *Foxp3* gene locus and is essential for FOXP3^{+} Treg cell induction (Burchill, Yang, Vogtenhuber, Blazar, & Farrar, 2007). On the other hand, IL-2 is also a potent inhibitor for Th17 cell program both *in vitro* and *in vivo*. STAT3 and STAT5 were shown to bind to similar gene loci in a competitive manner, and reciprocally antagonize each other's function (Laurence et al., 2007), suggesting that the relative amounts of surrounding IL-2 and IL-6, or their balance, is particularly important in dictating the fate between Th17 and Treg programs. Despite these studies, the detailed synergistic mechanism between IL-6 and TGF-β in inducing Th17 cell program is largely unclear.

1.2.1.2 Additional cytokines involved in Th17 cell differentiation and maturation

In Th17 cells, IL-21 is an essential downstream target of the IL-6/STAT3 signaling (Nurieva et al., 2007; Zhou et al., 2007). Similar to IL-6, IL-21 also activates STAT3, and can inhibit TGF-β induced *Foxp3* expression (Nurieva et al., 2007; Zhou et al., 2007). Interestingly, IL-21 can substitute IL-6 and induce Th17 cell differentiation *in vitro*, together with TGF-β (Zhou et al., 2007). Moreover, *Il21* can be induced by itself, and its deficiency caused severe defects in Th17 cell differentiation *in vitro* and *in vivo*, and resistance to EAE induction (Nurieva et al., 2007; Zhou et al., 2007). IL-21 is thus proposed as a T cell-derived autocrine cytokine critically promoting the expansion and development of Th17 cell program. Under *in vivo* condition, IL-6 deficient mice failed to induce Th17 cells and were completely resistant to EAE induction (Korn et al., 2007), indicating the induction of IL-21 is likely dependent on IL-6 *in vivo*.

IL-23 was first discovered in 2000 by scientists at the DNAX company. Interestingly, IL-23 belongs to the IL-12 cytokine family, and is a heterodimer composed of a unique p19 subunit and a common p40 subunit shared with IL-12, a cytokine crucial for inducing Th1 cell program (Oppmann et al., 2000). Early studies found targeting IL-12 was an efficient therapy for EAE (Constantinescu et al., 1998; Leonard, Waldburger, & Goldman, 1995, 1996), leading to the concept that antigen specific Th1 cells are responsible for autoimmunity. The elegant studies during 2003–2005 found that deficiency in the IL-23p19 subunit, but not the IL-12 unique subunit p35, failed to induce IL-17 producing T cells *in vivo* and EAE diseases (Cua et al., 2003; Langrish et al., 2005), shaking the foundation of Th1/Th2 binary concept of T helper cells. IL-23 was soon identified as a susceptible gene in many human autoimmune diseases including inflammatory bowel disease and psoriasis by GWAS studies since discovery (Cargill et al., 2007; Duerr et al., 2006; Liu et al., 2008). Though IL-23 is absolutely required for Th17 cell induction *in vivo*, it is dispensable for Th17 cell differentiation in *in vitro* cultures. IL-23 appears to have important function in inducing the expansion and mature of Th17 cells at later stage, when its receptor IL-23R is induced by IL-6 and IL-21 (Langrish et al., 2005; McGeachy et al., 2009; Zhou et al., 2007). Interestingly, IL-23 experienced Th17 cells are highly proinflammatory (McGeachy et al., 2007) and induce much more severe EAE disease in an adoptive T cell transfer model, than those induced with only IL-6 and TGF-β (Ghoreschi et al., 2010), suggesting an essential role of IL-23 in regulating the pathogenicity of Th17 cells.

IL-1 is an additional cytokine that critically regulates the differentiation and pathogenicity of Th17 cells (Chung et al., 2009). Like IL-23R, the IL-1 receptor is only induced post Th17 cell induction, suggesting it is not required at the initiation stage. IL-1 is believed to have an important role in reinforcing Th17 cell differentiation at both early and later stages, possibility through inducing expression of Th17-cell related transcription factors IRF4 and RORγt, as well as *via* antagonizing FOXP3-directed Treg program. Deficiency in IL-1 receptor not only significantly reduced Th17 cell induction but also greatly alleviated the disease symptoms in the EAE model (Chung et al., 2009). Notably, the combination of IL-1β, IL-23 and IL-6, in the absence of exogenous TGF-β, is sufficient to induce Th17 cells in *in vitro* cultures, featured with a highly increased proinflammatory activity in the adoptive T cell transfer EAE model (Ghoreschi et al., 2010).

Overall, it is now generally accepted that Th17 cells can exist at different states, with distinct gene expression patterns and physiological functions (Gaublomme et al., 2015; Ghoreschi et al., 2010; Lee et al., 2012; McGeachy et al., 2007; Wang, Yosef, et al., 2015). Th17 cells induced by IL-6 and TGF-β are regarded relatively non-pathogenic, characterized with elevated IL-10 production (McGeachy et al., 2007), and are likely generated under homeostatic condition *in vivo*, whereas those experienced IL-1β and IL-23 stimulations are highly pathogenic and express increased amount of T-bet, IFN-γ, GM-CSF, IL-22 and IL-23R and diminished expression of IL-10 (Ghoreschi et al., 2010). A recent study shows that TGF-β3, upregulated in an IL-23 dependent manner, could substitute the role of TGF-β1 and circumvent the requirement of IL-23 to induce pathogenic Th17 cells (Lee et al., 2012), further suggesting a complicated diversification of Th17 cell program. It is possible that these so called pathogenic Th17 cells are likely armed warriors in fighting against invading pathogens, and are associated with various autoimmune diseases due to uncontrolled responses. Therefore, it would be interesting to know if there is a reciprocal and reversible conversion between the non-pathogenic and pathogenic Th17 cell populations.

1.2.2 Transcription factors in regulation of Th17 cell differentiation

Lineage commitment of T helper subsets is initiated by the combined signals downstream of cytokine receptors and TCRs. Those signals then activate and integrate specific transcription factors to promote lineage-specific differentiation program, yet to suppress alternative differentiation pathways.

RAR-related orphan receptor gamma (RORγt), a steroid type receptor of the nuclear receptor family (Medvedev, Chistokhina, Hirose, & Jetten, 1997), is a transcriptional variant of RORγ encoded by *Rorc* (He, Deftos, Ojala, & Bevan, 1998). RORγ is broadly expressed in many tissues including liver, kidney and muscle, whereas RORγt expression appears to be limited to several cell types within the immune system, including thymocytes, Th17 cells and group 3 of the innate lymphoid cells (Jetten, 2009). RORγt is induced at the early stages of Th17 cell differentiation, up to 6 h post IL-6/TGF-β and TCR stimulation, and its expression is maintained throughout the different stages of Th17 cells (Yosef et al., 2013). RORγt directs Th17 cell differentiation mainly through direct binding to numerous Th17 cell-related gene loci, including the promoter or regulatory regions of the *Il17-Il17f* gene locus (Ciofani et al., 2012; Xiao et al., 2014), and its deficiency impaired Th17 cell differentiation *in vitro* and *in vivo* and dampened many Th17-related autoimmune diseases including EAE and colitis (Ivanov et al., 2006; Leppkes et al., 2009). In contrast, ectopic expression of RORγt in T cells is sufficient to induce IL-17 production under neutral or even Th1 or Th2 cell culture conditions (Ivanov et al., 2006). The sufficient and necessary roles in control of Th17 cell program thus characterize RORγt as the lineage-specific master transcription factor for Th17 cells.

It is noticed that RORγt deficiency could not completely abolish IL-17 production, indicating the presence of additional regulator (s). Interestingly, RORα, a family member of RORγt, is also highly and selectively expressed in Th17 cells. Similar to RORγt, RORα is induced by TGF-β and IL-6 and its overexpression is also sufficient to induce IL-17 expression under unfavorable culture conditions. RORα appears to play a less significant role than RORγt in Th17 cells, as its deficiency only led to ~20–50% reduction of IL-17 expression under various culture conditions, but deficiency in both RORγt and RORα completely abolished Th17 cell induction both *in vitro* and *in vivo* and resulted in fully resistance to EAE induction, suggesting RORα may complement the role of RORγt in Th17 cells (Yang, Pappu, et al., 2008). However, RORα clearly has its unique functions in the immune system, and the synergistic mechanism between RORα and RORγt remains largely unclear.

As stated above, STAT3 is absolutely required for Th17 cell differentiation, which is confirmed by the findings in human hyper IgE syndrome patients in which STAT3 mutations caused diminished IL-17 expression *in vivo* (Holland et al., 2007). As the immediate downstream target of IL-6 signaling, STAT3 is activated upstream of RORγt and RORα within minutes following Th17 cell polarization. Interestingly, STAT3 can be also activated by IL-21 and IL-23, indicating a persistent role throughout different stages of Th17 cell differentiation. ChIP-seq and RNA-seq studies show that STAT3 plays a crucial global effect on transcriptional induction of the Th17 cell program, through direct binding to numerous Th17 cell associated gene loci (Durant et al., 2010). Unlike RORγt and RORα, STAT3 is necessary but not sufficient for inducing Th17 cells. However, studies suggest STAT3 has a more profound effect on global epigenetic activation of Th17 cell program than RORγt, which is required for RORγt recruitment to the *Il17-17f* gene locus according to our recent study (Ciofani et al., 2012; Jiang et al., 2018), and it is yet interesting to know if STAT3 is required for RORγt binding to its target sites at genome-wide level.

In addition to the lineage-specific induced or activated transcription factors, such as STAT3, RORγt and RORα, Th17 cell differentiation also requires several other transcription factors that are expressed by multiple T helper cell subsets and have miscellaneous activities, including IRF4, BATF, c-Maf, IκBζ and RUNX1 (Bauquet et al., 2009; Brustle et al., 2007; Okamoto et al., 2010; Schraml et al., 2009; Wang et al., 2014; Zhang, Meng, & Strober, 2008). For example, IRF4 also regulates the differentiation of Th1, Th2, Th9 and Tfh cells *via* a T cell-intrinsic manner (Krishnamoorthy et al., 2017; Mahnke et al., 2016; Staudt et al., 2010; Zheng et al., 2009), whereas BATF is important for Th2 and Tfh cell differentiation (Betz et al., 2010). Deficiency of either of these transcription factors resulted in resistance to EAE, and nearly absence of Th17 cell induction (Brustle et al., 2007; Schraml et al., 2009).

Interestingly, these transcription factors, including STAT3, bind a large amount of common targets in Th17 cells, including the *Il17-17f* gene locus (Ciofani et al., 2012), and their defects could not be rescued by overexpression of RORγt, suggesting a cooperative effect of these factors together with RORγt in controlling Th17 cell differentiation. This is further supported by recent findings that Th17 cells develop a complex regulatory network during the progression of lineage commitment. A study in 2012 integrated high-throughput ChIP-seq and RNA-seq data of several essential Th17 cell related transcription factors, and found that the IRF4 and BATF complex, triggered by TCR signaling, serves as the first step to initiate epigenetic changes and chromatin accessibility at key Th17-related gene loci that allow subsequent binding of transcription factor complexes. Together with STAT3, those pioneer factors initiate a transcriptional program that is then orchestrated by lineage-specific transcription factors such as RORγt (Ciofani et al., 2012). In addition, another research in 2013 did transcriptional profiling of Th17 cells at high temporal resolution and found Th17 cells adopted a dynamic regulatory network with three distinct transcription waves starting from a naive-like state to a fully committed state of Th17 cell differentiation process, and are coordinately regulated by two self-reinforcing but mutually antagonistic modules composed of 72 densely correlated regulators (Yosef et al., 2013). However, their findings of the transcriptional network in Th17 cells still need to be further investigated and confirmed by more in-depth studies.

1.2.3 Epigenetic regulation of T helper cell differentiation

The recruitment of transcription factors to target DNA sequences is often affected by the status of chromatin structures and modifications, known as epigenetic regulation. This layer of regulation is dependent on nucleosome position and compaction, DNA-nucleosomes interactions, post-translational modifications of histones, DNA methylation status and so on. Unlike genetic control that is dependent on DNA sequences, epigenetic modifications are highly dynamic and plastic, and can be altered by a number of so called epigenetic "writers" and "erasers" in response to the various environmental and developmental stimuli (Chen, Li, Subramaniam, Shyy, & Chien, 2017).

Epigenetic regulation plays a profound role in cell fate determination, particularly when considering different types of cells derived from various tissues and organs in the same organisms share the same genetic information. It is also true for lineage commitment of different T helper cell subsets (Wilson, Rowell, & Sekimata, 2009). High-throughput ChIP-seq studies have revealed an interesting finding that the signature effector cytokines are generally marked with either permissive or non-permissive epigenetic markers in corresponding T helper cell subsets, whereas the loci of lineage-specific master transcription factors exhibit in a less cell-type specific manner (Ichiyama et al., 2015; Wei et al., 2009). In Th17 cells, for example, the *Il17-17f* locus is enriched with permissive histone marker H3K4Me3, and lacks of non-permissive histone marker H3K27Me3, whereas the *Ifng* and *Il4* loci are modified in the opposite manner in the same cell-type. In contrast, the gene locus of *Rorc* is marked with H3K4Me3 in Th17 cells but both H3K4Me3 and H3K27Me3 in Treg cells, and the *Ifng* and *Il4* loci bear both H3K4Me3 and H3K27Me3 in Th17 cells (Wei et al., 2009). The binary epigenetic status of key transcription factors are consistent with the findings of developmental plasticity among different T cell lineages, and may confer an evolutionary advantage for rapid response to changes of external and internal immune threats.

In view of the significance of epigenetic regulation, it is not surprising that disrupting histone and DNA modifying enzymes or chromatin organizers would cause dysregulated T helper cell programs. For instance, ablation of either Tet2 or Jmjd3, the enzymes catalyzing conversion of 5′-methylcytosine (5′mC) to 5-hydroxymethylcytosine (5′hmC) and histone H3K27 demethylation, respectively, led to impaired Th17 differentiation and protection from EAE diseases (Ichiyama et al., 2015; Liu et al., 2015). The microRNA MiR-155 critically controls Th17 cell effector cytokine gene expression, through inhibition of JARID2, the polycomb repressive complex 2 (PRC2) recruiting protein (Escobar et al., 2014). The BET family members, Brd2 and Brd4 transcriptionally regulate Th17 program by recruiting boundary protein CTCF and cohesin complex and supporting enhancer assembly, or by modulating RNA polymerase II activity, respectively (Cheung et al., 2017). Therefore, the chromatin accessibilities tightly control gene activation and inactivation during Th17 cell differentiation.

Cell-type specific transcription profiles are often controlled by integrating actions of serial transcription factors and epigenetic mechanisms. *Cis*-regulatory elements play an important role in this process by recruiting transcription factors and cofactors to form long range DNA–DNA interaction and undergo various epigenetic modifications (Lee, Kim, Spilianakis, Fields, & Flavell, 2006). In Th17 cells, there are eight conserved noncoding sequences (CNSs) identified in the *Il17-Il17f* locus, which are significantly enriched in lineage-specific permissive epigenetic markers (Akimzhanov, Yang, & Dong, 2007). Among them, CNS2 was genetically characterized by our group that serves as lineage-specific *cis*-regulatory element dictating

Il17 and *Il17f* expression selectively in Th17 cells, through chromosome looping and recruitment of key transcription factors and epigenetic modifiers (Wang et al., 2012). Recent genome occupancy studies revealed that other CNSs, particularly CNS3 and CNS5, are also bound by multiple transcription factors (Ciofani et al., 2012), suggesting a potential function in Th17 cells.

Enhancers, including the recently proposed super-enhancers (SEs), were reported to be associated with T cell fate determination (Vahedi et al., 2012, 2015). Genome-wide analysis of active enhancers, defined by heightened p300 binding or H3K27Ac modification, revealed distinct patterns in closely related T cell subsets (Kitagawa et al., 2017; Vahedi et al., 2015). Importantly, almost all known T helper cell-related transcription factors bind the so called super-enhancers, and their deficiencies dampen activation of enhancers with varying degrees. In Th1 and Th2 cells, deficiency of STATs resulted in a more profound defect of p300 recruitment than T-bet or GATA3 deficiency (Vahedi et al., 2012). Likewise, in Th17 cells, loss of STAT3, as well as the pioneer factors IRF4 and BATF, reduced global p300 binding intensity and the permissive histone marker H3K4Me3 at a greater degree than *Rorc* deficiency (Ciofani et al., 2012). Overall, STAT3 appears to be a more global regulator regulate chromatin accessibility and SE activation in Th17 cells.

Although accumulating data point an essential role of lineage-related transcription factors in regulating the epigenetic landscape of T cell subsets, it is largely unclear about the synchronizing working mechanisms between transcription factors and chromatin modifiers to control fate commitment of T cells, which likely involves in the helper functions coming from a number of cofactors based on recent studies.

1.3 Transcription factors and cofactors

1.3.1 General transcription factors and their cofactors

Gene transcription is initiated with core promoters, where general transcription factors form a complex called transcription preinitiation complex (PIC), together with RNA polymerase II to promote basal level of transcription. Efficient transcriptional events need the recruitment of gene-specific transcription factors to additional *cis*-regulatory elements, such as enhancers. Additionally, gene transcription can be further repressed *via* recruiting negative regulator(s) or repressor(s) to related gene locus. These coordinate actions are often mediated by participation of various transcription cofactors, another family of proteins involved in transcriptional regulation, which do not bind DNA directly, but are tethered to specific gene loci through protein–protein interactions, and transmit signals between basic transcription machinery and specific transcription factors (Reiter, Wienerroither, & Stark, 2017; Spitz & Furlong, 2012; Zabidi & Stark, 2016).

Transcriptional cofactors are often enzymes capable of catalyzing post-translational modifications. For instance, CDK8 of the Mediator complex is a serine/threonine phosphokinase, p300 and CBP are acetyltransferases, members of the MLL family as well as EHMTs and are methyltransferases (Hyun, Jeon, Park, & Kim, 2017; Malik & Roeder, 2010; Vo & Goodman, 2001). Some other cofactors may have weak or no enzymatic activities by themselves, but can function as histone readers or interact with other enzymes, and promote or inhibit gene transcription. Therefore, it is not surprising that cofactors are able to regulate gene transcription through post-translational modifications of various proteins including histones, transcription factors, RNA polymerase II and associated proteins. In addition, cofactors may also contribute to gene transcription by mediating protein–protein interactions and formation of multicomponent protein complex (Reiter et al., 2017). This is particularly important since gene regulation typically depends on combination of distinct transcription factors. Therefore, transcription cofactors have indispensable roles in regulating gene transcription.

1.3.2 Nuclear receptors and their coregulators

The nuclear receptor (NR) superfamily is a typical group of transcription factors frequently bound by cofactors. NR proteins are ligand-activated transcription factors responsible for the transduction of extra- and intracellular signals into distinct physiological responses. Their transcriptional activities are regulated by the steroid, thyroid and retinoid hormones and other hormone signals, as well as lipid metabolic products such as fatty acids and prostaglandins. Some of the NRs do not have known or validated ligands and are called as orphan receptors, such as the retinoid-related orphan receptors (RORs), which contain the key Th17 cell transcription factors RORγt and RORα (Cook, Kang, & Jetten, 2015).

NRs typically contain three main domains: a highly variable N-terminal AF-1 domain that is ligand independent and has several transactivation regions; a central C4 zinc finger DNA binding domain responsible for nuclear localization; and a conserved C-terminal ligand-binding AF2 domain.

NRs can function as a monomer or homo- or heterodimer following ligand binding and are recruited to target genes to regulate transcription positively or negatively, through context-dependent interaction with coactivators or corepressors, also known as coregulators. Following ligand binding, some NRs are released from cytoplasm anchoring chaperone proteins and then translocate into nucleus, interact with transcription coactivators, bind to and activate the transcription of target genes. In contrast, some other receptors are generally present in the nucleus, binding to target genes and associating with transcription corepressor complexes such as NCoR and SMRT. Ligand binding causes dissociation of corepressors from these NRs and association with coactivator complexes to activate downstream gene expression. In the transcriptional process, coactivators often serve as epigenetic activators, either possessing chromatin remodeling activities or able to recruit chromatin modifying enzymes, whereas corepressors often serve as epigenetic silencers, directly or indirectly (Dasgupta, Lonard, & O'Malley, 2014; Glass & Saijo, 2010; Lonard & O'Malley, 2012). These multiple layers of regulations ensure transcriptional events tightly controlled in a time, space and context dependent manner.

RORγt and RORα are members of the ROR subfamily which belongs to NR superfamily and contains four domains: a N-terminal domain, a highly conserved DNA binding domain, a hinge domain and a ligand binding domain. RORγt and RORα bind to similar conserved DNA motifs called ROREs in monomers (Cook et al., 2015). The endogenous ligands for RORγt and RORα have not yet been fully confirmed, but it appears that cholesterol or cholesterol-derived metabolic intermediates, including oxysterols and hydroxysterols, can bind to RORγt and significantly increase its transcription activities (Hu et al., 2015; Santori et al., 2015; Soroosh et al., 2014), and targeting RORγt through intervening ligand recruitment by small molecules has shown clinical benefits in treatment of murine models of Th17 cell-dependent autoimmune diseases (Huh et al., 2011; Solt et al., 2011; Xiao et al., 2014).

Current studies have mainly focused on the transcription factor regulation of Th17 cells, whereas less is known about their cofactor partners. With the recent discovery of several important cofactors in Th17 cells by our and other groups, it is found that cofactors definitely play critical roles. As we will summarize below, they not only act as bridging molecules between TFs and epigenetic activation, but also involved in signaling pathway and transcription network formation.

2. TRIM28: An essential epigenetic activator in Th17 cells downstream of IL-6

2.1 Introduction to TIF1 family proteins

Transcriptional intermediary factor I (TIF1) proteins are chromatin associated/related proteins and can function as either corepressors or coactivators. The TIF1 family contains four members, TIF1-α (TRIM24), TIF1-β (TRIM28), TIF1-γ (TRIM33) and TIF1-δ (TRIM66) (Friedman et al., 1996; Khetchoumian et al., 2004; Le Douarin et al., 1995; Venturini et al., 1999), and belong to the larger tripartite motif (TRIM) family proteins, among which most have E3 ubiquitin ligase activity, and have broad functions in various biological processes, including apoptosis, cell differentiation, carcinogenesis and immune responses (Hatakeyama, 2011; Jefferies, Wynne, & Higgs, 2011; Kawai & Akira, 2011; Ozato, Shin, Chang, & Morse, 2008).

TRIM proteins typically have an N-terminal RING domain, followed by one or two B boxes and an associated coiled-coil domain. Based on diverse structures of the C-terminal domains, TRIM proteins could be further classified into different groups. For example, the TIF1 group proteins are featured with a C-terminal PHD/bromodomain unit that can bind chromatins and are implicated in epigenetic regulation of transcription. All TIF1 proteins, except for TRIM66, have various regulatory functions in the immune system, including T and B cell development and functions (Ferri et al., 2015; Perez-Lloret et al., 2016; Tisserand et al., 2011; Wang, Kawaoka, et al., 2015; Weng et al., 2014). Among them, we have identified TRIM28 and TRIM33 as important co-regulators for Th17 cells and associated pathological functions (Jiang et al., 2018; Tanaka, Jiang, et al., 2018), which will be discussed further in details below.

2.2 TRIM28 functions in the immune system

TRIM28, also known as KRAB-associated protein 1 (KAP1), was initially characterized as a binding partner and also a corepressor for KRAB domain-containing zinc finger proteins (Friedman et al., 1996; Moosmann, Georgiev, Le Douarin, Bourquin, & Schaffner, 1996). TRIM28 is a multifunctional protein due to its diverse binding partners, such as heterochromatin-associated factors and members of histone modification complex, including Mi2α, CHD3 and SETDB1, and is therefore often regarded as a corepressor for transcription (Iyengar & Farnham, 2011).

TRIM28 is abundantly expressed in the immune system, and has important roles in regulating the development of B cells and NKT cells, as well as type I IFN dependent immune responses (Liang et al., 2011; Santoni de Sio et al., 2012; Zhou et al., 2012). In T cells, a recent study found that *Trim28*-deficient mice, generated by crossing *Trim28* floxed mice with the distal Lck-Cre mice, developed mild spontaneous autoimmune phenotypes when reaching to 16–22 weeks old, characterized by increased Th17 cell generation and enlargement of lymphoid organs. In addition, these mice showed exacerbated development of EAE disease, with elevated IL-17 but not IFN-γ production by $CD4^+$ T cells in the CNS. Further studies showed that *Trim28* deficiency did not affect the development of Treg cells, but selectively impaired their suppressive functions, since *Trim28*-deficeint Treg cells failed to control T cell dependent colitis in a transfer colitis model (Chikuma, Suita, Okazaki, Shibayama, & Honjo, 2012). However, this study did not evaluate the direct effect or T cell intrinsic effect of TRIM28 in Th17 cells.

2.3 TRIM28 intrinsically regulates Th17 cell development

To ascertain whether TRIM28 can directly regulate Th17 cell differentiation, we generated T cell-specific *Trim28* knockout mice *via* using the Cd4Cre mediated deletion strategy (Jiang et al., 2018). In contrast to the above *in vivo* findings, naive T cells isolated from these *Trim28*-deficient mice showed severe defect in Th17 cell differentiation in all tested culture conditions, characterized by impaired IL-17 production and increased Foxp3 expression. In addition, we did not observe autoimmune symptoms in those mice like in the *Trim28*$^{fl/fl}$Lckcre mice (Chikuma et al., 2012), suggesting a role of TRIM28 in the early stage of thymocyte development before CD4 expression, or due to different housing environments. To avoid the effect of TRIM28 on Treg cells, an adoptive T cell transfer colitis model was employed, in which the donor T cells barely express FOXP3 and turn into Treg cells in recipient mice. Consistent with our *in vitro* differentiation data, *Trim28*-deficent naive T cells expressed significantly reduced IL-17 and resulted in greatly ameliorated colitis in the *Rag1*$^{-/-}$ recipient mice, when compared with WT T cells. To further exclude the potential residue effect of TRIM28 on Treg cells, we generated Th17-specific *Trim28* knockout mice by crossing *Trim28*$^{fl/fl}$ mice with the Il17fcre mice generated by our lab recently (Ichiyama et al., 2015). As predicated, Th17-specific deletion of TRIM28 led to impaired Th17 differentiation *in vitro* and *in vivo*, and caused resistance to induction of EAE diseases, demonstrating an intrinsic role of TRIM28 in regulating Th17 cell developmental program.

2.4 TRIM28 acts as an epigenetic activator bridging STAT3 and RORγt

It is interesting that TRIM28 regulates Th17 cell development independent of Th17 related transcription factors, as indicated by ChIP-seq and RNA-seq experiments. TRIM28 could directly bind to the *Il17-Il17f* gene locus and regulate their expression, but did not control the expression of key T cell related transcription factors, including RORγt, RORα, STAT3, T-bet and GATA3. In addition, blockage of IL-2 diminished FOXP3 expression, but still couldn't rescue the IL-17 expression defect in *Trim28*-deficient T cells *in vitro*, suggesting TRIM28 regulates Th17 development independent of the direct effect on FOXP3 and other critical transcription factors.

In view of the presence of histone reading PhD-bromo domains in TRIM28, we examined the epigenetic function of TRIM28 in Th17 cells. Although TRIM28 was largely reported as a corepressor before, our observations strongly suggest it acts as a coactivator in driving Th17 cell development. *Trim28*-deficiency leads to reduced permissive epigenetic modifications, including H3K4Me3, H3K27Ac and 5hmc at the *Il17-Il17f* locus, and genome-wide TRIM28 binding sites are enriched with active but barely repressive epigenetic markers in Th17 cells, and overlap with almost all Th17-specific super-enhancers (SEs) (Vahedi et al., 2015), characterized by strong enrichment of p300 binding peaks and H3K27Ac modifications. In addition, *Trim28* deficiency significantly impaired p300 recruitment and Th17 specific SE-mediated transcriptional activities, including the expression of *Il17* and *Il17f*. Our study thus suggests a potential critical role of TRIM28 in establishing and activating Th17-specific SEs during the polarization and lineage commitment process of Th17 cells.

An interesting finding for TRIM28 is that it shares a large common binding sites with other Th17 cell related transcription factors, particularly RORγt and STAT3. Inspired by these observations, a series of ChIP experiments using the *IL17-IL17f* locus as a model were conducted in Th17 cells to determine if this is a correlative or causative binding phenomenon. Surprisingly, it was found that TRIM28 occupancy was abolished upon *Stat3* but not *Rorc* deficiency, whereas, RORγt recruitment, but not STAT3, were dramatically reduced upon *Trim28* deficiency. Additional studies showed that STAT3, RORγt and TRIM28 can interact with each other and collectively form a complex. These experimental evidences suggest the presence of causative sequential binding events among STAT3, TRIM28 and RORγt: STAT3 activation triggers the recruitment of TRIM28, likely through protein–protein interactions, which serves as an

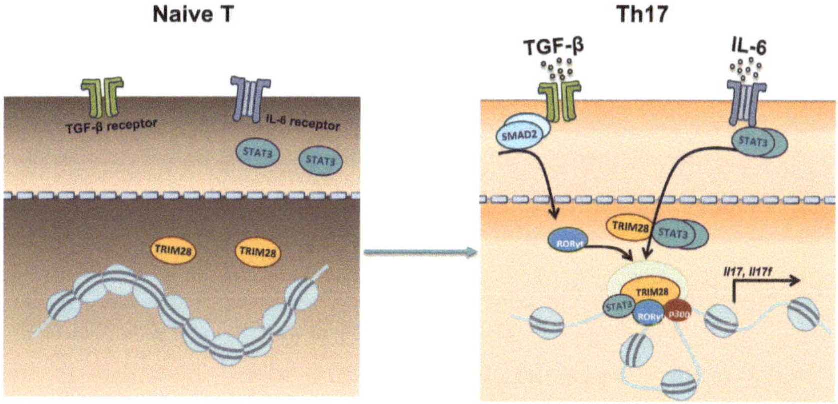

Fig. 1 TRIM28 epigenetically activates Th17 cell differentiation program. TRIM28, which is present in the nucleus of naive CD4$^+$ T cells and recruited to target gene loci following IL-6 stimulation, promotes deposition of permissive epigenetic markers and SE establishment, and facilitates the recruitment of RORγt, chromosome looping and following transcriptional events.

epigenetic activator to increase chromatin accessibility essential for RORγt recruitment (Fig. 1). As a result, RORγt overexpression couldn't restore defective Th17 differentiation in *Trim28* KO T cells, as well as in *Stat3* KO T cells. Notably, *Stat3* or *Trim28* deficiency dampened p300 recruitment at a much larger degree than *Rorc* deficiency in Th17 cells. Accordingly, loss of either STAT3 or TRIM28 impaired the interactions between *cis*-regulatory elements within the *Il17-17f* locus, suggesting a more important role of STAT3 and TRIM28 in epigenetic activation and chromosomal looping in Th17 cells, which is important for subsequent RORγt recruitment and following transcriptional events. TRIM28 thus functions as a transcriptional coactivator and plays an important role in bridging the gap between STAT3 and RORγt during the development of Th17 cells, despite the global effect of TRIM28 on RORγt binding activities need to be further investigated, as well as the involved detailed epigenetic mechanism.

3. TRIM33 regulates the proinflammatory activity of Th17 cells

3.1 Biological functions of TRIM33

TRIM33, also called TIF1γ, is the third member found in the TIF1 family. Like TRIM28, TRIM33 is also a multifunctional protein with many biological functions. It was initially discovered as a transcription co-repressor and exhibited a strong silencing activity when tethered to a promoter (Venturini et al., 1999). However, it can also promote transcription by recruiting transcription elongation factors p-TEFb and FACT to counteract RNA polymerase II pausing (Bai et al., 2010). In addition, genetic and biochemical evidences suggest it as a branch of the canonical transforming growth factor β signaling pathway through complexing with R-SMAD proteins and ubiquitylating SMAD4 (He et al., 2006). TRIM33 contains a PHD-Bromo domain which can function as a histone reader recognizing histone marks H3K9Me3 and H3K18ac (Xi et al., 2011).

In the immune system, TRIM33 has been reported to regulate hematopoiesis and innate immune responses, such as erythroid differentiation, maintenance of optimal HSC functions in transplantation assays, cytosolic RNA-induced NLRP3 inflammasome activation and so on (Bai et al., 2010; Ferri et al., 2015; He et al., 2006; Kusy et al., 2011; Wang, Kawaoka, et al., 2015; Weng et al., 2014). However, its role in T cells has not been reported before.

3.2 TRIM33 mediates proinflammatory Th17 cell development both *in vitro* and *in vivo*

As mentioned before, TGF-β is essential for the induction of both proinflammatory Th17 cells and anti-inflammatory iTreg cells. However, the underlying signaling mechanisms between these two subsets seem complicated. In the canonical TGF-β signaling pathway, binding of TGF-β to its receptor induces phosphorylation of R-SMAD proteins, which then interact with the common SAMD protein SMAD4 and translocate into nucleus to induce downstream gene expression. R-SMAD proteins are primarily composed of SMAD2 and SMAD3 (Massague, 2012). The relative contribution of SMAD proteins to Th17 and iTreg cell differentiation varies. Deletion of either SMAD2, SMAD3 or SMAD4, partially reduces TGF-β induced Foxp3 expression (Martinez et al., 2009, 2010; Yang, Nurieva, et al., 2008). In Th17 cells, SMAD4 is indispensable for their generation, whereas SMAD3 somehow negatively inhibits IL-17 induction, although there's also an argument that Smad3 deficiency didn't affect Th17 cell development (Martinez et al., 2009; Yang, Nurieva, et al., 2008). Studies from our group and others suggest a partial role of SMAD2 in direct regulation of IL-17 expression in Th17 cells (Lu et al., 2010; Martinez et al., 2010) and another report shows deficiency of both SMAD2 and SMAD3 nearly abolishes IL-17 expression and Th17 cell induction, likely due to augmented expression of IL-2 (Takimoto et al., 2010). These findings suggest involvement of multiple TGF-β signaling components in Th17 cell differentiation.

As a branch of TGF-β signaling (He et al., 2006), we evaluated the role of TRIM33 in Th17 cells (Tanaka, Jiang, et al., 2018). Like SMAD2 (Martinez et al., 2010), *Trim33*-deficiency also partially reduced Th17 cell differentiation in *in vitro* cultures, as evidenced by decreased IL-17 but increased IL-10 production. Further analysis suggest TRIM33 can directly bind to both the *Il17* and *Il10* gene loci, and promote IL-17 expression independent of IL-10, because blockage of IL-10 could not rescue defective IL-17 expression in *Trim33* deficient T cells. In addition, CCR6, the signature chemokine receptor of Th17 cells, was also downregulated after *Trim33* deletion, while expression of key transcription factors, including RORγt, STAT3, c-MAF, FOXP3 was comparable between WT and *Trim33* KO Th17 cells. Consistent with the above *in vitro* findings, T cell specific ablation of *Trim33* exhibited milder EAE diseases, with significantly fewer Th17 cells infiltrated into the central nervous system. Interestingly, TRIM33 deficiency resulted in increased IL-10 production in antigen-experienced T cells, both in EAE mice and KLH immunized mice, and IL-10 blockage was able to restore the susceptibility of *Trim33*-deficient mice to induction of EAE diseases and CNS-infiltrated Th17 cells, almost to WT mice. Together these data suggest TRIM33 regulates Th17 cell differentiation and pathogenicity mainly through IL-10, and less importantly through IL-17.

Despite the above findings, the differential roles of TRIM33 in control of *Il17* and *Il10* expression is not yet fully understood, although TRIM33 was found to alter the epigenetic status of these two gene loci in an opposite manner. Our further studies found that SMAD2 could interact with TRIM33 in response to TGF-β signaling, and was required for TRIM33 deposition to both the *Il17* and *Il10* gene loci. We also noticed a physical interaction between TRIM33 and RORγt based on co-IP experiment, although the physiological consequences of these interactions in terms of transcription regulations need to be further investigated.

3.3 TRIM33 and SMAD4 differentially regulate T cell development

In contrast to TRIM33, SMAD4, the classical downstream component of TGF-β signaling, is not required for Th17 cell differentiation, but regulate FOXP3 and IL-10 expression in iTreg cells. Interestingly, TRIM33 is known to have a E3 ubiquitin ligase RING domain that can cause ubiquitin and degradation of SMAD4 (Dupont et al., 2005). Indeed, we noticed elevated level of SMAD4 protein, but not its mRNA in *Trim33*-deficient Th17 cells. To our interest, further deletion of *Smad4* in *Trim33* deficient cells decreased *Il10* expression, suggesting binding of TRIM33 to the *Il10* gene locus may inhibit its expression indirectly through degrading and keeping SMAD4 away. In line with this, mutating the E3 ligase RING domain of TRIM33 partially attenuated TRIM33 mediated IL-10 suppression.

In view of these findings, we propose that TGF-β signaling promotes the formation of SMAD2/3/4 complex to drive the iTreg program, including inducing the expression of *Il10* and *Foxp3*. However, in the presence of IL-6 signaling, TRIM33 is somehow activated, causes SMAD4 degradation *via* its ubiquitin ligase activity and prevents the formation of SMAD2/3/4 complex, therefore inhibits IL-10 but promotes IL-17 production. On the other hand, TRIM33 interacts with SMAD2, as well as RORγt, promote *Il17, Il17f* and *Ccr6* in Th17 cells *via* binding to corresponding gene loci (Fig. 2). These results suggest multiple functions of TGF-β signaling in orchestrating the differentiation of Th17 cells.

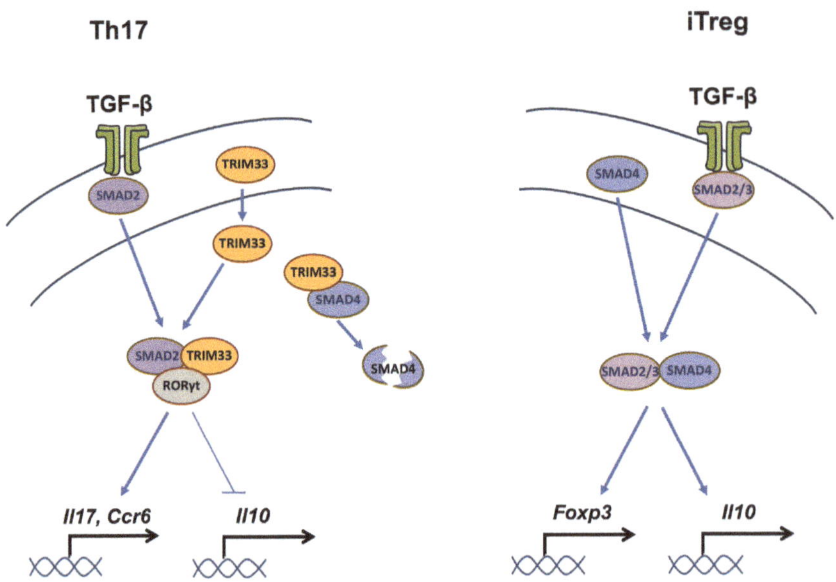

Fig. 2 TRIM33 and SMAD4 differentially regulate the generation of proinflammatory Th17 cells and anti-inflammatory iTreg cells. TGF-β signaling leads to formation of SMAD2/TRIM33/RORγt complex in Th17 cells and SMAD2/3/4 complex in iTreg cells, respectively. The SMAD2/TRIM33 axis is required for *Il17* and *Ccr6* expression, and for repression of *Il10,* likely through altering chromosomal structures and accessibilities, while SMAD4 promotes *Il10* expression. In Th17 cells, TRIM33 likely inhibits the formation of SMAD2/3/4 complex through promoting SMAD4 ubiquitination and degradation.

4. SRC-3 regulates RORγt activity in Th17 cells

4.1 SRC family proteins are coactivators for nuclear receptors

The steroid receptor coactivator (SRC) family proteins are the first discovered coactivators for NRs, composed of 3 members: SRC-1, SRC-2 and SRC-3, with more than 50% amino acid sequence similarities. The SRC proteins contain three distinct domains, including a b-HLH-PAS domain in the N terminus, a NR interacting domain composed of 3 LXXLL motifs in the middle and two activation domains, AD1 and AD2 in the C terminus. Among them, the b-HLH-PAS domain is the most conserved domain, and is responsible for interactions with transcription factors and cofactors, including SRCs, to activate gene transcription. The b-HLH-PAS domain contains several nuclear localization signals for subcellular localization. The central LXXLL motifs are essential for binding to and activating NRs. The C-terminal AD1 and AD2 domains are required to recruit additional cofactors for histone modification and chromatin remodeling to enhance gene transcription. The AD1 domain can interact with CBP and HAT to promote histone acetylation, while AD2 recruits several histone methyltransferases like CARM1 and PRMT1 (Johnson & O'Malley, 2012; York & O'Malley, 2010). The presence of multiple protein–protein interacting domains and different structural features of SRCs make them ideal platforms for coordinating various transcription factors and cofactors to modulate the complex functions of NRs.

4.2 SRC-3 mediates pathogenic Th17 generation

Early studies characterized SRC-1 and SRC2 as coactivators for RORγt, and have an important role in promoting survival of thymocytes (Xie, Sadim, & Sun, 2005). In Th17 cells, K446, a ubiquitination site in RORγt, was shown to negatively regulate Th17 cell differentiation by controlling interaction between RORγt and SRC-1(He et al., 2016). Mice with *Src*-1 deficiency were partially resistant to EAE induction, with decreased Th17 but increased Treg cell development *in vivo*. Accordingly, *Src*-1 deficient T cells showed severe Th17 differentiation defect and augmented Foxp3 expression *in vitro*. Mechanistically, SRC-1 enhances RORγt activity in a TCR dependent manner. TCR activated PKC-θ phosphorylates of SRC-1 and potentiates its interaction with RORγt and recruitment of CARM1, which deposits permissive H3417ame2 marker while suppressing the inhibitory H3K9me3 histone modifications at the *Il17* gene locus and

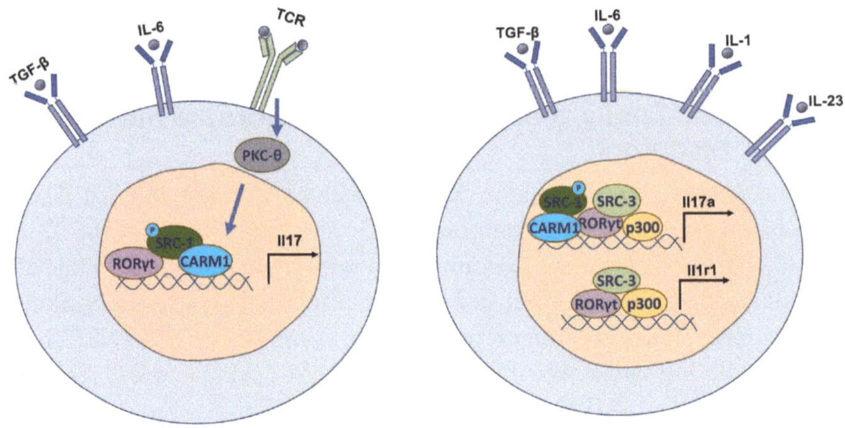

Fig. 3 SRCs promote Th17 differentiation by potentiating RORγt transcriptional activities. SRC-1 is phosphorylated by PKC-θ downstream of TCR signaling. Phosphorylation of SRC-1 promotes its recruitment of histone methyltransferase complex CARM1 and binding with RORγt, which then enhances *Il17* expression and Th17 induction. SRC-3 is involved in the pathogenic transcriptional program of Th17 cells. Although Th17 differentiation induced by TGF-β and IL-6 was not affected by SRC-3, SRC-3 promotes the pathogenic Th17 generation induced by IL-1, IL-6 and IL-23, mainly through enhancing Il1r1 expression. Mechanistically, SRC-3 binds and accelerates RORγt transcriptional activities by recruiting acetyltransferase p300 to increase chromatin accessibilities.

enhances its transcription in Th17 cells (Fig. 3). Interestingly, binding of SRC-1 to RORγt disrupts interaction between FOXP3 and RORγt and relieves the inhibition of RORγt by FOXP3. SRC-1 is therefore an important modulator in fate determination of Th17 vs iTreg programs through multiple mechanisms (Sen et al., 2018).

In addition to SRC-1, we have recently identified another SRC family member, SRC-3 as an essential cofactor in Th17 cells (Tanaka, Martinez, et al., 2018). Previous studies reported that germline deletion of *Src*-3 in mice alleviated EAE disease symptoms *in vivo* (Xiao et al., 2010), and SRC-3 could interact with RORα (Moraitis, Giguere, & Thompson, 2002), suggesting SRC-3 as a potential regulator for Th17 cell generation. To investigate T cell intrinsic role of SRC-3, we generated SRC-3 conditional knockout mice by crossing *Src3*$^{fl/fl}$ mice with Cd4cre mice. Unlike the Cd4Cre driven *Rorc* knockout mice, *Src*-3 conditional knockout mice looked grossly normal and exhibited similar lymphocyte proportions in both thymus and secondary lymphoid organs, indicating SRC-3 does not participate in RORγt-directed thymocyte development, which is in contrast to SRC-1 and SRC-2. Consistent with the previous report of germline KO mice, *Src*-3 conditional KO mice showed delayed onset of EAE diseases and alleviated disease severity following MOG immunization, and also reduced Th17 cells, but not Th1 cells, in both the CNS system and peripheral lymphoid organs.

To further investigate SRC-3 function in Th17 cells, naive WT and *Src-3* ablated T cells were sorted and induced for Th17 cells. A surprising finding is that during *in vitro* cultures, *Src*-3 deficiency did not affect Th17 cell differentiation induced by IL-6 and TGF-β, but selectively reduced pathogenic Th17 cell differentiation induced by IL-1, IL-6 and IL-23. On the contrary, *Src*-3 deficiency did not affect the differentiation of other T cell subsets. These evidence together suggest a selective role of SRC-3 in promoting pathogenic Th17 cell generation.

4.3 SRC-3 promotes Th17 cell pathogenicity through IL-1 signaling

Expression of several proinflammatory genes, including *Il17, Il17f, Il23r* and *Il1r1* was found to be downregulated by *Src-3* deficiency. Interestingly, those genes were directly bound by RORγt, indicating the critical role of SRC-3 in promoting RORγt transcriptional activity in Th17 cells. Importantly, we further discovered that overexpression of *Il1r1* could largely rescue defective IL-17 production in *Src*-3 deficient cells *in vitro* and their autoimmune functions *in vivo*, suggesting a unique role of SRC-3 in IL-1 signaling.

Mechanistically, SRC-3 was found to be recruited to the regulatory elements of *Il17a* and *Il1r1* genes, gene loci that were also bound by RORγt, and was required for their chromatin activation *via* recruiting p300. In addition, SRC-3 could interact with RORγt like the other SRC family members, and its recruitment to the target genes was dependent on RORγt (Fig. 3).

Interestingly, a subsequent study published recently show that SRC-3 only interacts with RORγt in Th17 cells, but not RORγt in thymocytes, and mutation of the lysine 313 amino acid in RORγt abolishes interaction between RORγt and SRC-3, but not RORγt and SRC-1 (He et al., 2019), whereas the lysine 446 in RORγt is required for interaction with SRC-1 (He et al., 2016). These findings suggest that different SRCs regulate the activity of RORγt *via* distinct mechanisms, which might be useful for differential control of Th17 cells in order to fulfill different physiological demands. However, the partial phenotypes of single SRC protein deficiency in terms of Th17 cell differentiation suggest potential synergistic or additional effect among SRC1/2/3 on RORγt transcriptional activity and associated Th17 cell response, which needs to be further investigated.

5. Conclusions and perspectives

Although our knowledge on transcriptional regulation in Th17 cells is rapidly expanding, the crosstalks among various trans-acting factors (such as transcription factors) and *cis*-acting elements are still largely unclear. Cofactors, often serving as posttranslational enzymes or scaffold proteins to recruit related epigenetic enzymes, are emerging as important intermediate modulators in orchestrating the transcriptional machinery in Th17 cells, through epigenetic or non-epigenetic mechanisms.

We and others have recently demonstrated a critical role of several cofactors in Th17 cells, including members of the TIF1 and SRC families (He et al., 2019; Jiang et al., 2018; Sen et al., 2018; Tanaka, Jiang, et al., 2018; Tanaka, Martinez, et al., 2018). In general, those transcription cofactors are able to modify chromatin structure and accessibilities, directly or indirectly, and each regulates Th17 cell program *via* distinct yet related mechanisms. For example, TRIM28 functions downstream of IL-6/STAT3 signaling and is essential for RORγt recruitment to its target sequences *via* regulating chromatin accessibility (Jiang et al., 2018), whereas TRIM33 functions downstream of TGF-β/SMAD2 signaling and is critical for antagonizing the SMAD4 dependent iTreg cell program in Th17 cells, through forming a complex with SMAD2 and RORγt (Tanaka, Jiang, et al., 2018). SRC-1 is particularly important in relieving RORγt from FOXP3 binding complex and FOXP3-mediated inhibition in a TCR dependent manner, and escorts Th17 cell differentiation toward the right direction, despite that it can also affect the chromatin status of the *Il17-17f* gene locus (Sen et al., 2018). Interestingly, SRC-3 seems to have a unique role in regulating cytokine signaling, *via* increasing *Il1r1* expression in a RORγt-dependent manner (Tanaka, Martinez, et al., 2018). The expression of RORγt is strictly cell-type specific, whereas cofactors or other transcription factors, including STAT3 and SMAD2, are broadly expressed, these findings highlight RORγt as a critical lineage-specific central hub in integrating various signals and orchestrating transcriptional control of Th17 program. Like RORγt, Th17 cells are also controlled *via* various NR family transcription factors (Park & Pan, 2015), including RORα, AHR, PPARγ, NR4A2, LXR and VDR (Bruce, Yu, Ooi, & Cantorna, 2011; Cui et al., 2011;

Klotz et al., 2009; Raveney, Oki, & Yamamura, 2013; Veldhoen et al., 2008; Yang, Pappu, et al., 2008). These NRs have miscellaneous binding activities with various cofactors, but the precise roles of these genes and how they crosstalk with RORγt in Th17 cells, remain largely unclear and need to be further investigated.

The role of RORγt is clearly beyond Th17 cells, and it also control the development and functions of several other immune cell subsets, including γδT cells and ILC3 cells, as well as the development of thymocytes (Eberl, 2017). Deficiency in RORγt impairs the development of peripheral lymphoid tissues and thymocytes, and can lead to thymoma (Kurebayashi et al., 2000; Sun et al., 2000; Ueda et al., 2002), which raises a significant safety issues in developing RORγt-targeting strategy in treatment of various Th17 cell related autoimmune syndromes. Our studies and others demonstrate that the transcription activity of RORγt is tightly controlled and fine-tuned by multiple cofactors or epigenetic modifiers through sophisticated mechanisms involving in formation of different RORγt binding complexes, which could be intervened and utilized to develop more specific RORγt targeting strategies to remain the beneficial function of RORγt whereas to restrict its pathogenic functions.

Acknowledgments

Our work was supported by grants from Ministry of Science and Technology (2016YFC 0906200 to C.D.), Beijing Municipal Science and Technology (Z171100000417005 to C.D.), National Natural Science Foundation of China (31570884 to X.W. and 31630022 to C.D.), and Beijing Natural Science foundation (5172017 to X.W.).

Author contributions

Y. J. wrote, X.W. revised, and C.D. instructed and revised the manuscript.

Reference

Akimzhanov, A. M., Yang, X. O., & Dong, C. (2007). Chromatin remodeling of interleukin-17 (IL-17)-IL-17F cytokine gene locus during inflammatory helper T cell differentiation. *The Journal of Biological Chemistry*, *282*, 5969–5972.

Aujla, S. J., & Kolls, J. K. (2009). IL-22: A critical mediator in mucosal host defense. *Journal of Molecular Medicine (Berlin, Germany)*, *87*, 451–454.

Bai, X., Kim, J., Yang, Z., Jurynec, M. J., Akie, T. E., Lee, J., et al. (2010). TIF1gamma controls erythroid cell fate by regulating transcription elongation. *Cell*, *142*, 133–143.

Bauquet, A. T., Jin, H., Paterson, A. M., Mitsdoerffer, M., Ho, I. C., Sharpe, A. H., et al. (2009). The costimulatory molecule ICOS regulates the expression of c-Maf and IL-21 in the development of follicular T helper cells and TH-17 cells. *Nature Immunology*, *10*, 167–175.

Bettelli, E., Carrier, Y., Gao, W., Korn, T., Strom, T. B., Oukka, M., et al. (2006). Reciprocal developmental pathways for the generation of pathogenic effector TH17 and regulatory T cells. *Nature, 441*, 235–238.

Betz, B. C., Jordan-Williams, K. L., Wang, C., Kang, S. G., Liao, J., Logan, M. R., et al. (2010). Batf coordinates multiple aspects of B and T cell function required for normal antibody responses. *The Journal of Experimental Medicine, 207*, 933–942.

Bruce, D., Yu, S., Ooi, J. H., & Cantorna, M. T. (2011). Converging pathways lead to overproduction of IL-17 in the absence of vitamin D signaling. *International Immunology, 23*, 519–528.

Brustle, A., Heink, S., Huber, M., Rosenplanter, C., Stadelmann, C., Yu, P., et al. (2007). The development of inflammatory T(H)-17 cells requires interferon-regulatory factor 4. *Nature Immunology, 8*, 958–966.

Burchill, M. A., Yang, J., Vogtenhuber, C., Blazar, B. R., & Farrar, M. A. (2007). IL-2 receptor beta-dependent STAT5 activation is required for the development of Foxp3 + regulatory T cells. *Journal of Immunology, 178*, 280–290.

Cargill, M., Schrodi, S. J., Chang, M., Garcia, V. E., Brandon, R., Callis, K. P., et al. (2007). A large-scale genetic association study confirms IL12B and leads to the identification of IL23R as psoriasis-risk genes. *American Journal of Human Genetics, 80*, 273–290.

Chen, W., Jin, W., Hardegen, N., Lei, K. J., Li, L., Marinos, N., et al. (2003). Conversion of peripheral CD4+CD25- naive T cells to CD4+CD25+ regulatory T cells by TGF-beta induction of transcription factor Foxp3. *The Journal of Experimental Medicine, 198*, 1875–1886.

Chen, Z., Li, S., Subramaniam, S., Shyy, J. Y., & Chien, S. (2017). Epigenetic regulation: A new frontier for biomedical engineers. *Annual Review of Biomedical Engineering, 19*, 195–219.

Cheung, K. L., Zhang, F., Jaganathan, A., Sharma, R., Zhang, Q., Konuma, T., et al. (2017). Distinct roles of Brd2 and Brd4 in potentiating the transcriptional program for Th17 cell differentiation. *Molecular Cell, 65*, 1068–1080.e1065.

Chikuma, S., Suita, N., Okazaki, I. M., Shibayama, S., & Honjo, T. (2012). TRIM28 prevents autoinflammatory T cell development in vivo. *Nature Immunology, 13*, 596–603.

Chung, Y., Chang, S. H., Martinez, G. J., Yang, X. O., Nurieva, R., Kang, H. S., et al. (2009). Critical regulation of early Th17 cell differentiation by interleukin-1 signaling. *Immunity, 30*, 576–587.

Ciofani, M., Madar, A., Galan, C., Sellars, M., Mace, K., Pauli, F., et al. (2012). A validated regulatory network for Th17 cell specification. *Cell, 151*, 289–303.

Constantinescu, C. S., Wysocka, M., Hilliard, B., Ventura, E. S., Lavi, E., Trinchieri, G., et al. (1998). Antibodies against IL-12 prevent superantigen-induced and spontaneous relapses of experimental autoimmune encephalomyelitis. *Journal of Immunology, 161*, 5097–5104.

Cook, D. N., Kang, H. S., & Jetten, A. M. (2015). Retinoic acid-related orphan receptors (RORs): Regulatory functions in immunity, development, circadian rhythm, and metabolism. *Nuclear Receptor Research, 2*, 101185.

Cua, D. J., Sherlock, J., Chen, Y., Murphy, C. A., Joyce, B., Seymour, B., et al. (2003). Interleukin-23 rather than interleukin-12 is the critical cytokine for autoimmune inflammation of the brain. *Nature, 421*, 744–748.

Cui, G., Qin, X., Wu, L., Zhang, Y., Sheng, X., Yu, Q., et al. (2011). Liver X receptor (LXR) mediates negative regulation of mouse and human Th17 differentiation. *The Journal of Clinical Investigation, 121*, 658–670.

Dasgupta, S., Lonard, D. M., & O'Malley, B. W. (2014). Nuclear receptor coactivators: Master regulators of human health and disease. *Annual Review of Medicine, 65*, 279–292.

Dong, C. (2008). TH17 cells in development: An updated view of their molecular identity and genetic programming. *Nature Reviews. Immunology, 8*, 337–348.

Duerr, R. H., Taylor, K. D., Brant, S. R., Rioux, J. D., Silverberg, M. S., Daly, M. J., et al. (2006). A genome-wide association study identifies IL23R as an inflammatory bowel disease gene. *Science*, *314*, 1461–1463.

Dupont, S., Zacchigna, L., Cordenonsi, M., Soligo, S., Adorno, M., Rugge, M., et al. (2005). Germ-layer specification and control of cell growth by Ectodermin, a Smad4 ubiquitin ligase. *Cell*, *121*, 87–99.

Durant, L., Watford, W. T., Ramos, H. L., Laurence, A., Vahedi, G., Wei, L., et al. (2010). Diverse targets of the transcription factor STAT3 contribute to T cell pathogenicity and homeostasis. *Immunity*, *32*, 605–615.

Eberl, G. (2017). RORgammat, a multitask nuclear receptor at mucosal surfaces. *Mucosal Immunology*, *10*, 27–34.

Escobar, T. M., Kanellopoulou, C., Kugler, D. G., Kilaru, G., Nguyen, C. K., Nagarajan, V., et al. (2014). miR-155 activates cytokine gene expression in Th17 cells by regulating the DNA-binding protein Jarid2 to relieve polycomb-mediated repression. *Immunity*, *40*, 865–879.

Ferri, F., Parcelier, A., Petit, V., Gallouet, A. S., Lewandowski, D., Dalloz, M., et al. (2015). TRIM33 switches off Ifnb1 gene transcription during the late phase of macrophage activation. *Nature Communications*, *6*, 8900.

Fontenot, J. D., Gavin, M. A., & Rudensky, A. Y. (2003). Foxp3 programs the development and function of CD4+CD25+ regulatory T cells. *Nature Immunology*, *4*, 330–336.

Fontenot, J. D., Rasmussen, J. P., Gavin, M. A., & Rudensky, A. Y. (2005). A function for interleukin 2 in Foxp3-expressing regulatory T cells. *Nature Immunology*, *6*, 1142–1151.

Friedman, J. R., Fredericks, W. J., Jensen, D. E., Speicher, D. W., Huang, X. P., Neilson, E. G., et al. (1996). KAP-1, a novel corepressor for the highly conserved KRAB repression domain. *Genes & Development*, *10*, 2067–2078.

Gaublomme, J. T., Yosef, N., Lee, Y., Gertner, R. S., Yang, L. V., Wu, C., et al. (2015). Single-cell genomics unveils critical regulators of Th17 cell pathogenicity. *Cell*, *163*, 1400–1412.

Ghoreschi, K., Laurence, A., Yang, X. P., Tato, C. M., McGeachy, M. J., Konkel, J. E., et al. (2010). Generation of pathogenic T(H)17 cells in the absence of TGF-beta signalling. *Nature*, *467*, 967–971.

Glass, C. K., & Saijo, K. (2010). Nuclear receptor transrepression pathways that regulate inflammation in macrophages and T cells. *Nature Reviews. Immunology*, *10*, 365–376.

Harrington, L. E., Hatton, R. D., Mangan, P. R., Turner, H., Murphy, T. L., Murphy, K. M., et al. (2005). Interleukin 17-producing CD4+ effector T cells develop via a lineage distinct from the T helper type 1 and 2 lineages. *Nature Immunology*, *6*, 1123–1132.

Harris, T. J., Grosso, J. F., Yen, H. R., Xin, H., Kortylewski, M., Albesiano, E., et al. (2007). Cutting edge: An in vivo requirement for STAT3 signaling in TH17 development and TH17-dependent autoimmunity. *Journal of Immunology*, *179*, 4313–4317.

Hatakeyama, S. (2011). TRIM proteins and cancer. *Nature Reviews. Cancer*, *11*, 792–804.

He, Y. W., Deftos, M. L., Ojala, E. W., & Bevan, M. J. (1998). RORgamma t, a novel isoform of an orphan receptor, negatively regulates Fas ligand expression and IL-2 production in T cells. *Immunity*, *9*, 797–806.

He, W., Dorn, D. C., Erdjument-Bromage, H., Tempst, P., Moore, M. A., & Massague, J. (2006). Hematopoiesis controlled by distinct TIF1gamma and Smad4 branches of the TGFbeta pathway. *Cell*, *125*, 929–941.

He, Z., Wang, F., Ma, J., Sen, S., Zhang, J., Gwack, Y., et al. (2016). Ubiquitination of RORgammat at lysine 446 limits Th17 differentiation by controlling coactivator recruitment. *Journal of Immunology*, *197*, 1148–1158.

He, Z., Zhang, J., Du, Q., Xu, J., Gwack, Y., & Sun, Z. (2019). SRC3 is a cofactor for RORgammat in Th17 differentiation but not thymocyte development. *Journal of Immunology*, *202*, 760–769.

Holland, S. M., DeLeo, F. R., Elloumi, H. Z., Hsu, A. P., Uzel, G., Brodsky, N., et al. (2007). STAT3 mutations in the hyper-IgE syndrome. *The New England Journal of Medicine*, *357*, 1608–1619.

Hori, S., Nomura, T., & Sakaguchi, S. (2003). Control of regulatory T cell development by the transcription factor Foxp3. *Science*, *299*, 1057–1061.

Hu, X., Wang, Y., Hao, L. Y., Liu, X., Lesch, C. A., Sanchez, B. M., et al. (2015). Sterol metabolism controls T(H)17 differentiation by generating endogenous RORgamma agonists. *Nature Chemical Biology*, *11*, 141–147.

Huh, J. R., Leung, M. W., Huang, P., Ryan, D. A., Krout, M. R., Malapaka, R. R., et al. (2011). Digoxin and its derivatives suppress TH17 cell differentiation by antagonizing RORgammat activity. *Nature*, *472*, 486–490.

Hyun, K., Jeon, J., Park, K., & Kim, J. (2017). Writing, erasing and reading histone lysine methylations. *Experimental & Molecular Medicine*, *49*, e324.

Ichiyama, K., Chen, T., Wang, X., Yan, X., Kim, B. S., Tanaka, S., et al. (2015). The methylcytosine dioxygenase Tet2 promotes DNA demethylation and activation of cytokine gene expression in T cells. *Immunity*, *42*, 613–626.

Ivanov, I. I., McKenzie, B. S., Zhou, L., Tadokoro, C. E., Lepelley, A., Lafaille, J. J., et al. (2006). The orphan nuclear receptor RORgammat directs the differentiation program of proinflammatory IL-17+ T helper cells. *Cell*, *126*, 1121–1133.

Iyengar, S., & Farnham, P. J. (2011). KAP1 protein: An enigmatic master regulator of the genome. *The Journal of Biological Chemistry*, *286*, 26267–26276.

Jefferies, C., Wynne, C., & Higgs, R. (2011). Antiviral TRIMs: Friend or foe in autoimmune and autoinflammatory disease? *Nature Reviews. Immunology*, *11*, 617–625.

Jetten, A. M. (2009). Retinoid-related orphan receptors (RORs): Critical roles in development, immunity, circadian rhythm, and cellular metabolism. *Nuclear Receptor Signaling*, *7*, e003.

Jiang, Y., Liu, Y., Lu, H., Sun, S. C., Jin, W., Wang, X., et al. (2018). Epigenetic activation during T helper 17 cell differentiation is mediated by Tripartite motif containing 28. *Nature Communications*, *9*, 1424.

Jin, W., & Dong, C. (2013). IL-17 cytokines in immunity and inflammation. *Emerging Microbes & Infections*, *2*, e60.

Johnson, A. B., & O'Malley, B. W. (2012). Steroid receptor coactivators 1, 2, and 3: Critical regulators of nuclear receptor activity and steroid receptor modulator (SRM)-based cancer therapy. *Molecular and Cellular Endocrinology*, *348*, 430–439.

Kawai, T., & Akira, S. (2011). Regulation of innate immune signalling pathways by the tripartite motif (TRIM) family proteins. *EMBO Molecular Medicine*, *3*, 513–527.

Khetchoumian, K., Teletin, M., Mark, M., Lerouge, T., Cervino, M., Oulad-Abdelghani, M., et al. (2004). TIF1delta, a novel HP1-interacting member of the transcriptional intermediary factor 1 (TIF1) family expressed by elongating spermatids. *The Journal of Biological Chemistry*, *279*, 48329–48341.

Kishimoto, T. (2005). Interleukin-6: From basic science to medicine—40 years in immunology. *Annual Review of Immunology*, *23*, 1–21.

Kitagawa, Y., Ohkura, N., Kidani, Y., Vandenbon, A., Hirota, K., Kawakami, R., et al. (2017). Guidance of regulatory T cell development by Satb1-dependent super-enhancer establishment. *Nature Immunology*, *18*, 173–183.

Klotz, L., Burgdorf, S., Dani, I., Saijo, K., Flossdorf, J., Hucke, S., et al. (2009). The nuclear receptor PPAR gamma selectively inhibits Th17 differentiation in a T cell-intrinsic fashion and suppresses CNS autoimmunity. *The Journal of Experimental Medicine*, *206*, 2079–2089.

Kolls, J. K., & Khader, S. A. (2010). The role of Th17 cytokines in primary mucosal immunity. *Cytokine & Growth Factor Reviews*, *21*, 443–448.

Korn, T., Bettelli, E., Gao, W., Awasthi, A., Jager, A., Strom, T. B., et al. (2007). IL-21 initiates an alternative pathway to induce proinflammatory T(H)17 cells. *Nature, 448*, 484–487.

Korn, T., Bettelli, E., Oukka, M., & Kuchroo, V. K. (2009). IL-17 and Th17 cells. *Annual Review of Immunology, 27*, 485–517.

Kretschmer, K., Apostolou, I., Hawiger, D., Khazaie, K., Nussenzweig, M. C., & von Boehmer, H. (2005). Inducing and expanding regulatory T cell populations by foreign antigen. *Nature Immunology, 6*, 1219–1227.

Krishnamoorthy, V., Kannanganat, S., Maienschein-Cline, M., Cook, S. L., Chen, J., Bahroos, N., et al. (2017). The IRF4 gene regulatory module functions as a read-write integrator to dynamically coordinate T helper cell fate. *Immunity, 47*, 481–497.e487.

Kurebayashi, S., Ueda, E., Sakaue, M., Patel, D. D., Medvedev, A., Zhang, F., et al. (2000). Retinoid-related orphan receptor gamma (RORgamma) is essential for lymphoid organogenesis and controls apoptosis during thymopoiesis. *Proceedings of the National Academy of Sciences of the United States of America, 97*, 10132–10137.

Kusy, S., Gault, N., Ferri, F., Lewandowski, D., Barroca, V., Jaracz-Ros, A., et al. (2011). Adult hematopoiesis is regulated by TIF1gamma, a repressor of TAL1 and PU.1 transcriptional activity. *Cell Stem Cell, 8*, 412–425.

Langrish, C. L., Chen, Y., Blumenschein, W. M., Mattson, J., Basham, B., Sedgwick, J. D., et al. (2005). IL-23 drives a pathogenic T cell population that induces autoimmune inflammation. *The Journal of Experimental Medicine, 201*, 233–240.

Laurence, A., Tato, C. M., Davidson, T. S., Kanno, Y., Chen, Z., Yao, Z., et al. (2007). Interleukin-2 signaling via STAT5 constrains T helper 17 cell generation. *Immunity, 26*, 371–381.

Le Douarin, B., Zechel, C., Garnier, J. M., Lutz, Y., Tora, L., Pierrat, P., et al. (1995). The N-terminal part of TIF1, a putative mediator of the ligand-dependent activation function (AF-2) of nuclear receptors, is fused to B-raf in the oncogenic protein T18. *The EMBO Journal, 14*, 2020–2033.

Lee, Y., Awasthi, A., Yosef, N., Quintana, F. J., Xiao, S., Peters, A., et al. (2012). Induction and molecular signature of pathogenic TH17 cells. *Nature Immunology, 13*, 991–999.

Lee, G. R., Kim, S. T., Spilianakis, C. G., Fields, P. E., & Flavell, R. A. (2006). T helper cell differentiation: Regulation by cis elements and epigenetics. *Immunity, 24*, 369–379.

Leonard, J. P., Waldburger, K. E., & Goldman, S. J. (1995). Prevention of experimental autoimmune encephalomyelitis by antibodies against interleukin 12. *The Journal of Experimental Medicine, 181*, 381–386.

Leonard, J. P., Waldburger, K. E., & Goldman, S. J. (1996). Regulation of experimental autoimmune encephalomyelitis by interleukin-12. *Annals of the New York Academy of Sciences, 795*, 216–226.

Leppkes, M., Becker, C., Ivanov, I. I., Hirth, S., Wirtz, S., Neufert, C., et al. (2009). ROR-gamma-expressing Th17 cells induce murine chronic intestinal inflammation via redundant effects of IL-17A and IL-17F. *Gastroenterology, 136*, 257–267.

Li, M. O., Wan, Y. Y., & Flavell, R. A. (2007). T cell-produced transforming growth factor-beta1 controls T cell tolerance and regulates Th1- and Th17-cell differentiation. *Immunity, 26*, 579–591.

Liang, Q., Deng, H., Li, X., Wu, X., Tang, Q., Chang, T. H., et al. (2011). Tripartite motif-containing protein 28 is a small ubiquitin-related modifier E3 ligase and negative regulator of IFN regulatory factor 7. *Journal of Immunology, 187*, 4754–4763.

Liu, Z., Cao, W., Xu, L., Chen, X., Zhan, Y., Yang, Q., et al. (2015). The histone H3 lysine-27 demethylase Jmjd3 plays a critical role in specific regulation of Th17 cell differentiation. *Journal of Molecular Cell Biology, 7*, 505–516.

Liu, Y., Helms, C., Liao, W., Zaba, L. C., Duan, S., Gardner, J., et al. (2008). A genome-wide association study of psoriasis and psoriatic arthritis identifies new disease loci. *PLoS Genetics*, *4*, e1000041.

Lonard, D. M., & O'Malley, B. W. (2012). Nuclear receptor coregulators: Modulators of pathology and therapeutic targets. *Nature Reviews. Endocrinology*, *8*, 598–604.

Lu, L., Wang, J., Zhang, F., Chai, Y., Brand, D., Wang, X., et al. (2010). Role of SMAD and non-SMAD signals in the development of Th17 and regulatory T cells. *Journal of Immunology*, *184*, 4295–4306.

Mahnke, J., Schumacher, V., Ahrens, S., Kading, N., Feldhoff, L. M., Huber, M., et al. (2016). Interferon regulatory factor 4 controls TH1 cell effector function and metabolism. *Scientific Reports*, *6*, 35521.

Malik, S., & Roeder, R. G. (2010). The metazoan mediator co-activator complex as an integrative hub for transcriptional regulation. *Nature Reviews. Genetics*, *11*, 761–772.

Mangan, P. R., Harrington, L. E., O'Quinn, D. B., Helms, W. S., Bullard, D. C., Elson, C. O., et al. (2006). Transforming growth factor-beta induces development of the T(H)17 lineage. *Nature*, *441*, 231–234.

Martinez, G. J., Zhang, Z., Chung, Y., Reynolds, J. M., Lin, X., Jetten, A. M., et al. (2009). Smad3 differentially regulates the induction of regulatory and inflammatory T cell differentiation. *The Journal of Biological Chemistry*, *284*, 35283–35286.

Martinez, G. J., Zhang, Z., Reynolds, J. M., Tanaka, S., Chung, Y., Liu, T., et al. (2010). Smad2 positively regulates the generation of Th17 cells. *The Journal of Biological Chemistry*, *285*, 29039–29043.

Massague, J. (2012). TGFbeta signalling in context. *Nature Reviews. Molecular Cell Biology*, *13*, 616–630.

McGeachy, M. J., Bak-Jensen, K. S., Chen, Y., Tato, C. M., Blumenschein, W., McClanahan, T., et al. (2007). TGF-beta and IL-6 drive the production of IL-17 and IL-10 by T cells and restrain T(H)-17 cell-mediated pathology. *Nature Immunology*, *8*, 1390–1397.

McGeachy, M. J., Chen, Y., Tato, C. M., Laurence, A., Joyce-Shaikh, B., Blumenschein, W. M., et al. (2009). The interleukin 23 receptor is essential for the terminal differentiation of interleukin 17-producing effector T helper cells in vivo. *Nature Immunology*, *10*, 314–324.

Medvedev, A., Chistokhina, A., Hirose, T., & Jetten, A. M. (1997). Genomic structure and chromosomal mapping of the nuclear orphan receptor ROR gamma (RORC) gene. *Genomics*, *46*, 93–102.

Moosmann, P., Georgiev, O., Le Douarin, B., Bourquin, J. P., & Schaffner, W. (1996). Transcriptional repression by RING finger protein TIF1 beta that interacts with the KRAB repressor domain of KOX1. *Nucleic Acids Research*, *24*, 4859–4867.

Moraitis, A. N., Giguere, V., & Thompson, C. C. (2002). Novel mechanism of nuclear receptor corepressor interaction dictated by activation function 2 helix determinants. *Molecular and Cellular Biology*, *22*, 6831–6841.

Nurieva, R., Yang, X. O., Martinez, G., Zhang, Y., Panopoulos, A. D., Ma, L., et al. (2007). Essential autocrine regulation by IL-21 in the generation of inflammatory T cells. *Nature*, *448*, 480–483.

Okamoto, K., Iwai, Y., Oh-Hora, M., Yamamoto, M., Morio, T., Aoki, K., et al. (2010). IkappaBzeta regulates T(H)17 development by cooperating with ROR nuclear receptors. *Nature*, *464*, 1381–1385.

Oppmann, B., Lesley, R., Blom, B., Timans, J. C., Xu, Y., Hunte, B., et al. (2000). Novel p19 protein engages IL-12p40 to form a cytokine, IL-23, with biological activities similar as well as distinct from IL-12. *Immunity*, *13*, 715–725.

Ouyang, W., & Valdez, P. (2008). IL-22 in mucosal immunity. *Mucosal Immunology*, *1*, 335–338.

Ozato, K., Shin, D. M., Chang, T. H., & Morse, H. C., 3rd. (2008). TRIM family proteins and their emerging roles in innate immunity. *Nature Reviews. Immunology, 8*, 849–860.
Park, H., Li, Z., Yang, X. O., Chang, S. H., Nurieva, R., Wang, Y. H., et al. (2005). A distinct lineage of CD4 T cells regulates tissue inflammation by producing interleukin 17. *Nature Immunology, 6*, 1133–1141.
Park, B. V., & Pan, F. (2015). The role of nuclear receptors in regulation of Th17/Treg biology and its implications for diseases. *Cellular & Molecular Immunology, 12*, 533–542.
Perez-Lloret, J., Okoye, I. S., Guidi, R., Kannan, Y., Coomes, S. M., Czieso, S., et al. (2016). T-cell-intrinsic Tif1alpha/Trim24 regulates IL-1R expression on TH2 cells and TH2 cell-mediated airway allergy. *Proceedings of the National Academy of Sciences of the United States of America, 113*, E568–E576.
Raveney, B. J., Oki, S., & Yamamura, T. (2013). Nuclear receptor NR4A2 orchestrates Th17 cell-mediated autoimmune inflammation via IL-21 signalling. *PLoS One, 8*, e56595.
Reiter, F., Wienerroither, S., & Stark, A. (2017). Combinatorial function of transcription factors and cofactors. *Current Opinion in Genetics & Development, 43*, 73–81.
Santoni de Sio, F. R., Massacand, J., Barde, I., Offner, S., Corsinotti, A., Kapopoulou, A., et al. (2012). KAP1 regulates gene networks controlling mouse B-lymphoid cell differentiation and function. *Blood, 119*, 4675–4685.
Santori, F. R., Huang, P., van de Pavert, S. A., Douglass, E. F., Jr., Leaver, D. J., Haubrich, B. A., et al. (2015). Identification of natural RORgamma ligands that regulate the development of lymphoid cells. *Cell Metabolism, 21*, 286–298.
Schraml, B. U., Hildner, K., Ise, W., Lee, W. L., Smith, W. A., Solomon, B., et al. (2009). The AP-1 transcription factor Batf controls T(H)17 differentiation. *Nature, 460*, 405–409.
Sen, S., Wang, F., Zhang, J., He, Z., Ma, J., Gwack, Y., et al. (2018). SRC1 promotes Th17 differentiation by overriding Foxp3 suppression to stimulate RORgammat activity in a PKC-theta-dependent manner. *Proceedings of the National Academy of Sciences of the United States of America, 115*, E458–E467.
Solt, L. A., Kumar, N., Nuhant, P., Wang, Y., Lauer, J. L., Liu, J., et al. (2011). Suppression of TH17 differentiation and autoimmunity by a synthetic ROR ligand. *Nature, 472*, 491–494.
Soroosh, P., Wu, J., Xue, X., Song, J., Sutton, S. W., Sablad, M., et al. (2014). Oxysterols are agonist ligands of RORgammat and drive Th17 cell differentiation. *Proceedings of the National Academy of Sciences of the United States of America, 111*, 12163–12168.
Spitz, F., & Furlong, E. E. (2012). Transcription factors: From enhancer binding to developmental control. *Nature Reviews. Genetics, 13*, 613–626.
Staudt, V., Bothur, E., Klein, M., Lingnau, K., Reuter, S., Grebe, N., et al. (2010). Interferon-regulatory factor 4 is essential for the developmental program of T helper 9 cells. *Immunity, 33*, 192–202.
Sun, Z., Unutmaz, D., Zou, Y. R., Sunshine, M. J., Pierani, A., Brenner-Morton, S., et al. (2000). Requirement for RORgamma in thymocyte survival and lymphoid organ development. *Science, 288*, 2369–2373.
Takimoto, T., Wakabayashi, Y., Sekiya, T., Inoue, N., Morita, R., Ichiyama, K., et al. (2010). Smad2 and Smad3 are redundantly essential for the TGF-beta-mediated regulation of regulatory T plasticity and Th1 development. *Journal of Immunology, 185*, 842–855.
Tanaka, S., Jiang, Y., Martinez, G. J., Tanaka, K., Yan, X., Kurosaki, T., et al. (2018). Trim33 mediates the proinflammatory function of Th17 cells. *The Journal of Experimental Medicine, 215*, 1853–1868.
Tanaka, K., Martinez, G. J., Yan, X., Long, W., Ichiyama, K., Chi, X., et al. (2018). Regulation of pathogenic T helper 17 cell differentiation by steroid receptor Coactivator-3. *Cell Reports, 23*, 2318–2329.

Thomas, L. W., Lee, E. B., & Wu, J. J. (2019). Systematic review of anti-drug antibodies of IL-17 inhibitors for psoriasis. *The Journal of Dermatological Treatment*, *30*, 110–116.

Tisserand, J., Khetchoumian, K., Thibault, C., Dembele, D., Chambon, P., & Losson, R. (2011). Tripartite motif 24 (Trim24/Tif1alpha) tumor suppressor protein is a novel negative regulator of interferon (IFN)/signal transducers and activators of transcription (STAT) signaling pathway acting through retinoic acid receptor alpha (Raralpha) inhibition. *The Journal of Biological Chemistry*, *286*, 33369–33379.

Ueda, E., Kurebayashi, S., Sakaue, M., Backlund, M., Koller, B., & Jetten, A. M. (2002). High incidence of T-cell lymphomas in mice deficient in the retinoid-related orphan receptor RORgamma. *Cancer Research*, *62*, 901–909.

Vahedi, G., Kanno, Y., Furumoto, Y., Jiang, K., Parker, S. C., Erdos, M. R., et al. (2015). Super-enhancers delineate disease-associated regulatory nodes in T cells. *Nature*, *520*, 558–562.

Vahedi, G., Takahashi, H., Nakayamada, S., Sun, H. W., Sartorelli, V., Kanno, Y., et al. (2012). STATs shape the active enhancer landscape of T cell populations. *Cell*, *151*, 981–993.

Veldhoen, M., Hirota, K., Westendorf, A. M., Buer, J., Dumoutier, L., Renauld, J. C., et al. (2008). The aryl hydrocarbon receptor links TH17-cell-mediated autoimmunity to environmental toxins. *Nature*, *453*, 106–109.

Veldhoen, M., Hocking, R. J., Atkins, C. J., Locksley, R. M., & Stockinger, B. (2006). TGFbeta in the context of an inflammatory cytokine milieu supports de novo differentiation of IL-17-producing T cells. *Immunity*, *24*, 179–189.

Veldhoen, M., Hocking, R. J., Flavell, R. A., & Stockinger, B. (2006). Signals mediated by transforming growth factor-beta initiate autoimmune encephalomyelitis, but chronic inflammation is needed to sustain disease. *Nature Immunology*, 7, 1151–1156.

Venturini, L., You, J., Stadler, M., Galien, R., Lallemand, V., Koken, M. H., et al. (1999). TIF1gamma, a novel member of the transcriptional intermediary factor 1 family. *Oncogene*, *18*, 1209–1217.

Vo, N., & Goodman, R. H. (2001). CREB-binding protein and p300 in transcriptional regulation. *The Journal of Biological Chemistry*, *276*, 13505–13508.

Wang, Y., Godec, J., Ben-Aissa, K., Cui, K., Zhao, K., Pucsek, A. B., et al. (2014). The transcription factors T-bet and Runx are required for the ontogeny of pathogenic interferon-gamma-producing T helper 17 cells. *Immunity*, *40*, 355–366.

Wang, E., Kawaoka, S., Roe, J. S., Shi, J., Hohmann, A. F., Xu, Y., et al. (2015). The transcriptional cofactor TRIM33 prevents apoptosis in B lymphoblastic leukemia by deactivating a single enhancer. *eLife*, *4*, e06377.

Wang, C., Yosef, N., Gaublomme, J., Wu, C., Lee, Y., Clish, C. B., et al. (2015). CD5L/AIM regulates lipid biosynthesis and restrains Th17 cell pathogenicity. *Cell*, *163*, 1413–1427.

Wang, X., Zhang, Y., Yang, X. O., Nurieva, R. I., Chang, S. H., Ojeda, S. S., et al. (2012). Transcription of Il17 and Il17f is controlled by conserved noncoding sequence 2. *Immunity*, *36*, 23–31.

Wei, G., Wei, L., Zhu, J., Zang, C., Hu-Li, J., Yao, Z., et al. (2009). Global mapping of H3K4me3 and H3K27me3 reveals specificity and plasticity in lineage fate determination of differentiating CD4+ T cells. *Immunity*, *30*, 155–167.

Weng, L., Mitoma, H., Trichot, C., Bao, M., Liu, Y., Zhang, Z., et al. (2014). The E3 ubiquitin ligase tripartite motif 33 is essential for cytosolic RNA-induced NLRP3 inflammasome activation. *Journal of Immunology*, *193*, 3676–3682.

Wilson, C. B., Rowell, E., & Sekimata, M. (2009). Epigenetic control of T-helper-cell differentiation. *Nature Reviews. Immunology*, *9*, 91–105.

Xi, Q., Wang, Z., Zaromytidou, A. I., Zhang, X. H., Chow-Tsang, L. F., Liu, J. X., et al. (2011). A poised chromatin platform for TGF-beta access to master regulators. *Cell*, *147*, 1511–1524.

Xiao, Y., Xu, J., Wang, S., Mao, C., Jin, M., Ning, G., et al. (2010). Genetic ablation of steroid receptor coactivator-3 promotes PPAR-beta-mediated alternative activation of microglia in experimental autoimmune encephalomyelitis. *Glia, 58*, 932–942.

Xiao, S., Yosef, N., Yang, J., Wang, Y., Zhou, L., Zhu, C., et al. (2014). Small-molecule RORgammat antagonists inhibit T helper 17 cell transcriptional network by divergent mechanisms. *Immunity, 40*, 477–489.

Xie, H., Sadim, M. S., & Sun, Z. (2005). RORgammat recruits steroid receptor coactivators to ensure thymocyte survival. *Journal of Immunology, 175*, 3800–3809.

Yang, X. O., Nurieva, R., Martinez, G. J., Kang, H. S., Chung, Y., Pappu, B. P., et al. (2008). Molecular antagonism and plasticity of regulatory and inflammatory T cell programs. *Immunity, 29*, 44–56.

Yang, X. O., Panopoulos, A. D., Nurieva, R., Chang, S. H., Wang, D., Watowich, S. S., et al. (2007). STAT3 regulates cytokine-mediated generation of inflammatory helper T cells. *The Journal of Biological Chemistry, 282*, 9358–9363.

Yang, X. O., Pappu, B. P., Nurieva, R., Akimzhanov, A., Kang, H. S., Chung, Y., et al. (2008). T helper 17 lineage differentiation is programmed by orphan nuclear receptors ROR alpha and ROR gamma. *Immunity, 28*, 29–39.

York, B., & O'Malley, B. W. (2010). Steroid receptor coactivator (SRC) family: Masters of systems biology. *The Journal of Biological Chemistry, 285*, 38743–38750.

Yosef, N., Shalek, A. K., Gaublomme, J. T., Jin, H., Lee, Y., Awasthi, A., et al. (2013). Dynamic regulatory network controlling TH17 cell differentiation. *Nature, 496*, 461–468.

Zabidi, M. A., & Stark, A. (2016). Regulatory enhancer-Core-promoter communication via transcription factors and cofactors. *Trends in Genetics, 32*, 801–814.

Zhang, F., Meng, G., & Strober, W. (2008). Interactions among the transcription factors Runx1, RORgammat and Foxp3 regulate the differentiation of interleukin 17-producing T cells. *Nature Immunology, 9*, 1297–1306.

Zheng, Y., Chaudhry, A., Kas, A., deRoos, P., Kim, J. M., Chu, T. T., et al. (2009). Regulatory T-cell suppressor program co-opts transcription factor IRF4 to control T(H)2 responses. *Nature, 458*, 351–356.

Zhou, L., Ivanov, I. I., Spolski, R., Min, R., Shenderov, K., Egawa, T., et al. (2007). IL-6 programs T(H)-17 cell differentiation by promoting sequential engagement of the IL-21 and IL-23 pathways. *Nature Immunology, 8*, 967–974.

Zhou, L., Lopes, J. E., Chong, M. M., Ivanov, I. I., Min, R., Victora, G. D., et al. (2008). TGF-beta-induced Foxp3 inhibits T(H)17 cell differentiation by antagonizing RORgammat function. *Nature, 453*, 236–240.

Zhou, X. F., Yu, J., Chang, M., Zhang, M., Zhou, D., Cammas, F., et al. (2012). TRIM28 mediates chromatin modifications at the TCRalpha enhancer and regulates the development of T and natural killer T cells. *Proceedings of the National Academy of Sciences of the United States of America, 109*, 20083–20088.

Zhu, J., Yamane, H., & Paul, W. E. (2010). Differentiation of effector CD4 T cell populations (*). *Annual Review of Immunology, 28*, 445–489.

CHAPTER SIX

T cell immune response within B-cell follicles

Qizhao Huang[a], Lifan Xu[b], Lilin Ye[b,*]

[a]Cancer Center, The General Hospital of Western Theater Command, Chengdu, China
[b]Institute of Immunology, Third Military Medical University, Chongqing, China
*Corresponding author: e-mail address: yelilinlcmv@tmmu.edu.cn

Contents

Abstract

B-cell follicle represents a functionally dynamic microstructure within second lymphoid tissues, predominantly consisting of B cells, follicular T cells and DCs. Through intimate interactions with cognate B cells, follicular helper T cells (Tfh) initiate and facilitate germinal center (GC) reactions by providing signals required for producing high-affinity antibodies, as well as for the generation of long-lived antibody-secreting plasma cells and memory B cells. Concomitantly, germinal center reaction needs to be fine controlled to avoid autoimmunity or B-cell malignancies. Among immune cells residing in follicles, follicular regulatory T cells (Tfr), converted from naïve Treg cells, are specifically assigned to repress excessive GC responses by suppressing Tfh and GC B cells within GC structure. Hence, through Yin and Yang (positive and negative) regulation of GC reaction, Tfh cells play concert with Tfr cells in maintaining immune homeostasis. Besides CD4$^+$ T cells, a small portion of CXCR5 expressing CD8$^+$ T cells, regarded as follicular cytotoxic T cells (Tfc), could migrate into B cell follicles during chronic viral infection and several types of cancers, and this population exhibit lower level of exhaustion than its CXCR5$^-$ counterparts. Besides, Tfc cells demonstrate a stem-cell like phenotype during chronic infection which could further differentiate into terminally differentiated CXCR5$^-$CD8$^+$ T cells. Collectively, in this review, we will discuss the recent advances in our understanding of the ontology and differentiation of B-cell follicle resident Tfh, Tfr and Tfc cells.

Advances in Immunology, Volume 144
ISSN 0065-2776
https://doi.org/10.1016/bs.ai.2019.08.008

1. Introduction

T cell immune responses, including $CD8^+$ T cell- and $CD4^+$ T cell-mediated immune responses, play critical roles in the adaptive immune system. At the initial phase, the invasive pathogens will be first processed by antigen presenting cells such as dendritic cells (DC), and then antigen peptides will be delivered to T cells in a MHC restricted manner. The binding of peptide-MHC (pMHC) complex to TCR, accompanied by costimulatory molecules and cytokines, provides stimulating signals which are vital for T cell activation. Upon activation, naïve $CD8^+$ T cells mainly differentiate into cytotoxic T lymphocytes (CTL) which mainly aim to eradicate intracellular infected or cancerous cells by directly killing and cytokine production. Upon antigen clearance, the majority of effector $CD8^+$ T cells die by apoptosis and less than 10% of them survive and differentiate into memory $CD8^+$ T cells, which are maintained long-term in the absence of antigens and can exert rapid effector functions in response to previously encountered antigens (Lewis, Williams, & Eisenbarth, 2019). For CD^+4 T cells, they mainly recognize invasive antigens in a MHC II restricted manner. When activated, naïve $CD4^+$ T cells differentiate into various subsets of helper T cells and regulatory T cells, depending on master transcription factors (TFs) and cytokine milieu, which will further orchestrate $CD8^+$ T cell and B cell immune responses (Huang, Hu, Tang, Xu, & Ye, 2019).

The generation of high-affinity antibodies is critical for the development of protective immunity to contain most infectious diseases. And the differentiation of antibody-secreting cells largely depends on optimized germinal center (GC) reactions (Basso & Dalla-Favera, 2015; Mesin, Ersching, & Victora, 2016). T cell has been confirmed to play a pivotal role during this process. During microbial infection, follicular helper T cells (Tfh) facilitate the formation of germinal centers (GCs) by intimate interactions with antigen-specific B cells, which are required for class-switch recombination, somatic hyper-mutation and the selection of B cells that produce high-affinity antibodies, as well as for the generation of long-lived antibody-secreting plasma cells and memory B cells (Qi, 2016; Vinuesa, Linterman, Yu, & MacLennan, 2016). However, although being critical for pathogen eradication, GC reaction needs to be intensively supervised to avoid autoimmune diseases or B-cell malignancies. In the near decades, scientists confirmed that follicular regulatory T (Tfr) cells, a special subset of $CD4^+$ regulatory T (Treg) cells, specializes in repressing excessive GC responses by suppressing Tfh and GC B cells within GC structure, and thus maintaining immune homeostasis (Sage & Sharpe, 2016).

Besides Tfh and Tfr cells, a subset of $CD8^+$ T cells expressing high level of CXCR5, first observed in human tonsils, have the ability to migrate into B-cell follicles (Quigley, Gonzalez, Granath, Andersson, & Sandberg, 2007). It is reported that $CXCR5^+CD8^+$ T cells displayed an activated and antigen-experienced phenotype, but lacked CCR7 expression which is characteristic of central memory cells. Recently, several groups including ours have confirmed that $CXCR5^+CD8^+$ T cells in second lymphoid organs, during chronic viral infection, exhibited a stem-cell like phenotype, which maintains a better proliferation capacity and can further differentiate into more terminally differentiated effector-like $CD8^+$ T cell progenies (He et al., 2016; Im et al., 2016; Leong et al., 2016). Besides, these $CXCR5^+CD8^+$ T cells exhibited lower levels of exhaustion, evidenced by less inhibitory receptors and more potent cytotoxicity than the $CXCR5^-$ subsets (He et al., 2016). More importantly, this subset functions as the major population to respond to PD-1 mediated immune checkpoint blockade in the context of both chronic viral infection and cancer (Im et al., 2016). Here we mainly review the recent advances in our understanding of Tfh, Tfr and $CXCR5^+CD8^+$ T cells.

2. Follicular helper T cell

2.1 The fate commitment of Tfh cells

The lineage commitment of Tfh cells are generally characterized as a multistage and multifactor involved process (Qi, 2016). Mechanistically, upon recognition of pMHC presented by DCs, some activated $CD4^+$ T cells augment Blimp1 (B lymphocyte-induced maturation protein 1) expression and differentiate to non-Tfh cells, including Th1, Th2, Th17, etc. (Xu et al., 2015). Meanwhile, naïve $CD4^+$ T cells adopting Tfh fate upregulate the "master regulator" Bcl6 (B cell lymphoma 6) (Choi, Yang, & Crotty, 2013; Nurieva et al., 2009; Takahashi & Yamanaka, 2006; Yu et al., 2009) within 2 or 3 days (Baumjohann, Okada, & Ansel, 2011; Haynes et al., 2007). Then early Tfh cells move to the T-B border by upregulating CXCR5 (CXC chemokine receptor 5) and down-regulating CCR7 (CC chemokine receptor 7) (Baumjohann et al., 2011; Haynes et al., 2007). Here, they interact with cognate B cells and get sufficient signals that further support them migrating into B-cell follicles and initiating GC reactions (Belanger & Crotty, 2016; Xu et al., 2013). During this process, the expression of Bcl6 is strengthened, propelling the maturation of fully functional Tfh cells (Choi et al., 2013). In acute viral infection, due to the strong type I inflammation, virus-specific $CD4^+$ T cells exhibit a bifurcate differentiation mode, i.e., either differentiating into Th1 cells or Tfh cells. Specifically, those activated CD4$^+$ T cells highly expressing Bcl6 will committee to Tfh fate. Otherwise, if they highly express Blimp1, they will differentiate into Th1 cells. Hence, the balance of Bcl6-Blimp1 axis dictates the dichotomous differentiation of Th1 versus Tfh in acute viral infection (Crotty, 2014; Qi, 2016; Vinuesa et al., 2016). But how Bcl6-Blimp1 axis is regulated for the optimal Tfh differentiation remained unclear. Many factors have been found to be involved in the induction of Bcl6 expression, including BATF, STAT1 (IL-6 signaling), STAT3 (IL-21 signaling) and STAT4 (IL-12 signaling) (Eto et al., 2011; Johnston, Choi, Diamond, Yang, & Crotty, 2012; Oestreich, Mohn, & Weinmann, 2012; Ray et al., 2014, 2015). Moreover, focusing on how the fate commitment of virus-specific Tfh cells is initiated during acute viral infection, Xu et al. (2015) demonstrated that much more TCF1 (T cell factor 1) was expressed in nucleus of early fate-committed Tfh cells, but not Th1 cells at day 2 after acute LCMV (Lymphocytic choriomeningitis virus, Armstrong strain) infection. And the expression of TCF1 positively correlated with Tfh-associated markers, such as CXCR5, Bcl6 and ICOS, but negatively correlated with Th1-related molecules, like Tim-3, CD25 and SLMA on both day 2 and 8 after infection, suggesting that TCF1 expression is maintained in Tfh, but not Th1 cells in response to acute viral infection. Next, using TCF1 conditional knock mice and shRNA-mediated TCF1 knockdown, they proved that TCF1 expression in CD4$^+$ T cells is required for Tfh differentiation, particularly for the early initiation of Tfh fate commitment. By screening *Bcl6* promoter, they found three putative conserved TCF1 binding sites and also three binding sites in 5′-regulatory region in *Prdm1*, which encodes transcription factor Blimp1. CHIP (Chromatin immunoprecipitation) assay further demonstrated that TCF1 can specifically bind to these sites in Tfh cells, but not in Th1 cells. Thus, by acting on Bcl6-Blimp1 axis, TCF1 expression dictated early commitment to the Tfh lineage versus Th1 cells during acute viral infection. These findings are further corroborated by other two studies (Choi et al., 2015; Wu et al., 2015). However, currently, the factors that are responsible for the reinforced TCF1 expression in early-fated Tfh cells remain to be determined.

Epigenetic modifications regulate differentiation fates of a wide variety of cell types (Henning, Roychoudhuri, & Restifo, 2018; Papalexi & Satija, 2017). Using ATAC-Seq (Assay for transposase-accessible chromatin with high throughput sequencing) technology, Chen et al. (2019) found that during acute viral infection, Tfh and Th1 cells exhibit largely distinct chromatin accession states. These unique chromatin states associated with Tfh-specified genes seem to be substantially regulated by H3K27me3 modifications. EZH2 (Enhancer of zeste homolog 2) functions as a methyl-transferase in the complex of PRC2 and specifically catalyze the methylation of K27 site in H3 (Gray, Amezquita, Guan, Kleinstein, & Kaech, 2017). In line with these points, Chen et al. (2019) observed newly differentiated virus-specific Tfh cells exhibited elevated levels of EZH2 expression and H3K27me3 modification relative to naïve T cells and Th1 counterparts in the early days after acute LCMV infection. Inactivation of EZH2 in virus-specific $CD4^+$ T cells led to a pronounced reduction in early Tfh cell commitment. They further identified that EZH2 was essential in remodeling the chromatin accessibility of Tfh lineage-associated genes during viral infection, including *Bcl6* and *Tcf7*, which are critical for the initiation of Tfh-cell differentiation in acute viral infection. Given that EZH2-mideated H3K27me3 is a canonical suppressive epigenetic marker and compresses the chromatin structures of corresponding gene loci (Schuettengruber, Chourrout, Vervoort, Leblanc, & Cavalli, 2007), it is a surprise to observe the open states of Tfh lineage specified genes when EZH2 is deleted in Tfh cells. Meanwhile, Li et al. (2018) found that Ezh2-mideated H3K27me3 repress Cdkn2a expression in Tfh cells, which participate in triggering Tfh cell apoptosis and inhibit Bcl6 function. Despite this, the mechanisms underlying Ezh2-mideated H3K27me3 in the regulation of TCF1 and Bcl6 expression in Tfh fate adoption need further investigations. Collectively, these studies suggest that the epigenetic modification following acute viral infection, specifically EZH2-mideated H3K27me3 deposition is crucial for priming early Tfh cell differentiation.

2.2 The functional maturation of Tfh cells

At the late stage of Tfh development, Tfh cells receive multiple intrinsic and extrinsic signals to guide their further differentiation and functional maturation, including transcription factors and environmental cues such as amino acids, stress, oxygen, etc. (Huang et al., 2019; Saxton & Sabatini, 2017). It is crucial to understand how these signals are integrated to guarantee Tfh maturation. mTORC1 (Mammalian target of rapamycin complex 1) activated by multiple nutrients was reported to inhibit Tfh development (Ray et al., 2015). On the contrary, mTORC2, which mainly responds to growth factor, was highly activated in Tfh cells when compared to Th1 cells. And mTORC2 was confirmed to be essential for Tfh differentiation by regulating mTORC2-AKT-TCF-1 axis and promoting glucose metabolism in Tfh cells through Foxo1 signaling (Yang et al., 2016; Zeng et al., 2016). Particularly, Hao et al. (2018) found that mTORC2 was specifically important for late stage of Tfh differentiation and effector function, but dispensable for early Tfh priming.

2.3 The maintenance of differentiated Tfh cells

Compared to an array of factors identified in the regulation of early Tfh fate commitment, it is much less known regarding the regulators involved in the maintenance of fully differentiated Tfh cells. Tfh differentiation is companied by Th1, Th2 or Th17 differentiation depending on the types of infection. Furthermore, it is interesting to notice that Tfh cells also express environmental specific TFs as their conventional counterparts do (such as T-bet, GATA-3 or ROR-γt in Type I, II or III immune response, respectively) (Jogdand, Mohanty, & Devadas, 2016). Such phenomenon indicates the complexity and environmental adaptability of Tfh cell response. Wang, Wang, et al. (2019) found that Tfh cells specifically in type I condition demonstrated consistent T-bet expression. Although slightly inhibits Tfh early fate commitment, T-bet was essential for optimal proliferation and maintenance of fully differentiated Tfh cells during acute viral infection. Besides, Microarray analysis showed comparable T-bet dependency in the transcriptome of Tfh and Th1 cells, although some important differences exist. Moreover, Fang et al. (2018) demonstrated that the short-term expression of T-bet at the early stage of $CD4^+$ T cells response is critical for IFN-γ production in Th1-like Tfh cell subset. Together, these data suggest the important role of T-bet in the maintenance of Tfh cells in the context of Th1 microenvironment.

3. Follicular regulatory T cells (Tfr)

In contrast to the positive role of Tfh in GC B cell responses, Tfr cells, negatively regulate the magnitude of GC reaction by directly suppressing Tfh and GC B cell responses. Tfr cells are differentiated from nature Treg cells, and mainly reside in germinal centers, which display a hybrid phenotype of Tfh and Treg cells (Sage et al., 2016). Similar to Tfh cells, Tfr cells express high levels of the master regulator Bcl6, PD-1, the costimulatory receptor ICOS and chemokine receptor CXCR5. Resembling Treg cells, Tfr cells express transcription factor Foxp3 and receptors CD25, GITR and CTLA4. The initial generation of Tfr needs TCR stimulation from APCs, including DCs for priming and B cells for optimal differentiation and/or expansion. Additionally, the differentiation of Tfr cells requires costimulatory signals including CD28, ICOS, and is negatively regulated by coinhibitory molecules, such as CTLA4 and PD-1 (Sage & Sharpe, 2016). Meanwhile, similar to Tfh, the strength and duration of TCR signaling also seem to be important for Tfr generation (Chung et al., 2011; Linterman et al., 2011; Wollenberg et al., 2011). The absence of TRAF3 related TCR downstream-ERK signaling in Treg cells leads to significant defects in Tfr development (Chang et al., 2014). These early molecular events coordinately induce the expression of transcription factors required for Tfr differentiation, such as Bcl6 (Chung et al., 2011) and NFAT2 (Vaeth et al., 2014). In addition, Tfr cells need SLAM-associated protein (SAP), which may be required for the interaction with B cells, for its functional maturation and maintenance (Linterman et al., 2011). On the other side, Blimp1 (Linterman et al., 2011), Id2/Id3 (Helix–loop–helix proteins inhibitor of DNA binding 2/3) (Miyazaki et al., 2014), IL2 (Botta et al., 2017) and IL21 (Jandl et al., 2017) negatively regulate Tfr differentiation. Thus, similar to Tfh differentiation program, Tfr differentiation is also a multi-step and multifactorial process orchestrated by various immune signals.

Despite these achievements, how nTreg cells recognize and integrate diverse environmental cues and being converted into Tfr cells remains unclear. We found that upon viral infection or protein immunization, Tfr cells exhibit elevated mTORC1 activity compared with Treg, Tfh and Th1 cells (Xu et al., 2017). Since Tfr cells are located in GC structure, a highly complex and dynamic microenvironment, and mTORC1 is the primary sensor and integrator of the cell's response to nutrient availability. It is reasonable to speculate that Tfr requires more mTORC1 related signaling for their differentiation and function. Consistent with this concept, we further confirmed that mTORC1^{hi} Tregs are more prone to be converted into Tfr cells during early phase, and the transient blocking of mTORC1 signaling by rapamycin inhibited early Tfr conversion from Tregs. Notably, without influencing the proliferation and maintenance of Treg cells, Rapamycin specifically inhibited Treg-to-Tfr conversion. We further demonstrated that, downstream of mTORC1, the STAT3-TCF-1-Bcl6 axis regulates expression of Tfr-associated proteins and the suppressive capacity of these cells in vivo, and overexpressing TCF1 or Bcl6 rescues Tfr differentiation in *Rptor* (the essential subunit of mTORC1) deficient Treg cells. Consistent with the requirement of mTOR signaling in Tfr differentiation,

Essig et al. (2017) found that Roquin, which upregulate Pten and thus inhibit PI3K-mTOR signaling, significantly suppresses the conversion from Treg to Tfr, and Treg cells deficient in Roquin exhibited upregulated mTOR activity as well as enhanced Tfr generation (Fig. 1).

4. Follicular cytotoxic CD8$^+$ T cells (Tfc)

Once activated, naïve CD8$^+$ T cells mainly differentiate into cytotoxic T lymphocytes (CTL), aiming to eradicate intracellular infected or cancerous cells. Upon antigen clearance during acute viral infection, the pool of effector CD8$^+$ T cells contracts and only a small portion of them survive and differentiate into memory CD8$^+$ T cells, which are maintained long-term in the absence of antigens and can exert rapid effector functions in response to previously encountered antigens (Kaech & Cui, 2012; Samji & Khanna, 2017). Currently, the pool of CD8$^+$ T cell subsets has been proved to be phenotypically and functionally heterogeneous. Several groups demonstrated the existence of a subset of CD8$^+$ T cells expressing high level of CXCR5 which could migrate into B cell follicles in response to the gradients of CXCL13 (Yu & Ye, 2018). This special population was first recorded in human tonsils more than 10 years ago (Quigley et al., 2007), and then another study described that CXCR5$^+$CD8$^+$ T cells may be involved in regulating autoimmunity in mice (Kim, Verbinnen, Tang, Lu, & Cantor, 2010).

Within the past 2 years or so, accumulating evidence during chronic viral infections (CL-13, HIV, SIV), in which the long-term persistence of antigen exposure drives virus-specific CD8$^+$ T cell exhaustion, identified CXCR5$^+$CD8$^+$ T cells as a unique subset of CD8$^+$ T cells with specialized functions and a distinct pattern of differentiation, which were termed as follicular cytotoxic T (Tfc) cells (He et al., 2016; Im et al., 2016; Leong et al., 2016; Mylvaganam et al., 2017; Snell et al., 2018; Xiao, Chen, He, & Ye, 2018). By using chronic LCMV infection (CL-13 strain), He et al. (2016) found that about 30% of virus-specific CD8$^+$ T cells in lymphoid tissues highly expressed CXCR5 and this population remained stable during the whole process of CL-13 infection while undetectable in acute LCMV infection models. And this population was also observed in HIV chronically infected patients. They confirmed that the virus-specific CXCR5$^+$CD8$^+$ subset is less exhausted and possesses higher antiviral potential in vivo than the CXCR5$^-$ subsets. When compared to their CXCR5$^-$countparts, virus-specific CXCR5$^+$CD8$^+$ T cells expressed lower levels of inhibitory

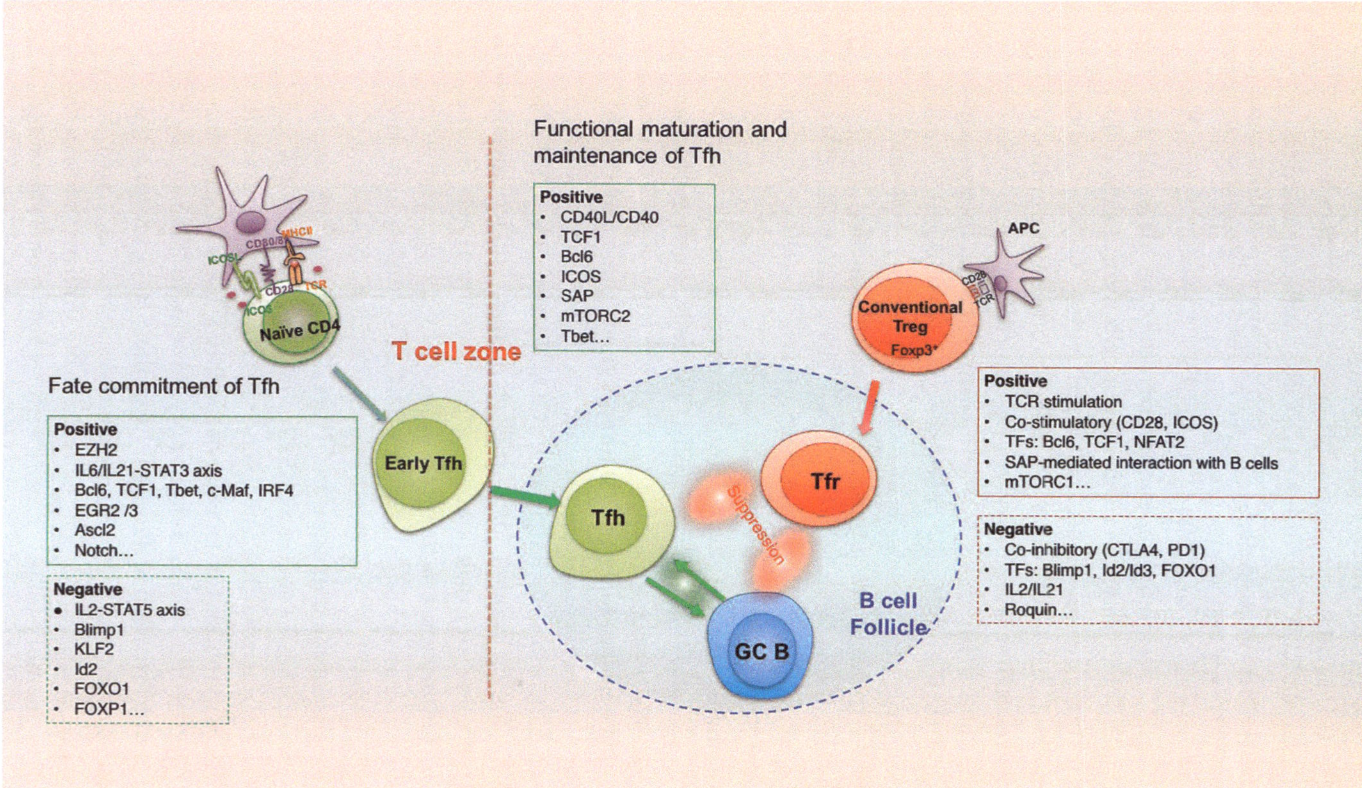

Fig. 1 The Yin and Yang regulation of germinal center B cells. The lineage commitment, functional maturation and maintenance of Tfh cells are generally characterized as a multistage and multifactor involved process. Naïve $CD4^+$ T cells adopting Tfh fate upregulate the "master regulator" Bcl6. Then early Tfh cells move to the T-B border by upregulating CXCR5 and down-regulating CCR7. Here, they interact with cognate B cells and get sufficient signals that further support them migrating into B-cell follicles and initiating GC reactions. In contrast, Tfr cells, negatively regulate the magnitude of GC reaction by directly suppressing Tfh and GC B cell responses. Tfr cells are differentiated from nature Treg cells, and mainly reside in germinal centers, which display a hybrid phenotype of Tfh and Treg cells. Similar to Tfh, the differentiation of Tfr cells is also a multi-step and multifactorial process orchestrated by various immune signals. Together, Tfh play concerts with Tfr cells in maintaining optimized GC reactions.

receptors, including PD-1(Programmed cell death 1), Tim-3 (Programmed cell death 1) and LAG3 (Lymphocyte activation gene 3), and higher levels of the stimulatory molecule KLRG1. And the $CXCR5^+$ subset seemed to be more polyfunctional than the $CXCR5^-$ counterparts upon re-stimulation with higher levels of IFN-γ and TNFα production. Moreover, by transferring sorted $CD44^{hi}CXCR5^+$ and $CD44^{hi}CXCR5^-$ $CD8^+$ T cells into CL-13 infected *Cd8*$^{-/-}$ recipients, they found that the viral loads in lungs and spleens of recipients receiving $CXCR5^+$ donor cells were almost 1000-fold lower than in tissues of recipients transferred with $CXCR5^-$ donor cells. Moreover, PD-$1^+CXCR5^+CD8^+$ T cells have been confirmed to be responsible for the proliferative burst after PD-1 blockade in both chronic viral infection and cancer (Im et al., 2016). In consistent with these observations, He et al. (2016) found that the cotransfer of $CD44^{hi}CXCR5^+$ cells, but not $CD44^{hi}CXCR5^-$ $CD8^+$ T cells into CL-13 infected recipients can synergize with PD-1 treatment to diminish viral load in animals.

Transcriptional profiling revealed (He et al., 2016; Im et al., 2016) that the PD-1^+ $CXCR5^+$ and PD-1^+ $CXCR5^-$ $CD8^+$ T cells in chronically infected mice had distinct gene signatures. PD-1^+ $CXCR5^+$ $CD8^+$ T cells expressed higher levels of several costimulatory molecules, such as *Cd28*, *Icos*, *Tnfsf14*, *Tnfrsf4*. Transcriptionally, Tfc cells expressed higher levels of *Bcl6*, *Tcf7* and *Plagl1* that are typically associated with Tfh cells while $CXCR5^-$ cells expressed *Prdm1* (Blimp-1) that is linked with Th1 cells. What's more, Tfc cells expressed higher levels of genes associated with memory cell formation, including *Sell* (CD62L) and *Il7r* (CD127). Collectively, the aforementioned data indicated that antigen-specific $CXCR5^+CD8^+$ T cells (Tfc) may function as memory stem cells during chronic infection. This notion was further confirmed by the fact that when transferred to infection-matched mice, the $CXCR5^+$ subsets not only undergo self-proliferation, but also give birth to $CXCR5^-CD8^+$ T cells. It has been confirmed that the transcription factors Blimp1 and E2A directly regulated *Cxcr5* expression (Leong et al., 2016). Our recent study (Wang, Hu, et al., 2019) demonstrated that the absence of *Tcf7* in antigen specific $CD8^+$T cells resulted in significant decrease of $CXCR5^+CD8^+$T cells during CL-13 infection. Besides, the E2A-inhibitory proteins Id2/Id3 and Bcl6 also participated in the formation of Tfc cells. All of these factors form a transcriptional circuit that governs Tfc cell development (He et al., 2016; Im et al., 2016; Leong et al., 2016). Given the remarkable similarities between Tfc cells and Tfh or memory $CD8^+$ T cells with regard to phenotype and differentiation, our knowledge of these lineages may strengthen our understanding of Tfc cells. However, the mechanism by which these different TFs are integrated to dictate the ontology and differentiation of Tfc cells remains largely unknown, especially in scenarios of chronic infection and tumorigenesis (Fig. 2).

5. Conclusion and perspectives

The "black box" of germinal center is complex and significantly involved in clinic application, such as autoimmune disease, vaccine design, chronic viral infection and tumor immune therapy. The overwhelmed Tfr responses often lead to immune tolerance, while uncontrolled Tfh and GC B cell responses are usually linked to autoimmune diseases or B-cell malignancy (Basso & Dalla-Favera, 2015; Tsou, Katayama, Ostrin, & Hanash, 2016). The balanced Tfh-Tfr ratio is essential for the optimal humoral immunity triggered by vaccine. Meanwhile, during chronic infection, the differentiation of effector $CD4^+$ T cells and Treg cells were skewed to Tfh-like (Fahey et al., 2011; Snell & Brooks, 2015) or Tfr phenotype (data not shown) respectively, together with upregulated CXCR5 expression in $CD8^+$ T cells, indicating a more dynamic activity within B-cell follicles which can be exploited as a potential therapeutic target. Notably, during HIV infection, Tfh cells are regarded as the major virus reservoir, and the anatomical isolation of latently infected Tfh cells might lay a major obstacle for exhausted HIV-specific $CD8^+$ T cells, which are normally excluded from B-cell follicles, to effectively eradicate HIV infection (Perreau et al., 2013; Sengupta & Siliciano, 2018; Xiao et al., 2018). The discovery of Tfc, which can migrate to B-cell follicles and exhibit better effector function, shed new lights on the efficient eradication of HIV infected Tfh cells. However, Tfc only occupies a very small proportion of $CD8^+$ T cells, and they will gradually lose the expression of CXCR5 during infection (He et al., 2016). Future attempts to expand this population and strengthen their follicular retention are of great significance. Additionally, a recent study found (using mouse model of spontaneous lymph node metastasis of breast cancer) that primary tumor induced B cells accumulate in draining LNs and promote the generation of pathogenic IgG that targeting glycosylated membrane protein HSPA4, resulting in enhanced lymph node metastasis (Gu et al., 2019). Given the important function of Tfh in supporting antibody production, it is urgent to evaluate the role of Tfh cells in this scenario.

Besides chronic viral infection, scientists confirmed the existence of $CXCR5^+CD8^+$ Tfc cells in blood, draining LNs and tumor tissues in

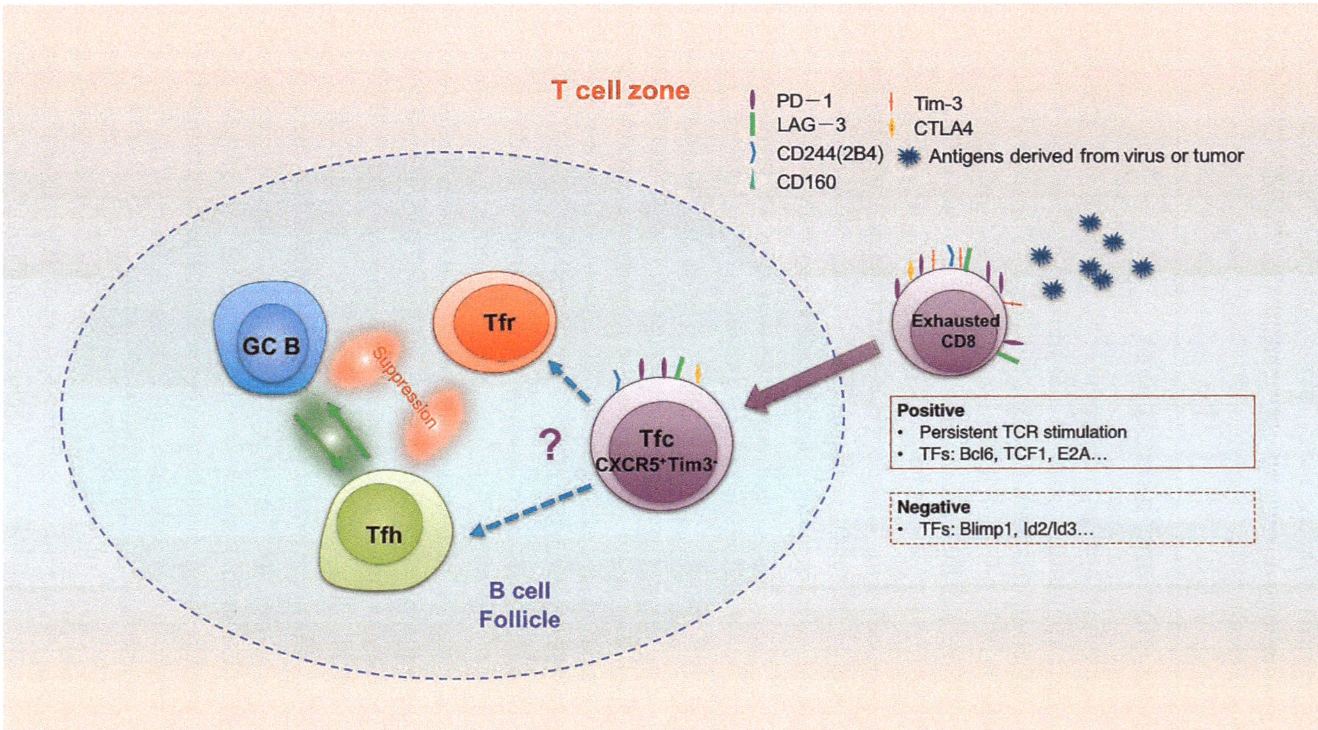

Fig. 2 Tfc: a unique subset of $CD8^+$ T cells. A subset of $CD8^+$ T cells have been observed to express high level of CXCR5 during chronic viral infections and tumorigenesis, which could migrate into B-cell follicles in response to the gradients of CXCL13. $CXCR5^+CD8^+$ T cells represent a unique subset of $CD8^+$ T cells with specialized functions and a distinct pattern of differentiation, which were termed as follicular cytotoxic T (Tfc) cell. Compared to their $CXCR5^-$ countparts, Tfc cells expressed lower levels of inhibitory receptors, including PD-1, Tim-3 and LAG3, and higher levels of the stimulatory molecule KLRG1. Tfc may function as memory stem cells during these cases and has been confirmed to be responsible for the proliferative burst after PD-1 blockade in both chronic viral infection and cancer.

patients with liver, lung, colorectal, pancreatic malignancies (Yu & Ye, 2018). And Tfc cells were also detected in mouse models with B-cell lymphoma (Leong et al., 2016). Moreover, these studies demonstrated that tumor-infiltrating Tfc-like cells positively correlated with the prognoses of several kinds of cancers (Bai et al., 2017; Brummelman et al., 2018; Jifu et al., 2018). Together these researches demonstrated that Tfc cells might play a critical role in the immuno-surveillance of tumorigenesis. Collectively, the underlying mechanisms as well as the regulatory circuits of ontology and differentiation of Tfh, Tfr and Tfc cells remain largely unsolved, especially in chronic infection and tumorigenesis. And whether Tfc cells interact with other two populations within B-cell follicles awaits further investigation. However, we are optimistic that unveiling the mysteries of T cell immune responses in B-cell follicles may lay a solid foundation for designing immunotherapies to treat certain infections and cancer.

Acknowledgments

This work is supported by funds from the National Natural Science Fund for Distinguished Young Scholars (No. 31825011 to L.Y.) and the National Natural Science Foundation of China (No. 31700774 to L.X.).

Conflict of interest disclosure

The authors declare no financial or commercial conflict of interest.

References

Bai, M., Zheng, Y., Liu, H., Su, B., Zhan, Y., & He, H. (2017). CXCR5(+) CD8(+) T cells potently infiltrate pancreatic tumors and present high functionality. *Experimental Cell Research*, *361*(1), 39–45. https://doi.org/10.1016/j.yexcr.2017.1009.1039. Epub 2017 Sep 1028.

Basso, K., & Dalla-Favera, R. (2015). Germinal centres and B cell lymphomagenesis. *Nature Reviews. Immunology*, *15*(3), 172–184. https://doi.org/10.1038/nri3814.

Baumjohann, D., Okada, T., & Ansel, K. M. (2011). Cutting edge: Distinct waves of BCL6 expression during T follicular helper cell development. *Journal of Immunology*, *187*(5), 2089–2092. https://doi.org/10.4049/jimmunol.1101393. Epub 1102011 Jul 1101329.

Belanger, S., & Crotty, S. (2016). Dances with cytokines, featuring TFH cells, IL-21, IL-4 and B cells. *Nature Immunology*, *17*(10), 1135–1136. https://doi.org/10.1038/ni.3561.

Botta, D., Fuller, M. J., Marquez-Lago, T. T., Bachus, H., Bradley, J. E., Weinmann, A. S., et al. (2017). Dynamic regulation of T follicular regulatory cell responses by interleukin 2 during influenza infection. *Nature Immunology*, *18*(11), 1249–1260. https://doi.org/10.1038/ni.3837.

Brummelman, J., Mazza, E. M. C., Alvisi, G., Colombo, F. S., Grilli, A., Mikulak, J., et al. (2018). High-dimensional single cell analysis identifies stem-like cytotoxic CD8+T cells infiltrating human tumors. *The Journal of Experimental Medicine*, *215*(10), 2520–2535. https://doi.org/10.1084/jem.20180684.

Chang, J. H., Hu, H., Jin, J., Puebla-Osorio, N., Xiao, Y., Gilbert, B. E., et al. (2014). TRAF3 regulates the effector function of regulatory T cells and humoral immune responses. *The Journal of Experimental Medicine*, *211*(1), 137–151. https://doi.org/10.1084/jem.20131019.

Chen, X., Cao, G., Wu, J., Wang, X., Pan, Z., Gao, J., et al. (2019). The histone methyltransferase EZH2 primes the early differentiation of follicular helper T cells during acute viral infection. *Cellular & Molecular Immunology*, *6*(10), 019–0219.

Choi, Y. S., Gullicksrud, J. A., Xing, S., Zeng, Z., Shan, Q., Li, F., et al. (2015). LEF-1 and TCF-1 orchestrate T(FH) differentiation by regulating differentiation circuits upstream of the transcriptional repressor Bcl6. *Nature Immunology*, *16*(9), 980–990. https://doi.org/10.1038/ni.3226.

Choi, Y. S., Yang, J. A., & Crotty, S. (2013). Dynamic regulation of Bcl6 in follicular helper CD4 T (Tfh) cells. *Current Opinion in Immunology*, *25*(3), 366–372. https://doi.org/10.1016/j.coi.2013.04.003.

Chung, Y., Tanaka, S., Chu, F., Nurieva, R. I., Martinez, G. J., Rawal, S., et al. (2011). Follicular regulatory T cells expressing Foxp3 and Bcl-6 suppress germinal center reactions. *Nature Medicine*, *17*(8), 983–988. https://doi.org/10.1038/nm.2426.

Crotty, S. (2014). T follicular helper cell differentiation, function, and roles in disease. *Immunity*, *41*(4), 529–542. https://doi.org/10.1016/j.immuni.2014.1010.1004.

Essig, K., Hu, D., Guimaraes, J. C., Alterauge, D., Edelmann, S., Raj, T., et al. (2017). Roquin suppresses the PI3K-mTOR signaling pathway to inhibit T helper cell differentiation and conversion of Treg to Tfr cells. *Immunity*, *47*(6), 1067–1082. https://doi.org/10.1016/j.immuni.2017.11.008.

Eto, D., Lao, C., DiToro, D., Barnett, B., Escobar, T. C., Kageyama, R., et al. (2011). IL-21 and IL-6 are critical for different aspects of B cell immunity and redundantly induce optimal follicular helper CD4 T cell (Tfh) differentiation. *PLoS One*, *6*(3), e17739. https://doi.org/10.11371/journal.pone.0017739.

Fahey, L. M., Wilson, E. B., Elsaesser, H., Fistonich, C. D., McGavern, D. B., & Brooks, D. G. (2011). Viral persistence redirects CD4 T cell differentiation toward T follicular helper cells. *The Journal of Experimental Medicine*, *208*(5), 987–999. https://doi.org/10.1084/jem.20101773. Epub 20102011 May 20101772.

Fang, D., Cui, K., Mao, K., Hu, G., Li, R., Zheng, M., et al. (2018). Transient T-bet expression functionally specifies a distinct T follicular helper subset. *The Journal of Experimental Medicine*, *215*(11), 2705–2714. https://doi.org/10.1084/jem.20180927.

Gray, S. M., Amezquita, R. A., Guan, T., Kleinstein, S. H., & Kaech, S. M. (2017). Polycomb repressive complex 2-mediated chromatin repression guides effector CD8 (+) T cell terminal differentiation and loss of multipotency. *Immunity*, *46*(4), 596–608. https://doi.org/10.1016/j.immuni.2017.1003.1012. Epub 2017 Apr 1011.

Gu, Y., Liu, Y., Fu, L., Zhai, L., Zhu, J., Han, Y., et al. (2019). Tumor-educated B cells selectively promote breast cancer lymph node metastasis by HSPA4-targeting IgG. *Nature Medicine*, *25*(2), 312–322. https://doi.org/10.1038/s41591-41018-40309-y. Epub 42019 Jan 41514.

Hao, Y., Wang, Y., Liu, X., Yang, X., Wang, P., Tian, Q., et al. (2018). The kinase complex mTOR complex 2 promotes the follicular migration and functional maturation of differentiated follicular helper CD4(+) T cells during viral infection. *Frontiers in Immunology*, *9*, 1127. https://doi.org/10.3389/fimmu.2018.01127. (eCollection 02018).

Haynes, N. M., Allen, C. D., Lesley, R., Ansel, K. M., Killeen, N., & Cyster, J. G. (2007). Role of CXCR5 and CCR7 in follicular Th cell positioning and appearance of a programmed cell death gene-1high germinal center-associated subpopulation. *Journal of Immunology*, *179*(8), 5099–5108. https://doi.org/10.4049/jimmunol.5179.5098.5099.

He, R., Hou, S., Liu, C., Zhang, A., Bai, Q., Han, M., et al. (2016). Follicular CXCR5-expressing CD8+ T cells curtail chronic viral infection. *Nature*, *537*(7620), 412–428. https://doi.org/10.1038/nature19317.

Henning, A. N., Roychoudhuri, R., & Restifo, N. P. (2018). Epigenetic control of CD8(+) T cell differentiation. *Nature Reviews. Immunology*, *18*, 340–356. https://doi.org/10.1038/nri.2017.146.

Huang, Q., Hu, J., Tang, J., Xu, L., & Ye, L. (2019). Molecular basis of the differentiation and function of virus specific follicular helper CD4(+) T cells. *Frontiers in Immunology*, *10*, 249. https://doi.org/10.3389/fimmu.2019.00249.

Im, S. J., Hashimoto, M., Gerner, M. Y., Lee, J., Kissick, H. T., Burger, M. C., et al. (2016). Defining CD8+ T cells that provide the proliferative burst after PD-1 therapy. *Nature*, *537*, 417–421. https://doi.org/10.1038/nature19330.

Jandl, C., Liu, S. M., Cañete, P. F., Warren, J., Hughes, W. E., Vogelzang, A., et al. (2017). IL-21 restricts T follicular regulatory T cell proliferation through Bcl-6 mediated inhibition of responsiveness to IL-2. *Nature Communications*, *8*(1), 14647. https://doi.org/10.1038/ncomms14647.

Jifu, E., Yan, F., Kang, Z., Zhu, L., Xing, J., & Yu, E. (2018). CD8(+)CXCR5(+) T cells in tumor-draining lymph nodes are highly activated and predict better prognosis in colorectal cancer. *Human Immunology*, *79*(6), 446–452. https://doi.org/10.1016/j.humimm.2018.1003.1003. Epub 2018 Mar 1012.

Jogdand, G. M., Mohanty, S., & Devadas, S. (2016). Regulators of Tfh cell differentiation. *Frontiers in Immunology*, *7*, 520. https://doi.org/10.3389/fimmu.2016.00520. (eCollection 02016).

Johnston, R. J., Choi, Y. S., Diamond, J. A., Yang, J. A., & Crotty, S. (2012). STAT5 is a potent negative regulator of TFH cell differentiation. *The Journal of Experimental Medicine*, *209*(2), 243–250. https://doi.org/10.1084/jem.20111174. Epub 20112012 Jan 20111123.

Kaech, S. M., & Cui, W. (2012). Transcriptional control of effector and memory CD8+ T cell differentiation. *Nature Reviews. Immunology*, *12*(11), 749–761. https://doi.org/10.1038/nri3307.

Kim, H. J., Verbinnen, B., Tang, X., Lu, L., & Cantor, H. (2010). Inhibition of follicular T-helper cells by CD8(+) regulatory T cells is essential for self tolerance. *Nature*, *467*(7313), 328–332. https://doi.org/10.1038/nature09370.

Leong, Y. A., Chen, Y., Ong, H. S., Wu, D., Man, K., Deleage, C., et al. (2016). CXCR5+ follicular cytotoxic T cells control viral infection in B cell follicles. *Nature Immunology*. https://doi.org/10.1038/ni.3543.

Lewis, S. M., Williams, A., & Eisenbarth, S. C. (2019). Structure and function of the immune system in the spleen. *Science Immunology*, *4*(33), eaau6085. https://doi.org/10.1126/sciimmunol.aau6085.

Li, F., Zeng, Z., Xing, S., Gullicksrud, J. A., Shan, Q., Choi, J., et al. (2018). Ezh2 programs TFH differentiation by integrating phosphorylation-dependent activation of Bcl6 and polycomb-dependent repression of p19Arf. *Nature Communications*, *9*(1), 5452. https://doi.org/10.1038/s41467-41018-07853-z.

Linterman, M. A., Pierson, W., Lee, S. K., Kallies, A., Kawamoto, S., Rayner, T. F., et al. (2011). Foxp3+ follicular regulatory T cells control the germinal center response. *Nature Medicine*, *17*(8), 975–982. https://doi.org/10.1038/nm.2425.

Mesin, L., Ersching, J., & Victora, G. D. (2016). Germinal center B cell dynamics. *Immunity*, *45*(3), 471–482. https://doi.org/10.1016/j.immuni.2016.09.001.

Miyazaki, M., Miyazaki, K., Chen, S., Itoi, M., Miller, M., Lu, L. F., et al. (2014). Id2 and Id3 maintain the regulatory T cell pool to suppress inflammatory disease. *Nature Immunology*, *15*(8), 767–776. https://doi.org/10.1038/ni.2928.

Mylvaganam, G. H., Rios, D., Abdelaal, H. M., Iyer, S., Tharp, G., Mavinger, M., et al. (2017). Dynamics of SIV-specific CXCR5 + CD8 T cells during chronic SIV infection. *Proceedings of the National Academy of Sciences of the United States of America*, *114*, 1976–1981. https://doi.org/10.1073/pnas.1621418114.

Nurieva, R. I., Chung, Y., Martinez, G. J., Yang, X. O., Tanaka, S., Matskevitch, T. D., et al. (2009). Bcl6 mediates the development of T follicular helper cells. *Science*, *325*(5943), 1001–1005. https://doi.org/10.1126/science.1176676. Epub 1172009 Jul 1176623.

Oestreich, K. J., Mohn, S. E., & Weinmann, A. S. (2012). Molecular mechanisms that control the expression and activity of Bcl-6 in TH1 cells to regulate flexibility with a TFH-like gene profile. *Nature Immunology*, *13*(4), 405–411. https://doi.org/10.1038/ni.2242.

Papalexi, E., & Satija, R. (2017). Single-cell RNA sequencing to explore immune cell heterogeneity. *Nature Reviews. Immunology*, *18*, 35–45. https://doi.org/10.1038/nri.2017.76.

Perreau, M., Savoye, A. L., De Crignis, E., Corpataux, J. M., Cubas, R., Haddad, E. K., et al. (2013). Follicular helper T cells serve as the major CD4 T cell compartment for HIV-1 infection, replication, and production. *The Journal of Experimental Medicine*, *210*(1), 143–156. https://doi.org/10.1084/jem.20121932.

Qi, H. (2016). T follicular helper cells in space-time. *Nature Reviews. Immunology*, *16*(10), 612–625. https://doi.org/10.1038/nri.2016.94.

Quigley, M. F., Gonzalez, V. D., Granath, A., Andersson, J., & Sandberg, J. K. (2007). CXCR5 + CCR7- CD8 T cells are early effector memory cells that infiltrate tonsil B cell follicles. *European Journal of Immunology*, *37*(12), 3352–3362. https://doi.org/10.1002/eji.200636746.

Ray, J. P., Marshall, H. D., Laidlaw, B. J., Staron, M. M., Kaech, S. M., & Craft, J. (2014). Transcription factor STAT3 and type I interferons are corepressive insulators for differentiation of follicular helper and T helper 1 cells. *Immunity*, *40*(3), 367–377. https://doi.org/10.1016/j.immuni.2014.1002.1005. Epub 2014 Mar 1013.

Ray, J. P., Staron, M. M., Shyer, J. A., Ho, P. C., Marshall, H. D., Gray, S. M., et al. (2015). The Interleukin-2-mTORc1 kinase Axis defines the signaling, differentiation, and metabolism of T Helper 1 and follicular B Helper T Cells. *Immunity*, *43*(4), 690–702. https://doi.org/10.1016/j.immuni.2015.1008.1017. Epub 2015 Sep 1022.

Sage, P. T., Ron-Harel, N., Juneja, V. R., Sen, D. R., Maleri, S., Sungnak, W., et al. (2016). Suppression by TFR cells leads to durable and selective inhibition of B cell effector function. *Nature Immunology*, *17*, 1436–1446. https://doi.org/10.1038/ni.3578.

Sage, P. T., & Sharpe, A. H. (2016). T follicular regulatory cells. *Immunological Reviews*, *271*(1), 246–259. https://doi.org/10.1111/imr.12411.

Samji, T., & Khanna, K. M. (2017). Understanding memory CD8(+) T cells. *Immunology Letters*, *185*, 32–39. https://doi.org/10.1016/j.imlet.2017.02.012.

Saxton, R. A., & Sabatini, D. M. (2017). mTOR signaling in growth, metabolism, and disease. *Cell*, *168*(6), 960–976. https://doi.org/10.1016/j.cell.2017.1002.1004.

Schuettengruber, B., Chourrout, D., Vervoort, M., Leblanc, B., & Cavalli, G. (2007). Genome regulation by polycomb and trithorax proteins. *Cell*, *128*(4), 735–745. https://doi.org/10.1016/j.cell.2007.1002.1009.

Sengupta, S., & Siliciano, R. F. (2018). Targeting the latent reservoir for HIV-1. *Immunity*, *48*(5), 872–895. https://doi.org/10.1016/j.immuni.2018.04.030.

Snell, L. M., & Brooks, D. G. (2015). New insights into type I interferon and the immunopathogenesis of persistent viral infections. *Current Opinion in Immunology*, *34*, 91–98. https://doi.org/10.1016/j.coi.2015.03.002.

Snell, L. M., MacLeod, B. L., Law, J. C., Osokine, I., Elsaesser, H. J., Hezaveh, K., et al. (2018). CD8(+) T cell priming in established chronic viral infection preferentially directs differentiation of memory-like cells for sustained immunity. *Immunity*, *49*(4), 678–694. https://doi.org/10.1016/j.immuni.2018.1008.1002. Epub 2018 Oct 1019.

Takahashi, K., & Yamanaka, S. (2006). Induction of pluripotent stem cells from mouse embryonic and adult fibroblast cultures by defined factors. *Cell, 126*(4), 663–676. https://doi.org/10.1016/j.cell.2006.07.024.

Tsou, P., Katayama, H., Ostrin, E. J., & Hanash, S. M. (2016). The emerging role of B cells in tumor immunity. *Cancer Research, 76*(19), 5597–5601. https://doi.org/10.1158/0008-5472.CAN-16-0431.

Vaeth, M., Muller, G., Stauss, D., Dietz, L., Klein-Hessling, S., Serfling, E., et al. (2014). Follicular regulatory T cells control humoral autoimmunity via NFAT2-regulated CXCR5 expression. *The Journal of Experimental Medicine, 211*(3), 545–561. https://doi.org/10.1084/jem.20130604.

Vinuesa, C. G., Linterman, M. A., Yu, D., & MacLennan, I. C. (2016). Follicular helper T cells. *Annual Review of Immunology, 34*, 335–368. https://doi.org/10.1146/annurev-immunol-041015-055605.

Wang, Y., Hu, J., Li, Y., Xiao, M., Wang, H., Tian, Q., et al. (2019). The transcription factor TCF1 preserves the effector function of exhausted CD8 T cells during chronic viral infection. *Frontiers in Immunology, 10*, 169. https://doi.org/10.3389/fimmu.2019.00169.

Wang, P., Wang, Y., Xie, L., Xiao, M., Wu, J., Xu, L., et al. (2019). The transcription factor T-bet is required for optimal type I follicular helper T cell maintenance during acute viral infection. *Frontiers in Immunology, 10*, 606. https://doi.org/10.3389/fimmu.2019.00606. (eCollection 02019).

Wollenberg, I., Agua-Doce, A., Hernandez, A., Almeida, C., Oliveira, V. G., Faro, J., et al. (2011). Regulation of the germinal center reaction by Foxp3+ follicular regulatory T cells. *Journal of Immunology, 187*(9), 4553–4560. https://doi.org/10.4049/jimmunol.1101328. Epub 1102011 Oct 1101327.

Wu, T., Shin, H. M., Moseman, E. A., Ji, Y., Huang, B., Harly, C., et al. (2015). TCF1 is required for the T follicular helper cell response to viral infection. *Cell Reports, 12*(12), 2099–2110. https://doi.org/10.1016/j.celrep.2015.08.049.

Xiao, M., Chen, X., He, R., & Ye, L. (2018). Differentiation and function of follicular CD8 T cells during human immunodeficiency virus infection. *Frontiers in Immunology, 9*, 1095. https://doi.org/10.3389/fimmu.2018.01095.

Xu, L., Cao, Y., Xie, Z., Huang, Q., Bai, Q., Yang, X., et al. (2015). The transcription factor TCF-1 initiates the differentiation of T(FH) cells during acute viral infection. *Nature Immunology, 16*(9), 991–999. https://doi.org/10.1038/ni.3229.

Xu, L., Huang, Q., Wang, H., Hao, Y., Bai, Q., Hu, J., et al. (2017). The kinase mTORC1 promotes the generation and suppressive function of follicular regulatory T cells. *Immunity, 47*(3), 538–551. https://doi.org/10.1016/j.immuni.2017.08.011.

Xu, H., Li, X., Liu, D., Li, J., Zhang, X., Chen, X., et al. (2013). Follicular T-helper cell recruitment governed by bystander B cells and ICOS-driven motility. *Nature, 496*(7446), 523–527. https://doi.org/10.1038/nature12058.

Yang, J., Lin, X., Pan, Y., Wang, J., Chen, P., Huang, H., et al. (2016). Critical roles of mTOR complex 1 and 2 for T follicular helper cell differentiation and germinal center responses. *Elife, 5*, e17936. https://doi.org/10.17554/eLife.17936.

Yu, D., Rao, S., Tsai, L. M., Lee, S. K., He, Y., Sutcliffe, E. L., et al. (2009). The transcriptional repressor Bcl-6 directs T follicular helper cell lineage commitment. *Immunity, 31*(3), 457–468. https://doi.org/10.1016/j.immuni.2009.1007.1002. Epub 2009 Jul 1023.

Yu, D., & Ye, L. (2018). A portrait of CXCR5(+) follicular cytotoxic CD8(+) T cells. *Trends in Immunology, 39*, 965–979. https://doi.org/10.1016/j.it.2018.10.002.

Zeng, H., Cohen, S., Guy, C., Shrestha, S., Neale, G., Brown, S. A., et al. (2016). mTORC1 and mTORC2 kinase signaling and glucose metabolism drive follicular helper T cell differentiation. *Immunity, 45*(3), 540–554. https://doi.org/10.1016/j.immuni.2016.08.017.

CHAPTER SEVEN

Autoimmune diseases in China

Ru Li[a,b,*], Xing Sun[a,b], Xu Liu[a,b], Yue Yang[a,b], Zhanguo Li[a,b,*]
[a]Department of Rheumatology & Immunology, Peking University People's Hospital, Beijing, China
[b]Beijing Key Laboratory for Rheumatism Mechanism and Immune Diagnosis (BZ0135), Beijing, China
*Corresponding author: e-mail address: doctorliru123@163.com

Contents

Abstract

Autoimmune diseases, such as rheumatoid arthritis, systematic lupus erythematosus and Sjögren's syndrome, are a group of diseases characterized by the activation of immune cells and excessive production of autoantibodies. Although the pathogenesis of these diseases is still not completely understood, studies have shown that multiple factors including genetics, environment and immune responses play important roles in the development and progression of the diseases. In China, there are great achievements in the mechanisms of autoimmune diseases during the last decades. These studies provide new insight to understand the diseases and also shed light on the development of novel therapy.

Advances in Immunology, Volume 144
ISSN 0065-2776
https://doi.org/10.1016/bs.ai.2019.09.002

The pathogenesis of autoimmune diseases is complex and largely remains unknown. Abnormal responses of immune system against self-antigens account for the main mechanisms of these diseases. Both environment and genetic background contribute to the development of autoimmunity. In the past decades, research in autoimmune diseases has developed rapidly in China. Numerous studies have been published in recent years, mainly focused on epidemiology, mechanisms, early diagnosis and interventions. Here we presented the discoveries in the pathogenesis and novel therapy of autoimmune diseases, including rheumatoid arthritis (RA), systematic lupus erythematosus (SLE), Sjögren's syndrome (SS) and several other disorders.

1. Rheumatoid arthritis

Rheumatoid Arthritis (RA) is the most common chronic multisystem disease of unknown etiology. There are a variety of systemic manifestations of RA, and the characteristic feature is persistent inflammatory synovitis involving peripheral joints in a symmetric distribution.

In the past 20 years, rheumatologists and immunologists in China have made great progress in the epidemiology, early diagnosis, treatment, and basic research including genetics, mechanisms and novel therapeutic targets of RA. In this part, we focus on the major advances in the epidemiology, etiology, pathogenesis and treatment of RA.

1.1 Epidemiology

The prevalence of RA is about 0.5–1% around the world regardless of geography and ethnics. Although higher in some groups of North America (~5%), prevalence of RA in China is about 0.28% with the peak of onset in median or older age, and comorbids with other autoimmune diseases such as systemic lupus erythematosus (SLE) and Sjögren's syndrome (SS) (Li et al., 2012; Zeng et al., 2008, 2015). Women are affected approximately three times more often than men.

The work functioning impairment rate of Chinese RA patients are 48% (Zhang, Mu, et al., 2015). Another study shows that the remission rate of RA patients in China is about 10.9% according to the 28-joint Disease Activity Score (DAS-28) (Zhu et al., 2018). Recently, Clinical deep remission (CliDR) has been proposed to evaluate RA remission efficiently and simply, which has been proved achievable in a large cohort of Chinese RA patients (Liu et al., 2019). The early RA (ERA) criteria, with

72.3–78.4% sensitivity and 86.3–87.8% specificity, has been confirmed better for the early RA classification nationwide (Ye et al., 2016; Zhao, Su, et al., 2014). Moreover, quantities of efforts including the etiology, diagnosis and therapy, have been made in the past decades.

1.2 Etiology and pathogenesis

The precise cause of RA remains uncertain. It has been suggested that RA might be a manifestation of the response to an infectious agent in a genetically susceptible host. In the past 20 years, Chinese rheumatologists and immunologists have made great progress and provided more clues in understanding of the etiology and pathogenesis of RA.

1.2.1 Genetics and environmental risks

Enormous basic researches have been carried out in China to elucidate the pathogenesis of RA and have identified several genetic risk loci and different epigenetics (Du et al., 2014; Guo et al., 2019; He et al., 2019; Jiang et al., 2014; Li, Mu, Guo, et al., 2014; Lu et al., 2011; Yang et al., 2019; Zhao et al., 2017; Zhu et al., 2019). Genome-wide screens have implicated more than 100 genes all over the world, many of which were involved with immune function. Chinese researchers have expanded the list of RA risk alleles and added new insights into genetics of RA over time. In 2017, Zhao et al. reported a missense variant (g.74779296G>A; p.Arg90His) in NCF1, which encoded the $p47^{phox}$ subunit of the phagocyte NADPH oxidase (NOX2), suggesting that the reduction of NOX2-derived ROS levels played a pathogenic role in autoimmune diseases such as SLE and RA (Zhao et al., 2017). Guo et al. provide the first evidence that HLA-DQ-α1:160D, instead of HLA-DRB1*0405, is the strongest and independent genetic risk for ACPA-positive RA in Han Chinese (Guo et al., 2019).

Infections could also initiate RA through a variety of mechanisms, including directly infecting the synovium, activating immunity by pattern-recognition receptors, especially the Toll-like receptor, or inducing autoreactive adaptive immune response by molecular mimicry. The gut and oral microbiota are environmental factors that influences metabolic and immune homeostasis, and the composition of them are stable in individuals but different among individuals. A metagenomic shotgun sequencing and a metagenome-wide association study (MGWAS) of fecal, dental and salivary samples from RA patients elucidated that RA represents the state of chronic inflammation triggered or aggravated by the overgrowth of pathogenic bacteria (Lactobacillus salivarius) or lack of immune-modulating commensal bacteria (Haemophilus spp.). This study established specific alterations in the gut and oral microbiomes in RA patients and provided potential ways of using microbiome composition for the prognosis and diagnosis of RA (Zhang, Zhang, Jia, et al., 2015). Human Cytomegaloviruses (hCMV) was also reported to participate in the mechanism of autoimmune disease. In 2016, an autoantibody recognizing a group of peptides with conserve motif matching Pp150 protein of hCMV was identified, which could induce death of $CD56^{bright}$ NK cells via both antibody dependent cellular cytotoxicity (APCC) and complement-dependent cytotoxicity (CDC) mechanisms and was observed in several autoimmune diseases such as RA, SLE and pSS (Liu et al., 2016).

1.2.2 Autoimmunity

Autoimmunity can be present several years before the onset of clinical arthritis, through the production of autoantibodies recognizing common molecules derived from specific proteins including normal constituents such as fibrinogen, vimentin, and fibronectin, as well as xenoproteins such as EBV or CMV-derived peptides. Autoantibodies and other biomarkers reflect the immune dysregulation and play pathological roles in the pathogenesis of RA. Rheumatologists in China have been focusing on varieties of new autoantibodies and biomarkers, including anti-citrullinated human papilloma virus (HPV)-47 $E2_{345-362}$ (Shi, Sun, Zhao, Zhao, & Li, 2008), anti-cyclic citrullinated collagen type II (CII) (Liang et al., 2019), 14-3-3η protein (Zeng & Tan, 2018), serum connective tissue growth factor (SCTGF) (Yang et al., 2017), and etc. Secondary SS-specific peptide (3S-P) and elevated antibody of 3S-P specific for secondary SS was identified in autoimmune disease such as RA (Li, Gao, et al., 2018). In addition, Wang et al. showed a glycomic approach to detect N-glycan biomarkers for the classification of both ACPA/RF positive and negative RA, which could be applied to other autoimmune and infectious diseases (Wang et al., 2017).

T cells, including IL-17 producing $CD4^+$ T (Th17) cells and forkhead box protein $P3(FOXP3)^+$ regulatory T (Treg) cells, have been implicated in the pathogenesis of RA. The collagen-induced arthritis (CIA) could be exacerbated by leptin treatment, which could increase the generation of Th17 cells in joint tissue and draining lymph nodes (Deng et al., 2012). Jiao et al. showed that Notch signaling played a promoting role in Th1 and Th17 differentiation and facilitated the blockage of Notch signaling as a novel therapeutic strategy for RA treatment (Jiao et al., 2014). Ye et al. reported the first case-control study of the $CD4^+$ T cell transcriptome profile in RA, and provided the evidence that $CD4^+$ T cells had abnormal functional networks in STAT3 and Wnt signaling in RA patients (Ye et al., 2015).

A subset of helper T cells has been characterized in previous studies, termed as follicular B helper T (Tfh) cells with a distinct gene expression profile and a specialized role in facilitating the autoimmune responses. He et al. found that the circulating $CCR7^{lo}PD\text{-}1^{hi}CXCR5^+$ Tfh precursor cells in active RA patients could circulate to the nondraining lymphoid organs, differentiate into mature Tfh cells and facilitate the germinal centers(GCs) formation, which suggested that Tfh precursors were generated primarily in the early phase of inflammatory response but not derived from Tfh cells in GCs, and better than other $CD4^+$ T cell subsets in providing B helper function in vitro culture (He et al., 2013).

One previous study showed that the function of Treg cells was impaired through TNF-induced FOXP3 dephosphorylation by protein phosphatase 1 (PP1) overexpression (Nie et al., 2013). IL-17-producing CD4 $FOXP3^+$ Treg cells were reported in RA patients by Wang et al. in 2014. The frequency of this subsets were significantly increased in peripheral blood and remained their inhibition to autoimmunity, whereas they were decreased in the synovium of RA patients and could be pathogenic due to the lack of suppression function (Wang, Sun, et al., 2015). Another study showed that maresin 1 (MaR1) could effectively ameliorate the progression of RA through retrieving the balance of Th17/Treg cells by upregulating FOXP3 expression via miR-21 (Jin et al., 2018).

CD147 was expressed on different immune cells, even higher on activated T cells such as memory T (Tm) cells, and promoted the progression of RA through the endothelial growth factor (EGFR) and Hif-1α pathway (Wang et al., 2012). Researchers in our country have conducted series studies and developed a humanized monoclonal antibody (mAb) against CD147, 5A12, which exerted a significant immunosuppressive function in vitro (Luan et al., 2017). The same group subsequently identified that CD147 expression silencing or blockage with mAb could inhibit the activation and proliferation of Tm cells and genesis of osteoclasts through suppressing ZAP70-LAT-ERK signaling. Then they resolved the crystal structure of $CD147_{ecto}$-$5A12_{Fab}$ complex and revealed that Tm cells could be specifically inhibited via the mutation of K63A/D65A in the binding epitope, which was similar to 5A12 (Guo, Ye, et al., 2019).

Hyperactivated B cells are one of the most important participants in the initiation and development of RA. Human CD27 + IgD + B cells, also termed as unswitched memory B (Bm) cells, producing natural antibody-like

IgM, were found negatively correlated with disease activity and clinical manifestations of RA patients. Modulating the status of CD27+IgD+ B cells could provide novel therapeutic strategies for RA (Hu et al., 2018).

IL-10-producing CD1d^{hi}CD5^{+}B cells, known as B10 cells and regulatory B (Breg) cells, have been proved to play critical roles in negatively regulating autoimmune responses. In previous studies of B10 cells, a novel function of B-cell activating factor (BAFF) in the induction of B10 cells has been reported to inhibit the proliferation of T cells (Yang et al., 2010). Then the same group reported that the development of CIA was effectively suppressed by BAFF-induced B10 cells, and expanded B10 cells could inhibited Th17 cells differentiated from naive CD4+ T cells through reducing STAT3 phosphorylation and retinoid-related orphan receptor γt (RORγt) expression. B10 cells could be detected in vivo 3 weeks after transfer. All these results may provide a new cellular therapy for RA (Yang et al., 2012). A subset of B10 cells that could release granzyme B (GrB) and negatively regulate Th1 and Th17 cells, were numerically and functionally impaired in RA (Xu, Liu, et al., 2017). In addition, several studies have demonstrate that B10 cells could not only lose their immunosuppression capacity but also convert into RANKL-producing cells pathogenically in RA patients, which could facilitate the progression of RA (Hu et al., 2017).

γδ T cells have two main subsets including Vγ9/Vδ2 and Vδ1 T cells. Vγ9/Vδ2 T cells accounts for the major population of peripheral blood γδ T cells and can produce high levels of interferon (IFN)-γ, tumor necrosis factor (TNF)-α and IL-17. One recent study has demonstrated that Vδ2 T cells were lower in peripheral blood and accumulated in the synovium of RA which resulted from the upregulation of CCR5 and CXCR3 induced by TNF-α via NF-κB signaling pathway. TNF-α antagonists could repopulated the Vδ2 T cells in the peripheral blood of RA (Mo et al., 2017).

Hypoxia relates to the innate immunity mainly in macrophages, and the innate immunity mediated by Toll-like receptors (TLRs) was associated with hypoxia through NF-κB pathway. Hypoxia-induced 1α (Hif-1α), as the key regulator of hypoxia, may control the Th17/Treg balance and plays a pivotal role in the pathogenesis of RA, of which the upregulated expression was shown in RA synovial tissues. Hypoxia was shown to potentiate TLR signaling-induced inflammation in RA via HIF-1α, which could be a new therapeutic target for overcoming the persistent and chronic inflammatory disease (Hu et al., 2014).

Fibroblast-like synoviocytes (FLSs), as unique cells proliferating along with the intimal lining of the RA synovium, play an important role in the onset and development of RA. Discoidin domain receptor 2 (DDR-2)/MMP signaling is involved in the cartilage destruction of RA. The activation of annexin A2, identified as a DRR-2 binding protein for the first time, could promote FLSs invasion to the joints and joint destruction (Zhao, Zhang, et al., 2014). GATA4, a critical regulator of cardiac differentiation-specific gene expression, was demonstrated for the first time that it played a key role in regulating VEGF secretion from FLSs of RA by directly binding to the promoter and enhancing transcription. The knockdown of GATA4 prevented RA-enhanced angiogenesis (Jia et al., 2018). The inhibition of sonic hedgehog (SHH) could decrease the proliferation and migration of RA-FLS via mitogen-activated protein kinases/extracellular signal-regulated kinases (MAPK/ERK) pathway (Liu, Feng, et al., 2018). LERFS (lowly expressed in rheumatoid fibroblast-like synoviocytes), as a long non-coding RNA (lncRNA), was identified to negatively regulate the migration, invasion, the proliferation of FLSs and might contribute to synovial aggression and joint destruction in RA (Zou et al., 2018). Recently, lncRNA metastasis associated lung adenocarcinoma transcript 1 (MALAT1) was reported to inhibit the proliferation and inflammation of FLSs by promoting CTNNB1 methylation and inhibiting the Wnt signaling pathway (Li, Fang, et al., 2019). Sorting nexin (SNX) 10, a member of the SNX family which participates in the regulation of endosomal sorting, plays a role in malignant osteopetrosis. Chinese researchers found that the deficiency of SNX10 prevented bone loss through impairing the maturation of osteoclasts rather than osteogenesis in CIA mice, which was induced by accelerating the degradation of NFATc1 through inhibiting of integrin β3-Src-PYK2 signaling. (Zhou et al., 2016).

1.3 Immunotherapy

RA affects about 0.3% of Chinese population and continues to be one of the major health problems influencing the quality of life and consuming healthcare resources in China. It have been found that 77.6% of Chinese RA patients had physical disability, 39% of whom had moderate to severe disabilities, and this results suggested the loss of work capacity and cost of illness (Zhou et al., 2018). The progression of RA has been delayed by efficient disease control and management through the use of disease-modifying anti-rheumatic drugs (DMARDs) over the past 2 decades in China. The current treatment strategy for RA involves a treat-to-target approach which is based on regular and tight evaluation of disease activity and modification of management if not reaching the treatment goal. Several Chinese groups have also investigated novel therapeutic methods and strategies in RA.

1.3.1 DMARDs

DMARDs includes conventional synthetic DMARDs (csDMARDs), biological DMARDs (bDMARDs) and targeted synthetic DMARDs (tsDMARDs). Conventional synthetic DMARDs are small chemical drugs with anti-inflammatory function such as methotrexate, leflunomide, etc., while targeted synthetic DMARDs (tsDMARDs) could target small molecules specifically like JAKs. In contrast to csDMARDs and tsDMARDs, bDMARDs are the monoclonal antibodies or receptor constructs targeting soluble extracellular and cell-membrane associated proteins with high specificity, and could be biological originator or biosimilar DMARDs. And the composition of DMARDs has been developed due to increasing novel therapeutic targets of RA.

One randomized-control trial (RCT) in China has shown that 54.1% of patients receiving methotrexate (MTX) as an anchor drug of RA, combined with leflunomide (LEF) and hydroxychloroquine (HCQ), also known as prolonged intensive DMARDs therapy (PRINT), achieved a good EULAR response after 36 weeks of treatment. In addition, LEF was suggested a good maintenance treatment as single treatment in RA (Li et al., 2016). Then the evidence was cited into the 2018 update of the APLAR recommendation of RA treatment.

Iguratimod (IGU), a new synthetic small-molecule DMARD, was suggested effective and well tolerated in RA treatment in a Chinese RCT (Lu et al., 2009). Then lots of studies showed that IGU combined with MTX appeared to have a good efficacy and safety for active RA. IGU became an effective option in combination with MTX-CsA-HCQ-prednisone of step-up strategies for refractory RA (Duan, Zhang, Mao, Shang, & Shi, 2015; Zheng, Guo, & Wu, 2018).

The routine clinical practice of bDMARDs in China was shown in a real-world large-scale study. There are 89.5% of RA patients enrolled from 15 teaching hospitals nationwide received a combination of bDMARDs and csDMARDs, whereas 10.5% received bDMARDs monotherapy. In our country, Etanercept was most common bDMARDs, including Enbrel® and local brandYiSai Pu®and Qiangke®, accounting for 66.6% of the total, while tocilizumab, adalimumab, and infliximab were used by 17.0%, 7.5%, and 6.6% of RA patients, respectively. Longer duration of bDMARDs usage and combination with csDMARDs showed a better prognosis of RA (An et al., 2017).

Because there are large population of infectious disease such as tuberculosis (TB), hepatitis B virus (HBV), hepatitis C virus (HCV) and human immunodeficiency viruses (HIV) infections in China, there are more infectious risks when using bDMARDs. There are evidence for RA patients with previous exposure to HBV but negative HBsAg and normal liver function at baseline that Infliximab therapy showed no correlation with liver impairments in China (Zhang, Zhang, et al., 2013). Rituximab was reported to enhance the HCV activity in RA through decreasing exosomal microRNA-155 (*exo*-miR-155), which suggested that *exo*-miR-155 became a potential diagnostic biomarker or therapeutic target in RA patients accompanied with HCV (Liao et al., 2018).

In a Phase 3 RCT, tofacitinib, an oral JAK inhibitor for the treatment of RA, was reported to improve quality of life, physical function and relieve pain in Chinese RA patients who had not responded to csDMARDs previously (Li, An, et al., 2018).

Dasatinib is a second-generation tyrosine kinase inhibitor (TKI) that is used for the treatment of chronic myeloid leukemia or Philadelphia chromosome-positive acute lymphoblastic leukemia. Chinese researchers have demonstrated that dasatinib exhibited not only treatment effects on CIA mice but also inhibition to the RA-FLS migration and proliferation and promotion of FLS apoptosis, which provided a promising and powerful strategy for RA treatment (Guo, Bu, et al., 2018).

1.3.2 Traditional Chinese medicine

According traditional Chinese medicine (TCM), RA can be defined as a "Bi" syndrome. Different kinds of TCM has been established and approved to treat RA in China during the past decades. Tripterygium wilfordii Hook F (TwHF), as traditional Chinese medicine, monotherapy was not inferior to, and combined to MTX was better than, MTX monotherapy in treating RA safely in Tripterygium wilfordii Hook F with methotrexate in the treatment of active rheumatoid arthritis (TRIFRA) RCT (Lv et al., 2015). Then almost half of these patients were followed up to 2 years. The results showed that TwHF monotherapy was not inferior to MTX in controlling disease activity and retarding radiological progression in patients with active RA.

Sinomenine (SIN), as the prescription drug approved for RA treatment in China, was showed that it could suppress RA progression and became an alternative cost-effective agent along with MTX in the treatment of RA (Liu, Zhang, et al., 2018).

Polyphyllin I (PPI), one of the main components in the Rhizoma of Paris polyphyllin, was demonstrated effectively ameliorating synovial inflammation in the joints of CIA mice by suppressing NF-κB signaling pathway in activated macrophages (Wang, Zhou, et al., 2018).

1.3.3 Mesenchymal stem cells

Mesenchymal stem cells (MSCs) have the capacity to regulate the immune response by suppressing T and B lymphocyte proliferation in a non-major histocompatibility complex (non-MHC)-restricted manner. The disease activity of refractory RA could reduce after allogeneic MSCs transplantation (Liang et al., 2012). And in 2015, the same group in this country found that umbilical cord (UC)-MSCs transplantation into CIA mice prevented arthritis progression both in the number and function of Tfh cells in vivo, which suggested MSCs inhibited Tfh cell differentiation through the indoleamine 2,3-dioxygenase (IDO) production in response to IFN (Liu, Li, et al., 2015).

1.3.4 Other therapies

Apremilast, a novel phosphodiesterase 4 (PDE4) inhibitor suppressing immune and inflammatory responses, was suggested effective in treating autoimmune arthritis and prevent bone erosion in the CIA model, implicating its therapeutic potential in patients with RA (Chen, Wang, et al., 2018).

Biphosphonates, such as alendronate, bind to mineralized bone and inhibit osteoclasts function at sites of bone resorption. However, Aminobisphosphonates (N-BPs) promote the activation and proliferation Vδ2 T cells that N-BPs probably play an unfavorable role in the treatment of RA (Mo, Yin, Chen, & Zhang, 2018).

Denosumab, a circulating humanized monoclonal antibody, can reduce the number and function osteoclast at any sites and decrease the bone resorption by inhibiting human RANKL pathway. One study has suggested that denosumab could induce partial repair of erosions in RA patients (Yue et al., 2017).

Melatonin was identified to ameliorate RA by inhibiting TNF-α and IL-1β production through downregulation of the PI3K/AKT, ERK, NF-κB signaling pathways, as well as miR-3150a-3p overexpression (Huang et al., 2019).

Cell-free DNA (cfDNA) released from damaged or dead cells can activate the DNA sensors related to RA pathogenesis. Cationic nanoparticles (cNP) could scavenger nucleic acid (NA) such as cfDNA to limit inflammation. Liang et al. showed that ~40 nm cNP could scavenge cfDNA derived from RA patients and inhibit the activation of primary synovial fluid monocytes and fibroblast-like synoviocytes, and suggested a new nanomedicine therapy in treating RA (Liang, Peng, et al., 2018). $Cu_{7.2}S_4$ nanoparticles (NPs) combined with near infrared (NIR) light could not only inhibit bone resorption but also inhibit the inflammation in the synovial tissue, which might be a novel potential RA treatment (Lu et al., 2018).

An altered hemagglutinin 308–317 ($HA^{308-317}$) peptide (Sun et al., 2012), a Tylophorine analog (NK-007) (Wen et al., 2012) and T cell vaccination (Chen, Li, Zang, et al., 2007) were found to be potentially important in the treatment of RA.

In conclusion, csDMARDs combined with or without biologics or TCM, are the main therapeutic choice for RA patients in our country, whereas LEF and MTX are the two "anchor" drugs. Moreover, bDMARDs are quite effective with lower risk of side effects than csDMARDs and has been used nationwide, which is consistent with the international guidelines. There is also a great interest in other new promising therapeutic targets.

2. Systemic lupus erythematosus

SLE is characterized by production of antibodies to cellular components, with activation of innate and the adaptive immune system. Disease manifestations of lupus are heterogeneous, ranging from detectable laboratory abnormalities to multi-organ inflammation and failure. Clinical manifestation is characterized by multisystem involvement including skin, joints, kidney, heart, and neuropsychiatric system. Reported prevalence of SLE ranges from 20 to 240 per 100,000 persons. In China, Li et al. have reported the prevalence rate of 30 per 100,000 persons (Li et al., 2012). Peak disease incidence occurred during reproductive years.

2.1 Autoantibodies in SLE

Autoantibodies that recognize cellular components, particularly cell nuclei, were present in the sera of lupus patients. Isolation of complexes of antibody with DNA-binding proteins, such as histones, was an important factor in the classification of SLE. The hallmark serologic feature is the presence of ANAs. Extractable nuclear antigens (ENAs) refer to a heterogeneous mixture of non-DNA nuclear antigens which can be "extracted" from cells in the laboratory.

Studies using protein array technologies have demonstrated the presence of over 100 different autoantibodies in patients with SLE. Autoantibodies to blood components can be responsible for hemolytic anemia, neutropenia, or thrombocytopenia. Rheumatoid factor can be found in SLE, as well as ACPA and ANCA.

As one of the most valuable markers in the diagnosis of SLE, anti-nucleosome antibody (AnuA) was introduce to China in 2007 (Su, Jia, Han, & Li, 2007). The study also indicated that AnuA was valuable in patients lacking of anti-DNP, anti-Sm and anti-dsDNA antibodies. Other novel autoantibodies in Chinese lupus patients have been found including anti-cmDNA, anti-Histones antibody and anti-Lymphocyte antibody etc. Approximate 30% patients were anti-Histones antibodies positive in 144 SLE patients lacking anti-nucleosome, anti-cmDNA, anti-Sm, and anti-dsDNA (Sun, Shi, Han, Su, & Li, 2008). There was close correlation of anti-Histone and anti-H1 antibodies with SLE disease activity. Anti-cmDNA (cell-membrane associated DNA) was also informative in diagnosis of SLE (Chen, Guo, & Li, 2008). Skin rash, alopecia, oral ulcer, and joint pain are more common in patients with anti-cmDNA antibodies. Anti-lymphocyte antibody (ALA) was reported highly specific in SLE. The sensitivity and specificity of ALA IgG in SLE were 42.3% and 96.7%, respectively, (Li, Mu, Lu, et al., 2014). ALA occurred more frequently in patients with active SLE and was independently associated with lymphopenia, higher SLEDAI scores, and increased risk for lupus nephritis.

Autoantibodies against the major acute-phase reactant C-reactive protein (CRP) are found in patients with lupus nephritis. Li et al. found that amino acids 35–47 constitute the major epitope recognized by anti-CRP autoantibodies in patients with lupus nephritis (Li, Li, et al., 2017). The results also provide evidence for the in vivo generation of monomeric CRP (mCRP) and suggest that mCRP is actively involved in pathogenesis of lupus nephritis by regulating complement activation. Another new autoantibody in complement activation pathway is the antibody against the linear 08 epitope of C1q A chain. Previous study has shown that antibodies to complement C1q appear to be prevalent in patients with active lupus nephritis. In a study that included 210 active lupus nephritis patients, antibody against linear 08 epitope of C1q A chain was correlated better with disease relapse than that of antibodies to either the intact or the collagen-like region of C1q (Pang et al., 2016).

An autoantibody that is induced by the Phosphoprotein 150 (anti-Pp150) of human cytomegalovirus (hCMV) was identified among several autoimmune diseases including SLE. Anti-Pp150 induces the death of CD56bright NK cells by recognizing the single-pass membrane protein CIP2A. The number of circulating CD56bright NK cells in lupus patients was negatively correlated with anti-Pp150 concentration. The finding helps to uncover the role of hCMV infection in the pathogenesis of SLE (Liu et al., 2016).

2.2 Etiology and pathogenesis

Rapid progress has been made in defining interaction of genetic factors with environmental triggers. Type I interferon (IFN) is a critical pathogenic factor in activation of innate immune system during the progression of SLE. Studies were undertaken to identify the important microRNAs in the IFN pathway in SLE. Several important microRNAs have been indicated as critical factors that controls SLE through stabilizing and modulating immune homeostasis (Han et al., 2016; Pan et al., 2015; Wang, Dai, et al., 2018; Wu et al., 2016). MiR-31 is a novel enhancer of IL-2 production during T cell activation. Dysregulation of miR-31 could be a novel molecular mechanism underlying the IL-2 deficiency in patients with SLE. MiR-146a maturation in type I IFN pathway contributes to the uncontrolled inflammation and excessive inflammatory gene expression in SLE. MiR-155 promotes pristane-induced lung inflammation and contributes to ectopic activation of NF-κB signaling pathways by targeting multiple negative regulators. MiR-130b is a novel negative regulator of the type I IFN pathway in renal cells. Overexpression of miR-130b could inhibit IFNα-accelerated LN.

Adaptive immune system has also been extensively studied in SLE. Epigenetics studies demonstrated that gene regulatory regions in $CD4^+$ T cells are abnormally regulated by demethylation and methylation which contributes to the development of autoreactivity and overstimulation of autoantibodies (Zhao et al., 2016). MicroRNAs were identified to regulate DNA methylation in $CD4^+$ T cells and contributes to T cell autoreactivity in SLE by directly targeting Dnmt1 (Zhao et al., 2011). Growth arrest and DNA damage-induced 45α (GADD45α) reduces epigenetic silencing of genes by removing methylation. Recently, gadd45α was proved to contribute to lupus autoimmune reaction by promoting DNA demethylation in SLE $CD4^+$ T cells (Zhao et al., 2018).

B cell and antigen presentation cell also play important roles in balancing immune-protection and immune-pathology. The receptors for the Fc portion of IgG molecules (FcγRs) was one of the regulatory strategies. A single-nucleotide polymorphism in the transmembrane domain of FcγRIIB, FcγRIIB-T232, is associated with lupus (Xu, Xia, et al., 2016). Pathogenic mechanism of FcγRIIB-T232 at both functional and structural levels were investigated. The Result showed that single-residue polymorphism T232 enforces the inclination of the transmembrane domain and thereby reduces the lateral mobility and inhibitory functions of FcγRIIB in lupus. Similarly, the hIgG1-G396R variant was also important in autoimmune response of SLE (Chen, Sun, et al., 2018).

The importance of plasma cells and autoantibodies in SLE has been well established. However, the underlying molecular mechanisms which control autoantibody production remains unclear. Peli1 has a B cell-intrinsic function to protect against lupus-like autoimmunity. A study published in 2018 showed that in humans, Peli1 negatively correlate with disease severity in SLE patients (Liu, Huang, et al., 2018). Furthermore, Peli1 is a negative regulator of the noncanonical NF-κB pathway in the context of restraining the pathogenesis of lupus-like disease.

Due to development of genome-wide association studies (GWAS) in the past decade, at least 80 genetic loci with susceptibility to SLE have been confirmed. The first Chinese GWAS of SLE was in 2009 by genotyping 1047 cases and 1205 controls using Illumina Human610-Quad Bead Chips (Han et al., 2009). Nine new susceptibility loci and seven previously reported loci were identified. Comparison with previous GWAS findings, this study highlighted the genetic heterogeneity of SLE susceptibility between Chinese Han and European populations.

I In 2 Chinese populations (Zhang, Zhang, Zhang, et al., 2015), Lau and Yang et al. performed GWAS and identified ANXA6 as a novel SLE susceptibility gene with multiple independently contributing variants. Using a custom exome array, large-scale exome-wide study was performed in 5004 SLE cases and 8179 healthy controls in a Han Chinese population (Wen et al., 2018). This study identified four new susceptibility gene regions for SLE including LCT, TPCN2, AHNAK2 and TNFRSF13B.

Population-based candidate gene strategy has also been widely used in genetic study. A large population based study identified that Polymorphism of leucocyte immunoglobulin-like receptor A3 (LILRA3) and Deletion of LCE3C_LCE3B were associated with systemic lupus erythematosus in the Chinese Han population (Du et al., 2015; Lu et al., 2011). Functional LILRA3 is highly predisposes to certain phenotypes such as leucopenia and thrombocytopenia in SLE, and may confer increased disease activity in SLE. Zhou et al. conducted a genetic association study in more than 10,000 Han Chinese and observed a genetic association between light chain 3B, a widely used marker for autophagy, and susceptibility to SLE (Qi et al., 2018).

In the post-GWAS era, refinement of these associated genes is required, and their potential roles in gene–gene interactions need to be further investigated. Recently, gene–gene interaction was investigated in B cell/T cell responses pathway. The results of this study provide evidence of the possible gene–gene interactions in SLE, which may represent a synergic effect of T cells and B cells through the NF-κB pathway in determining immunologic aberration (Zhou et al., 2012).

2.3 New therapeutic strategy

Treatment of moderate or severe SLE requires induction immunosuppressive therapy followed by maintenance therapy. Corticosteroid, antimalarials and immunosuppressive therapy were broadly used in these patients.

Cyclophosphamide (CYC) has long been considered a gold standard in inducing renal remission and preventing renal flares for patients with lupus nephritis. However, the rational use of CYC has not reached a consensus, such as the timing and length of treatment, the route of administration, and the ideal dosage. A 1-year trial was taken to compare High-dose (6 monthly pulses followed by two quarterly pulses at a dose of 0.5–1.0 g/m2) and short-interval lower-dose (SILD, 12 fortnightly pulses at a fixed dose of 400 mg followed by 6 monthly pulses) intravenous CYC (Zhang, Li, et al., 2014). The result showed that efficacy of SILD iv CYC regimen in the treatment of lupus nephritis is equivalent to that of the high-dose regimen, whereas the incidence of adverse events is much lower in the SILD group.

Multi-target therapy (steroid, mycophenolate mofetil and tacrolimus) was first used in the induction treatment of class V + IV LN, in comparison with iv CYC therapy (Bao et al., 2008). The result showed that multitarget therapy is superior to iv CYC for inducing complete remission of class V + IV lupus nephritis and is well tolerated.

Another trial of combination immunosuppressive therapy was carried in 2018. A large-scale, multi-centered trial was conducted to compare affordable triple strategy that combined CYC with another immunosuppressive agent plus hydroxychloroquine (HCQ) to CYC only as a remission-inducing treatment for lupus nephritis. At week 24, both the rate of complete remission and total response was higher in the combined group with less treatment failure (An et al., 2019).

A prospective observational multi-center study was carried to investigate the efficacy and safety profile of leflunomide compared with cyclophosphamide in the treatment of patients with biopsy-proven proliferative lupus nephritis. The remission rate in the leflunomide group was the same as in the cyclophosphamide group (Wang et al., 2008). Therefore, compared with cyclophosphamide, leflunomide was effective in the induction therapy of proliferative lupus nephritis and was generally well-tolerated.

Novel biologic therapy is proved to be effective in active SLE patients. Belimumab is a fully human anti-BLyS (BLyS, also known as B cell activation factor [BAFF]) monoclonal antibody. A phase III placebo-controlled RCT was carried out in North-east Asia. Belimumab treatment resulted in a modest, although significant, reduction in disease activity (Zhang et al., 2018).

Another promising biologic therapy of lupus is low-dose interleukin (IL)-2. Since the homeostasis of $CD4^+$ T cell subsets is regulated by IL-2, and reduced production of IL-2 by T cells is observed in individuals with SLE. He et al. demonstrated that treatment with low-dose recombinant human IL-2 selectively modulated the abundance of regulatory T cells, follicular helper T cells and IL-17-producing helper T cells, accompanied by marked reductions of disease activity in patients with SLE (He et al., 2016). They also showed that interleukin-2 deficiency associated with renal impairment in SLE (Shao et al., 2019). Patients with exogenous low-dose IL-2 supplement demonstrated better improved nephritis and higher remission rate.

It was reported that in lupus patients, immunization with inactivated autoreactive T cells could induce idiotype anti-idiotypic reaction and deplete specific subsets of autoreactive T cells. In a study, six SLE patients with active disease index were treated with T cell vaccination. Autoreactive T cell clones were derived from peripheral blood mononuclear cells of the patients and irradiated T cells were inoculated subcutaneously at 0, 2, 6 and 8 weeks, respectively. The enrolled patients were followed up for 32–40 months at an interval of 3–6 months. The clinical characteristics and laboratory abnormalities improved after inoculation without increasing the dose of corticosteroids and immunosuppressants in most patients. Moreover, SLEDAI score was also decreased after T cell vaccination (Li, Mu, Dai, & Gao, 2005).

At last, allogeneic mesenchymal stem cells (MSCs) exhibit therapeutic effects in human autoimmune diseases including SLE. Umbilical cord-derived

MSCs (UC-MSCs) results in amelioration of disease activity, serologic changes, and stabilization of proinflammatory cytokines (Sun et al., 2010). Ongoing works are about mechanisms of MSCs mediating immunosuppression in lupus patients (Feng et al., 2014; Li et al., 2005).

3. Sjögren's syndrome

Sjögren's syndrome (SS) is a systemic autoimmune disease characterized by lymphocytic infiltration of exocrine glands and epithelia at multiple sites. It mainly attacks lacrimal and salivary glands, causing dry eyes (keratoconjunctivitis sicca) and dry mouth (xerostomia). In addition, SS may also affect many extraglandular organs and systems. Hendrik Sjögren was the first to establish the disease spectrum in 1993. Subsequent studies in the mid-twentieth century further confirmed the association of SS with other autoimmune diseases and with hematologic malignancies. SS is further classified as either primary or secondary. Primary SS (pSS) presents alone, whereas secondary SS (sSS) occurs in the presence of another autoimmune disease, such as rheumatoid arthritis (RA), systemic lupus erythematosus (SLE), systemic sclerosis (SSc), or primary biliary cholangitis (PBC).

In China, the concept of SS can be traced back to around 500 BC. A condition of severe dry eyes and dry mouth with glandular swelling was described in the ancient medical book *The Yellow Emperor's Classic of Internal Medicine* as "Zao Bi," meaning "dryness impediment" literally. For over a 1000 years, traditional Chinese medicine (TCM) was used with the aim of relieving symptoms. It is likely that these herbal remedies have similar cholinergic and anti-inflammatory properties to pilocarpine and salicylates in the West. In the past generation, however, the landscape of epidemiology, diagnosis and treatment of SS has changed dramatically, along with the increased introduction of western medicine in China. Large-scale population-based surveys were initiated to generate reliable prevalence estimates; high-quality basic research studies were performed to elucidate the mechanisms of pathogenesis; observational studies and clinical trials were conducted to assess unique features of SS in Chinese population and to evaluate effective approach to treatment.

3.1 Epidemiology and clinical features

In 1995, a survey of 2066 pSS patients was conducted in Beijing. As shown in the survey, the prevalence of pSS was 0.77% by the Copenhagen criteria and 0.33% by the modified San Diego criteria (Zhang et al., 1995). This was the first known population-based survey of pSS in China. In subsequent surveys, the reported prevalence using the Copenhagen criteria was 0.58% and 0.39%, respectively (Xiang & Dai, 2009). There was a female predominance with a female to male ratio of 2:1 in the surveys. After correcting for the sex bias, the overall prevalence of pSS was estimated at 0.45%. The peak age of onset was between 40 and 50 years.

Compared with previous studies performed in other countries, SS patients in China showed some unique clinical and laboratory features. In a recent multi-center study, 483 consecutive patients who fulfilled the 2002 classification criteria for pSS were registered from 16 Chinese medical centers nationwide from 2009 to 2011 (Xiang & Dai, 2009). The cohort included 456 women and 27 men (ratio 17:1), with the mean age at onset 42 ± 11 years and the median age at diagnosis 49 years (range 41–56 years). Male patients showed a lower frequency of xerophthalmia and a higher frequency of arthritis. Young-onset patients showed a higher frequency of low C3 levels and pancytopenia. Patients with systemic involvement had a higher frequency of immunoglobulin A (IgA) and immunoglobulin M (IgM). Patients with pulmonary involvement had a higher parotid enlargement, purpura and higher anti-La/SSB, immunoglobulin G (IgG) and IgA levels. Patients with anti-Ro/SSA antibodies had more frequent exocrine gland symptoms.

The spectrum of clinical manifestations of pSS in Chinese population was also assessed in several other retrospective and cohort studies. It was suggested that Chinese patients with pSS probably experienced more severe organ diseases. In a retrospective study, 42.3% (221/522) patients were reported to have developed certain form of pulmonary complications after a median follow-up of 48 months from the onset of disease (Yan, Zhao, Zeng, Zhang, & Dong, 2008). A recent case-control study conducted by our group involved 853 hospitalized patients with pSS, 165 (19.34%) among whom were identified with interstitial lung disease (ILD) (Gao et al., 2018). Of these patients with pSS-ILD, 91.5% were women. The mean age was 61.25 ± 9.79 years, and the median disease duration was 84 (24–156) months. Non-specific interstitial pneumonia (NSIP) was the predominant (39.1%) pattern on high-resolution computed tomography (HRCT). The 5-year survival rate for all patients with pSS-ILD was 88.5%. Age, rheumatoid factor (RF), and C-reactive protein (CRP) were independent predictors of ILD after adjustment for confounders. Except for ILD, pulmonary arterial hypertension (PAH) was also recognized as a leading cause of mortality in patients with pSS. In a case-control study, 29 pSS hospitalized patients from 2007 to 2015 with right heart catheterization (RHC)-confirmed PAH were included (mean age at onset 38.4 ± 8.3 years, mean pSS duration 54.6 months) (Yan et al., 2018). PAH was the initial clinical presentation of pSS in 12 (41.4%) patients. Raynaud's phenomenon, rheumatoid factor $\geq$200 U/mL, hepatic injury and pericardial effusion were identified as independent risk factors for the development of PAH in pSS. Further cohort studies demonstrated that the predictors of mortality in patients with pSS-PAH include delayed onset of PAH in pSS, red blood cell distribution width (RDW) >15%(Hui et al., 2019) and worse cardiac function (cardiac index $< 2\,L/min/m^2$) (Liu, Yang, et al., 2018). Immunosuppressants were proved to effectively improve the prognosis of pSS-PAH (Liu, Wang, et al., 2018).

Besides pulmonary and cardiac involvement, renal injuries have also been suggested to be common in Chinese patients. In a retrospective study including 130 pSS patients, 95 (73.1%) patients developed renal tubular acidosis (RTA) (Ren et al., 2008). Of these patients, 91 were diagnosed distal RTA (dRTA). There was a correlation between hypergammaglobulinemia and dRTA. The combination of corticosteroids and immunosuppressant drugs significantly improved the renal function of the patients. Another study reported 103 biopsy-proven cases with renal involvement among 2096 pSS inpatients from 2005 to 2015 (Yang, Wang, et al., 2018). Tubulointerstitial was the prominent (51.5%) pathologic pattern, whereas glomerulonephritis (GN) was present in 48.5% of the patients. The patterns of GN lesions included membranous nephropathy (35.9%), mesangial proliferative glomerulonephritis (5.8%), IgA nephropathy (2.9%), minimal change disease (3.9%) and focal segmental glomerulosclerosis (2.9%). In another study with 192 pSS patients, histological positivity for labial salivary gland biopsy (LSGB), anti-SSA/Ro52-positivity, reduced C3 levels, hypoalbuminemia and anemia indicated significant association with renal involvement (Luo et al., 2019).

Complications of SS can affect both the peripheral (PNS) and the central nervous systems (CNS). In a cross-sectional study, 32.5% (184/566) patients had neurologic involvement (Ye, Chen, et al., 2018). The various manifestations were categorized into 5 subgroups: PNS presentations, neuropsychiatric symptoms (depression, cognitive dysfunction), unspecific neurological complains (headache, dizziness, muscular weakness), paroxysmal disease (epilepsy), and CNS radiological results (cerebral hemorrhage, infarction, demyelination, cerebral tumor, etc.). Of note, the prevalence of depression (36.9%) and anxiety (33.8%) was high in adult pSS patients (Cui et al., 2018).

The Hospital Anxiety Scale (HAS) and Hospital Depression Scale (HDS) scores of the pSS patients were significantly higher than that of patients with other internal diseases (Liu, Dong, et al., 2017). Therefore, rheumatologists should pay attention to the potential mental comorbidities in order to identify effective strategies for preventing and treating depression and anxiety among pSS patients.

Of the various organs and systems involved in pSS, Chinese pSS patients may also present with some rare manifestations such as protein-losing enteropathy and autoimmune hemolytic anemia (AIHA) (Liao et al., 2015; Mok & Lau, 1997; Wen et al., 2015). Except for the close association with lymphoma as extensively discussed previously, the development of plasma cell dyscrasia including multiple myeloma has also gained attention in SS patients with higher disease activity (Yang, Chen, et al., 2018).

3.2 Mechanisms

A new era has emerged during the past two decades in the understanding of human genomes and the technical capacity to detect genetic variation. The development of genome-wide association study (GWAS) technology has advanced the understanding of disease pathogenesis through the successful identification of new genetic susceptibility loci. Contributions from genetic factors to the etiology of SS were discovered by Chinese researchers. In 2013, a three-stage GWAS of pSS was carried out in Han Chinese (Li, Zhang, et al., 2013). In the discovery stage, 556,134 autosomal single-nucleotide polymorphisms (SNPs) in 542 cases and 1050 controls were analyzed. Subsequently, promising associations were validated in two replication stages comprising 1303 cases and 2727 controls. The combined analysis identified *GTF2I* at 7q11.23 (rs117026326) as a new susceptibility locus for pSS. The analysis also confirmed previously reported associations in Europeans in the regions of *STAT4*, *TNFAIP3* and the major histocompatibility complex (MHC). Fine mapping of the region around *GTF2I* showed that rs117026326 in *GTF2I* had the most significant association, with associated SNPs extending from *GTF2I* to *GTF2IRD1-GTF2I*. Subsequent study reported a missense variant (g.74779296G > A; p.Arg90His) in *NCF1*, encoding the $p47^{phox}$ subunit of the phagocyte NADPH oxidase (NOX2) (Zhao et al., 2017). The p.Arg90His substitution, as the cause of reduced reactive oxygen species (ROS) production, predisposes to pSS, further explains the association of rs117026326 with SS in Chinese. Other loci involved in various innate and adaptive immune processes have also been shown to be substantially associated with SS. Examples are *DCIR* (Liu, Wu, et al., 2015), *LILRA3* (Du et al., 2015), *MUC19*, *MUC5AC* (Yu et al., 2008), *RBMS3* (Song et al., 2016), *IKZF1* and *GTF2I* (Qu et al., 2017). These results provided new insight into the pathogenesis of SS.

Several types of immune cells have been demonstrated to have pathological roles in the development of SS. Currently, T helper 17 cells (Th17) have been recognized as an important effector cell subtype in various autoimmune diseases. When immunized with salivary glands (SG) proteins to induce experimental SS (ESS) in wildtype and IL-17 knockout (IL-17 KO) C57BL/6 mice, it was notably that IL-17 KO mice were completely resistant for SS induction. Adoptive transfer of Th17 cells rapidly induced the onset of ESS in immunized IL-17 KO mice (Lin et al., 2015). In patients with SS, Th17 have been detected in inflamed salivary glands and are associated with tissue damage (Bikker et al., 2010). Overexpressed interleukin-17 (IL-17) is thought to contribute to the abnormal T cell and B cell response and to play a crucial role in the autoimmune epithelitis. In a recent study, IL-17 secreted by Th17 was diffusely detected in the renal proximal tubule of pSS patients with renal Fanconi syndrome, with a negative correlation of IL-17 and megalin expression. The expression of the orphan nuclear receptor retinoic acid-related receptor α (RORα), a critical receptor in the development of Th17, was significantly increased in the labial salivary gland (LSG) of pSS patients (Weng, Liu, Cui, & Cheng, 2018). This indicated the importance of RORα in controlling pathologic lymphocytic infiltration of the salivary glands and suggested that RORα may be a druggable target in treating pSS. Besides, proteasome inhibition has been demonstrated to effectively ameliorate ESS by suppressing the Th17 response, which may as well contribute to the development of a novel therapeutic strategy for the treatment of SS (Xiao et al., 2017). In addition to Th17, T follicular helper (Tfh) cells were also involved in the ESS development. T follicular regulatory (Tfr) cells, a new subset of regulatory T (Treg) cells, which also express CXCR5, ICOS, PD-1 and Bcl6, while coexpress typical Treg cell markers such as Foxp3, GITR, Blimp-1 and CTLA-4, was proved to play a critical protective role in the development ESS by controlling the germinal center and antibody response in a recent study (Fu et al., 2018).

A variety of cytokines have been recognized to participate in the pathogenesis of SS as well, among which the role of interleukin 35 (IL-35) was explored by Chinese researchers. As a newly discovered immunoregulatory cytokine that possesses the ability to inhibit $CD4^+$ effector T cells and alleviate autoimmune diseases, IL-35 has been found in one study to be significantly decreased in pSS patients, in together with lower P35 and EBI3 mRNA levels, decreased percentages of $CD4^{+}EBI3^{+}$ T cells and increased percentages of $CD19^{+}EBI3^{+}$ B cells (Guo, Gu, et al., 2018). However, the aberrant serum IL-35 levels in patients with pSS showed different trends associated with disease durations in another study (M. Han et al., 2018). Strikingly, the serum IL-35 levels in pSS patients with short disease duration (<1year) were significantly lower compared with healthy controls (HCs). However, the serum IL-35 levels in pSS patients with medium (1–2year) and long disease duration (>2years) were higher compared with HCs. Furthermore, a positive correlation between expression of IL-35 and erythrocyte sedimentation rate, IgG, EULAR SS disease activity index (ESSDAI) was observed. These findings may suggest that IL-35 could play a key role in pSS pathogenesis and act as a biomarker of disease activity, although further studies are still needed to elucidate the exact role of this cytokine.

3.3 Novel diagnostic tests

Early treatment in SS is important as it can prevent irreversible damage of glands and organs. The biological complexity of pSS determines that conventional biomarkers such as anti-SSA and anti-SSB antibodies are limited in diagnostic sensitivities and specificities. Thus, the diagnosis is difficult when these antibodies are negative, and the patient is reluctant to receive a LSGB. To solve the problem, novel diagnostic biomarkers were pursued. The role of anti-α-fodrin antibody (Chen, Li, He, et al., 2007; He, Chen, & Li, 2006; He, Zhao, & Li, 2008) and anti-muscarinic acetylcholine type-3 receptor (M3R) antibody in diagnosing SS has been studied extensively by our group and others in China (He et al., 2011, 2012). Other autoantibodies, such as anti-3S-P antibody (Li, Gao, et al., 2018), anti-SP-1 antibody (Xuan et al., 2018), anti-mouse double minute 2 (MDM2) antibody (Liu, Liao, et al., 2017), anti-Lamin A/C antibodies (Zhang et al., 2016), have also been investigated. Several biomarkers were identified to be associated with certain form of organ involvements or complications in SS patients. Increased levels of serum galectin-3 (Gal-3) (Zhang, Sun, Song, Zuo, & Xiao, 2014), nerve grow factor (NGF) and brain-derived neurotrophic factor (BDNF) (Li, Yang, Lei, et al., 2014) were associated with the development of interstitial lung disease in pSS patients. The combination of 3 autoantibodies including anti-cofilin-1, anti-α-enolase and anti-RGI2 yielded high sensitivity (95%) and specificity (94%) in distinguishing pSS patients who progressed to mucosal-associated lymphoid tissue lymphoma (MALT) (Cui et al., 2017).

Imaging modalities as well have had rapid progress throughout the last decade. Technetium-99methyl cysteinate dimer (^{99m}Tc ECD) SPECT was proven a sensitive tool for detecting regions of hypoperfusion in the brains of patients with neuropsychiatric presentations and normal findings on brain MRI (Chang, Shiau, Wang, Ho, & Kao, 2002). Recent studies showed that salivary gland ultrasonography (SGUS) was valuable for assessing major salivary gland involvement in SS (Cornec et al., 2013; Tzioufas & Moutsopoulos, 2008), but a consensus has not been reached regarding the typical SGUS changes and 2 proposed scoring systems (De Vita, Lorenzon, Rossi, Sabella, & Fossaluzza, 1992; Hocevar, Ambrozic, Rozman, Kveder, & Tomsic, 2005). In 2015, a study was conducted by our group to compare the usefulness of the two scoring systems for pSS (Zhang, Zhang, He, et al., 2015). It was shown that SGUS is a feasible method for pSS diagnosis with higher sensitivity using the 0–48 system (Hocevar et al., 2005) and better specificity using the 0–16 (De Vita et al., 1992) system. SGUS scores are related to RF and γ-globulin%.

Except for SGUS, other methods such as magnetic resonance imaging (MRI) have also been found to be superior to X-ray sialography for noninvasively evaluating the parotid parenchyma. Diffusion-weighted imaging (DWI), which quantifies water molecular diffusion with an apparent diffusion coefficient (ADC) value, has been shown to be sensitive for detecting early injury to the parotid glands in pSS. Nevertheless, only the mean ADC value has been obtained from one or several regions of interest (ROIs) in most previous studies, introducing a sampling error and neglecting the heterogeneity of the parotid injury (Xu, Su, et al., 2017). A recent study has been designed to compare the differences between whole-volume ADC histogram and texture analyses for parotid glands in pSS patients with different activities and to explore the potential of these indexes in predicting disease activity in pSS patients (Chu et al., 2018). It was shown that the entropy value derived from whole-volume ADC histogram and texture analyses of the parotid glands had great potential for predicting the disease activity of pSS. The diagnostic performance of whole-volume ADC histogram and texture analyses can be further improved by combining parotid entropy with anti-SSB and the MRI morphology, which can serve as an imaging biomarker of pSS disease activity.

3.4 Therapy

For the management of sicca symptoms, tear substitution therapy consisting of high-viscosity eye drops and gels is commonly used. A short-term course of topical anti-inflammatory agents including cyclosporin A (CsA), and non-steroidal anti-inflammatory drugs might also be required for SS patients with severe or refractory keratoconjunctivitis sicca (Perry et al., 2008). However, persistent burning after the application of ophthalmic solutions of CsA may reduce medication adherence. A randomized clinical trial (RCT) was conducted to evaluate the efficacy of an ophthalmic solution containing 0.1% fluorometholone (FML) and 0.1% sodium hyaluronate (HA) for the treatment of ocular dryness in SS patients (Lin & Gong, 2015). It was shown that treatment using topical 0.1% FML provided faster improvement in the symptoms of ocular dryness in SS patients compared with topical 0.5% CsA.

Regarding management of systemic involvement, only a few clinical trials have been done, and evidence-based guidelines are still lacking. Non-biological therapies are still the mainstay of treatment. A retrospective study compared between the combination of cyclophosphamide and glucocorticoids alone in the treatment of pSS patients with chronic tubulointerstitial nephritis (TIN) (Shen et al., 2017). Combination therapy has been proven with better tolerability and effectiveness for patients with pSS-associated TIN, especially those with higher IgG levels and poor baseline renal function.

Previously, increased frequency of circulating Tfh cells was found in pSS patients and was positively correlated with the ESSDAI score (Szabo et al., 2013). Mesenchymal stem cells (MSCs), which are pluripotent stem cells with the capacity to differentiate into different cell lineages and to modulate T and B lymphocytes, dendritic cells and natural killer cells, have been used for the treatment of various autoimmune diseases including SS. In 2012, researchers in China revealed, for the first time, that bone marrow MSCs in SS-like NOD/Ltj mice and human SS patients were defective in immunoregulatory functions. Treatment with allogeneic MSCs suppressed autoimmunity and restored salivary gland secretory function in both mouse models and SS patients. It was shown that MSC treatment directed T cells toward Treg and Th2, while suppressing Th17 and Tfh responses, and alleviating disease symptoms (Xu et al., 2012). Afterwards, umbilical cord MSCs were also suggested to have an inhibitory effect on the differentiation of cTfh cells in pSS patients via the secretion of indoleamine 2,3-dioxygenase (IDO) (Liu, Su, et al., 2015).

In recent years, the rise of low-dose IL-2 therapy as a novel biologic treatment for autoimmune diseases has gained broad interest in the field of Rheumatology and Immunology (Li, He, & Yu, 2017). In our previous studies, we demonstrated that low-dose IL-2 therapy could suppress Tfh and Th17 cells in humans (He et al., 2016). In addition, using a mouse model, we revealed that suppression of Tfh and Th17 cells was as sensitive to low-dose IL-2 as the promotion of Treg cells. In patients with pSS, the absolute number of circulating CD4 Treg cells has been shown significantly lower than that in healthy patients. Notably, low-dose IL-2 treatment restored CD4 Treg cells and the ratio of Th17/Treg which are helpful for controlling disease activity (Miao et al., 2018). In our recent randomized, double-blind, placebo-controlled clinical trial with low-dose IL-2 in the treatment of pSS patients, disease activity assessed by the ESSDAI, the EULAR SS Patient Reported Index (ESSPRI), and the multidimensional fatigue inventory (MFI-20) were decreased significantly in IL-2 group compared to the placebo group. The resolution of systemic manifestations was observed after IL-2 treatment, including decreased pulmonary and renal tubular abnormalities, arthritis, thrombocytopenia, leukopenia and fatigue. Immunological analyses revealed expansion of Treg and B10 cells, with reduction of serum IL-17A and IFNα in IL-2 group. These findings strengthen the concept of immunoregulation in the treatment of SS.

In China, TCM is a common complementary and alternative medicine (CAM) therapy widely accepted by patients. TCM therapy followed traditional treatment principles to nourish *yin*, moisten dryness and generate body fluids, replenish *qi* and blood. The herbal medicines include multicomponent decoctions, concentrated herbal granules, herbal injections, and patent medicines. A variety of RCTs and population-based studies have been performed in treating SS (Chang et al., 2015; Wu, Li, Fan, Yu, & Chen, 2013). In 2012, a systemic review analyzed 52 RCTs, testing various TCMs in the treatment of pSS (Luo, Li, Liu, Andrew, & George, 2012). The findings from these trials suggested that TCM, delivered either in conjunction with conventional medicine or as a sole treatment, may be more effective than conventional medicine in managing pSS symptoms, with particular reference to lacrimal and salivary gland function. However, a high risk of bias in these studies and the heterogeneity of the TCM intervention and outcome assessment suggested that these positive findings must be interpreted with considerable caution. Since then, more studies have been done to assess the effectiveness and safety of TCM therapies in the treatment of SS. Among these TCM, total glucosides of peony (TGP) is one with the most evidence.

TGP is extracted from the root of *Paeonia lactiflora* pall. It has been demonstrated to have immunomodulatory effects by inhibiting dendritic cell maturation and selectively blocking TLR4/5 activation, sequentially leading to the impairment of Th1 and Th17 differentiation and of associated cytokines in vivo. In non-obese diabetic (NOD) mice model, saliva flow rate (SFR), submandibular glands (SMG) index, and the ration of Treg were significantly higher in TGP group compared to normal saline group (Li, He, Li, Zheng, & Hua, 2013). TGP improves pathological damage of submandibular glands of NOD mice with SS by upregulating Aquaporin-5 (AQP-5) and its mRNA expression in submandibular glands (Wu, Pu, Yu, & Li, 2015). In patients with pSS, TGP increases the expression of programmed cell death protein 1 (PD-1) and its relevant ligand PD-L1 in the peripheral blood mononuclear cells. In a recent RCT, the ESSPRI, dry eyes/throat/vagina visual analog scale (VAS), fatigue VAS, mental discomfort VAS, patient global assessment (PGA), Schirmer's test, and ESR were all improved more in the TGP group than in the placebo group.

4. Other autoimmune diseases

Other autoimmune diseases (AIDs), such as systemic sclerosis (SSc), polymyositis (PM)/dermatomyositis (DM) and Primary biliary cholangitis (PBC), et al., are also multifactorial diseases, characterized by activation of abnormal autoimmune responses. Genetic susceptibility, environmental and infectious factors are important in the development of these diseases. Recent findings revealed novel biomarkers and therapeutic targets.

4.1 Pathogenesis

4.1.1 Genetic predisposition

Genetic susceptibility in systemic sclerosis(SSc) has been investigated in a Chinese SSc patient cohort. HLA-DRB1*15:02 and *16:02 were identified as the major SSc-risk allele subtypes in China. The susceptible genes had been linked with different antibody patterns. HLA-DRB1*15:02 was significantly associated with anti-centromere autoantibodies (ACA), and HLA-DRB1*16:02 with anti-topoisomerase I autoantibodies (ATA). Another study showed that the frequency of HLA-DRB1*11:04 alleles was significantly increased in SSc patients with ATA. However, HLA-DRB1*01:01 *04:06, *07:01 and *13:02 were protective alleles in Chinese SSc patients (He et al., 2014; Xu et al., 2019). As reported, HLA-DPB1*03:01 significantly increased in Chinese SSc patients and was associated with the development of pulmonary fibrosis. DPB1*04 was also highly expressed in SSc patients with ACA (Wang, Guo, et al., 2014). In addition, Non-HLA genes such as polymorphisms in interferon regulatory factor (IRF) genes had been proved to be associated with SSc (Xu, Wang, Tian, Liu, & Yang, 2016). Copy number variation (CNV) of HLA-DQA1 and APOBEC3A/B were shown to contribute to the SSc susceptibility in a Chinese Han population (Guo et al., 2016). These findings promote the knowledge of genetics of SSc in China.

Lin et al. performed a two-stage genome-wide association study (GWAS) in Han Chinese ankylosing spondylitis (AS) patients. They identified two new loci between EDIL3 and HAPLN1 at 5q14.3 and within ANO6 at 12q12. It was shown that rs13202464 within the MHC region mainly represented the risk effect of HLA-B*27 variants in Chinese (Lin et al., 2011). Liu et al. also found six loci non-MHC region associated with AS in Chinese population (Liu, Pu, et al., 2019). These newly discovered loci suggested the potential involvement in the etiology of AS.

In GWAS and functional studies conducted in Chinese Behçet's disease (BD) patients, STAT4 was identified as a novel locus associated with BD. STAT4 upregulated the production of inflammatory cytokines, such as IL-17, suggesting a potential pathway in the pathogenesis of BD (Hou et al., 2012). IL-23R, LACC1, CEBPB-PTPN1, ADO-EGR2, RIPK2, CD6 and CD11c had also been reported to play important roles in the susceptibility of BD in China (Hou et al., 2012; Jiang et al., 2010; Zheng et al., 2016). In addition, Hou et al. found that a high copy number of C4A increased risk for BD by enhancing IL-6 production (Hou et al., 2013).

IgG4-related disease (IgG4-RD) is a systemic autoimmune disease involving multiple manifestations, characterized by elevated serum IgG4 and infiltration of $IgG4^+$ plasma cells in tissues and mass formation of organs. Higgs et al. used whole transcriptomic sequencing to identify both cell and pathway-associated activation in IgG4-RD patients with salivary gland lesions (RD-SG), without SG lesions (RD-nonSG) and retroperitoneal fibrosis (RF). It was shown that the mRNA levels of IgG4 and IgE, genes specific for Th2 cells, eosinophils, and neutrophils were over-expressed in RD-SG and RD-nonSG. B-cell signature was suppressed in patients group vs controls, while Th1, Th2, Treg, and eosinophil gene signatures increased in patients without treatment. The results suggested the imbalance of immune and inflammatory cells in IgG4-related disease (Higgs et al., 2017).

Primary biliary cholangitis (PBC) is an autoimmune liver disease. Qiu et al. conducted a GWAS study and found 14 PBC risk loci including

6p21 (HLA-DRA and DPB1), 17q12 (ORMDL3), 3q13.33 (CD80), 2q32.3 (STAT1/STAT4), 3q25.33 (IL12A), 4q24 (NF-κB) and 22q13.1 (RPL3/SYNGR1). They also identified variants in IL21, IL21R, CD28/CTLA4/ICOS, CD58, ARID3A and IL16 as novel PBC risk loci (Qiu et al., 2017). Yin et al. identified PTPN1 as a susceptible gene for psoriasis, which might affect the risk of psoriasis via modulating the function of TYK2 kinase (Yin et al., 2017).

4.1.2 Epigenomics and autoimmunity

Epigenetic studies in SSc had been published involving histone post-translational modifications, DNA methylation, microRNAs and long non-coding RNAs. Hypomethylation had been reported in patients with scleroderma, especially in fibroblasts and T cells. Overexpression of JMJD3 might led to demethylation of H3K27me3 in $CD4^+$ T cells from patients with SSc (Wang, Xiao, et al., 2015). Demethylation of CD11a regulatory elements and CD70 promoter region might contribute to the over-expression of CD11a and CD70 in $CD4^+$ T cells, thus mediate autoimmune responses and fibrosis in SSc (Jiang et al., 2012; Wang, Shu, et al., 2014). Demethylation of CD40L regulatory elements on the inactive X chromosome also increased the expression of CD40L in $CD4^+$ T cells from female patients with SSc (Lian et al., 2012).

There was growing evidence that specific microRNAs played their roles in the pathogenesis of idiopathic inflammatory myopathy. Study showed that the expression of miR-196a-5p was negatively associated with polymyositis (PM). In addition, miR-193b-3p was negatively associated with dermatomyositis (DM) and PM. The study pave the way on further diagnostic and mechanistic studies of DM and PM (Gao et al., 2019).

Psoriasis is characterized by aberrant keratinocyte proliferation and differentiation in the epidermis. T cells play important role in the pathogenesis of psoriasis. Wu et al. found that miR-210 was highly expressed in psoriasis patients. MiR-210 might inhibit the expression of STAT6 and LYN, subsequently induce the differentiation of Th1/Th17, however, inhibit Th2 differentiation. Wu et al. also found that HIF-1α recruited P300 and promoted histone H3 acetylation in the miR-210 promoter region, which induced the production of TGF-β and IL-23, and enhanced miR-210 expression. The study suggested that miR-210 might be a potential therapeutic target for psoriasis (Wu et al., 2018). In previous studies, DNA methylation was involved in the pathogenesis of psoriasis. Zhang et al. characterized whole-genome DNA methylation patterns in skin lesions from psoriasis patients. They identified differentially methylated regions (DMRs) and showed that the number of hypermethylated DMRs were markedly higher than that of hypomethylated DMRs in psoriatic skin. In this study, the genes PDCD5 and TIMP2 were confirmed the methylation status (Zhang, Zhao, et al., 2013).

Interleukin-17 (IL-17) plays important role in the development of many inflammatory autoimmune diseases (Huang et al., 2017). It had been reported that IL-17 downregulated miR-23b in inflammatory lesions of autoimmune diseases such as multiple sclerosis. In turn, miR-23b suppressed NF-κB activation induced by IL-17, tumor necrosis factor α (TNF-α) or IL-1β and downregulated the expression of inflammatory cytokine, thus inhibited the development of autoimmune diseases (Zhu et al., 2012).

4.1.3 Infections

Microbiota are main environmental factor and have been considered to contribute to the pathogenesis of Behçet's disease (BD). High level of Bilophila spp., a sulfate-reducing bacteria (SRB) and several opportunistic pathogens (e.g., Parabacteroides spp. and Paraprevotella spp.) were shown in fecal samples from active BD patients, along with a reduced level of butyrate-producing bacteria (BPB) Clostridium spp. and methanogens (Methanoculleus spp. Methanomethylophilus spp.) (Ye, Zhang, et al., 2018). Ye et al. also found the BD-enriched SRB and opportunistic pathogens were positively associated with each other, but negatively correlated with BPB and methanogens. It was shown that fecal microbiota transplantation from BD patients to mice significantly exacerbated EAU activity and increased the production of IL-17 and IFN-γ.

Evidence revealed that the interaction between bacteria and fungi might play an important role in AS development (Li, Dai, et al., 2019). In a quantitative metagenomics study in China, the amount of Prevotella melaninogenica and Prevotella copri were increased in AS patients (Wen et al., 2017). In addition, the Bifidobacterium genus also accumulated in AS patients. These results suggested the association of gut microbiome with development of AS.

Recent evidence indicated that indigenous Clostridium species induced the differentiation of colonic regulatory T cells (Tregs). Supplement of probiotics Clostridium butyricum CGMCC0313.1 (CB0313.1) could inhibit the onset of diabetes by upregulating pancreatic Tregs and rebalancing Th1/Th2/Th17 cells differentiation in non-obese diabetic (NOD) mice (Jia et al., 2017). In addition, dysbiosis was also found in the gut microbiome in PBC, suggesting a potential therapeutic target and diagnostic biomarker for PBC (Tang et al., 2018).

4.2 Biomarkers for diagnosis

Biomarkers including autoantibodies and specific serum soluble mediators are important in diagnosis and disease monitoring in autoimmune diseases. Based on serum profiling analysis using a human proteome microarray, Hu et al. reported six novel PBC autoantigens with high sensitivities and specificities, including hexokinase-1, Kelch-like protein 7, Kelch-like protein 12, zinc finger, BTB domain-containing protein 2, and eukaryotic translation initiation factor 2C, subunit 1 (Hu et al., 2012). Yuan et al. found that anti-LL-37 and ADAMTS-L5 antibodies were markedly increased in patients with psoriasis and correlated with disease activities. Notably, patients with psoriatic arthritis (PsA) had significantly higher anti-ADAMTS-L5 and anti-LL-37 autoantibody levels, compared to those without PsA (Yuan et al., 2019). Cheng et al. screened novel autoantigens or autoantibodies in circulating immune complexes (CICs) from BD patients, and identified 17 potential antigens. Among these candidates, anti-tubulin-α-1c antibody was proved to be a promising biomarker in diagnosis and severity evaluation of BD, correlating with the risk of deep venous thrombosis and erythema nodosum (Cheng et al., 2018).

Recently, Wang et al. identified two N-glycans as biomarkers with high sensitivity and specificity for AS. These specific N-glycans of IgG provided new insight into the pathogenesis of AS and might be potentially diagnostic tool in future (Wang et al., 2019). It was observed in a study that patients with type 1 diabetes (T1D) had increased levels and enzymatic activities of neutrophil elastase (NE) and proteinase 3 (PR3), which might serve as biomarkers for the diagnosis of T1D (Wang, Xiao, et al., 2014). In addition, serum β-Defensin 2 (BD-2) had been found to be a biomarker of IL-17-driven skin pathology in psoriasis patients (Kolbinger et al., 2017).

4.3 Novel treatments

Mesenchymal stromal cells (MSC) are multipotent cell population with self-renewal and the ability to differentiate into different cells. It had been reported that mesenchymal stem cell transplantation (MSCT) was effect and safe in the treatment of autoimmune diseases, including SLE, SS and SSc. It was shown that MSCT could effectively mitigate osteopenia in SSc mice by transferring miR-151-5p to the recipient bone marrow MSCs in SSc mice and inhibiting IL4Rα expression, thus downregulating mTOR pathway activation and enhancing osteogenic differentiation. The study provided a specific target for the treatment of SSc (Chen et al., 2015, 2017; Liang, Zhang, et al., 2018).

Thioredoxin (Trx)-1 is one of the principal intracellular redox protein mediating the redox regulatory function. In a recent study in China, mice with bleomycin-induced SSc were subcutaneously injected with Trx-1-overexpressing BMSCs in hypoxic conditions. The study showed that Trx-1-overexpressing BMSCs alleviated hypoxia-induced apoptosis and fibrosis by inhibiting the production of TGF-β. In addition, Trx-1-overexpressing BMSCs could promote the formation of tubular-like structures and angiogenesis in SSc. The study suggested the therapeutic potential of engineered BMSCs in SSc patients (Jiang et al., 2017).

All-trans RA (atRA) is the active derivative of vitamin A. Lu et al. found that atRA sustained the expression of Foxp3 and the suppressive function of human natural Tregs (nTregs) by suppressing the upregulation of IL-1 receptor (IL-1R), accelerating IL-6R downregulation, preventing the upregulation of STIP1 homology and U-Box containing protein 1 on $Foxp3^+$ cells and also increasing histone acetylation and CpG demethylation in Foxp3 locus. Lu et al. pretreated human nTregs with atRA and transferred them to xenograft-vs-host disease mice. The results showed nTregs pretreated with atRA significantly upregulated the suppressive effects, suggesting that atRA might be used for the treatment of autoimmune diseases. Sun et al. also reported atRA as a novel therapy of SSc (Sun et al., 2018).

Multiple sclerosis (MS) is characterized by autoimmune damage to the central nervous system. Du et al. found that activation of kappa opioid receptor (KOR) alleviates the symptoms of MS. As reported, KOR promoted the differentiation oligodendrocyte and myelination both in vitro and in vivo. The study provided a new treatment target of MS (Du et al., 2016). In addition, anti-human CD6 monoclonal antibody and polysaccharide from *Eclipta prostrata* had been administrated to EAE mice and showed significant effect on EAE treatment, suggesting which might potentially become new therapies in MS (Li, Shi, et al., 2018; Li, Singer, et al., 2017).

References

An, Y., Liu, T., He, D., Wu, L., Li, J., Liu, Y., et al. (2017). The usage of biological DMARDs and clinical remission of rheumatoid arthritis in China: A real-world large scale study. *Clinical Rheumatology*, *36*(1), 35–43.

An, Y., Zhou, Y., Bi, L., Liu, B., Wang, H., Lin, J., et al. (2019). Combined immunosuppressive treatment (CIST) in lupus nephritis: A multicenter, randomized controlled study. *Clinical Rheumatology*, *38*(4), 1047–1054.

Bao, H., Liu, Z. H., Xie, H. L., Hu, W. X., Zhang, H. T., & Li, L. S. (2008). Successful treatment of class V+IV lupus nephritis with multitarget therapy. *Journal of the American Society of Nephrology*, *19*(10), 2001–2010.

Bikker, A., van Woerkom, J. M., Kruize, A. A., Wenting-van Wijk, M., de Jager, W., Bijlsma, J. W., et al. (2010). Increased expression of interleukin-7 in labial salivary glands of patients with primary Sjogren's syndrome correlates with increased inflammation. *Arthritis and Rheumatism*, *62*(4), 969–977.

Chang, C. M., Chu, H. T., Wei, Y. H., Chen, F. P., Wang, S., Wu, P. C., et al. (2015). The core pattern analysis on Chinese herbal medicine for Sjogren's syndrome: A nationwide population-based study. *Scientific Reports*, *5*, 9541.

Chang, C. P., Shiau, Y. C., Wang, J. J., Ho, S. T., & Kao, A. (2002). Abnormal regional cerebral blood flow on 99mTc ECD brain SPECT in patients with primary Sjogren's syndrome and normal findings on brain magnetic resonance imaging. *Annals of the Rheumatic Diseases*, *61*(9), 774–778.

Chen, C., Akiyama, K., Wang, D., Xu, X., Li, B., Moshaverinia, A., et al. (2015). mTOR inhibition rescues osteopenia in mice with systemic sclerosis. *The Journal of Experimental Medicine*, *212*(1), 73–91.

Chen, H. Y., Guo, J. L., & Li, Z. G. (2008). Significance of anti-cell membrane-associated DNA (mDNA) antibodies in systemic lupus erythematosus. *Clinical Rheumatology*, *27*(2), 183–187.

Chen, Q., Li, X., He, W., Zhang, H., Gao, A., Cheng, Y., et al. (2007). The epitope study of alpha-fodrin autoantibody in primary Sjogren's syndrome. *Clinical and Experimental Immunology*, *149*(3), 497–503.

Chen, G., Li, N., Zang, Y. C., Zhang, D., He, D., Feng, G., et al. (2007). Vaccination with selected synovial T cells in rheumatoid arthritis. *Arthritis and Rheumatism*, *56*(2), 453–463.

Chen, X., Sun, X., Yang, W., Yang, B., Zhao, X., Chen, S., et al. (2018). An autoimmune disease variant of IgG1 modulates B cell activation and differentiation. *Science*, *362*(6415), 700–705.

Chen, C., Wang, D., Moshaverinia, A., Liu, D., Kou, X., Yu, W., et al. (2017). Mesenchymal stem cell transplantation in tight-skin mice identifies miR-151-5p as a therapeutic target for systemic sclerosis. *Cell Research*, *27*(4), 559–577.

Chen, W., Wang, J., Xu, Z., Huang, F., Qian, W., Ma, J., et al. (2018). Apremilast ameliorates experimental arthritis via suppression of Th1 and Th17 cells and enhancement of CD4(+)Foxp3(+) regulatory T cells differentiation. *Frontiers in Immunology*, *9*, 1662.

Cheng, Y., Zhao, X., Chen, Y., Li, Y., Jia, R., Zhu, L., et al. (2018). Circulating immune complexome analysis identified anti-tubulin-alpha-1c as an inflammation associated autoantibody with promising diagnostic value for Behçet's disease. *PLoS One*, *13*(6), e0199047.

Chu, C., Wang, F., Zhang, H., Zhu, Y., Wang, C., Chen, W., et al. (2018). Whole-volume ADC histogram and texture analyses of parotid glands as an image biomarker in evaluating disease activity of primary Sjogren's syndrome. *Scientific Reports*, *8*(1), 15387.

Cornec, D., Jousse-Joulin, S., Pers, J. O., Marhadour, T., Cochener, B., Boisrame-Gastrin, S., et al. (2013). Contribution of salivary gland ultrasonography to the diagnosis of Sjogren's syndrome: Toward new diagnostic criteria? *Arthritis and Rheumatism*, *65*(1), 216–225.

Cui, L., Elzakra, N., Xu, S., Xiao, G. G., Yang, Y., & Hu, S. (2017). Investigation of three potential autoantibodies in Sjogren's syndrome and associated MALT lymphoma. *Oncotarget*, *8*(18), 30039–30049.

Cui, Y., Xia, L., Li, L., Zhao, Q., Chen, S., & Gu, Z. (2018). Anxiety and depression in primary Sjogren's syndrome: A cross-sectional study. *BMC Psychiatry*, *18*(1), 131.

De Vita, S., Lorenzon, G., Rossi, G., Sabella, M., & Fossaluzza, V. (1992). Salivary gland echography in primary and secondary Sjogren's syndrome. *Clinical and Experimental Rheumatology*, *10*(4), 351–356.

Deng, J., Liu, Y., Yang, M., Wang, S., Zhang, M., Wang, X., et al. (2012). Leptin exacerbates collagen-induced arthritis via enhancement of Th17 cell response. *Arthritis and Rheumatism*, *64*(11), 3564–3573.

Du, Y., Cui, Y., Liu, X., Hu, F., Yang, Y., Wu, X., et al. (2014). Contribution of functional LILRA3, but not nonfunctional LILRA3, to sex bias in susceptibility and severity of anti-citrullinated protein antibody-positive rheumatoid arthritis. *Arthritis & Rhematology*, *66*(4), 822–830.

Du, C., Duan, Y., Wei, W., Cai, Y., Chai, H., Lv, J., et al. (2016). Kappa opioid receptor activation alleviates experimental autoimmune encephalomyelitis and promotes oligodendrocyte-mediated remyelination. *Nature Communications*, *7*, 11120.

Du, Y., Su, Y., He, J., Yang, Y., Shi, Y., Cui, Y., et al. (2015). Impact of the leucocyte immunoglobulin-like receptor A3 (LILRA3) on susceptibility and subphenotypes of systemic lupus erythematosus and Sjogren's syndrome. *Annals of the Rheumatic Diseases*, *74*(11), 2070–2075.

Duan, X. W., Zhang, X. L., Mao, S. Y., Shang, J. J., & Shi, X. D. (2015). Efficacy and safety evaluation of a combination of iguratimod and methotrexate therapy for active rheumatoid arthritis patients: A randomized controlled trial. *Clinical Rheumatology*, *34*(9), 1513–1519.

Feng, X., Che, N., Liu, Y., Chen, H., Wang, D., Li, X., et al. (2014). Restored immunosuppressive effect of mesenchymal stem cells on B cells after olfactory 1/early B cell factor-associated zinc-finger protein down-regulation in patients with systemic lupus erythematosus. *Arthritis & Rhematology*, *66*(12), 3413–3423.

Fu, W., Liu, X., Lin, X., Feng, H., Sun, L., Li, S., et al. (2018). Deficiency in T follicular regulatory cells promotes autoimmunity. *The Journal of Experimental Medicine*, *215*(3), 815–825.

Gao, H., Zhang, X. W., He, J., Zhang, J., An, Y., Sun, Y., et al. (2018). Prevalence, risk factors, and prognosis of interstitial lung disease in a large cohort of Chinese primary Sjogren syndrome patients: A case-control study. *Medicine (Baltimore)*, *97*(24), e11003.

Gao, S., Zhang, H., Zuo, X., Xiao, Y., Liu, D., Zhu, H., et al. (2019). Integrated comparison of the miRNAome and mRNAome in muscles of dermatomyositis and polymyositis reveals common and specific miRNA-mRNAs. *Epigenomics*, *11*(1), 23–33.

Guo, K., Bu, X., Yang, C., Cao, X., Bian, H., Zhu, Q., et al. (2018). Treatment effects of the second-generation tyrosine kinase inhibitor dasatinib on autoimmune arthritis. *Frontiers in Immunology*, *9*, 3133.

Guo, J., Gu, M., Zhang, W., Liu, Y., Qian, C., & Deng, A. (2018). Aberrant IL-35 levels in patients with primary Sjogren's syndrome. *Scandinavian Journal of Immunology*, *88*(5), e12718.

Guo, S., Li, Y., Wang, Y., Chu, H., Chen, Y., Liu, Q., et al. (2016). Copy number variation of HLA-DQA1 and APOBEC3A/3B contribute to the susceptibility of systemic sclerosis in the Chinese Han population. *The Journal of Rheumatology*, *43*(5), 880–886.

Guo, N., Ye, S., Zhang, K., Yu, X., Cui, H., Yang, X., et al. (2019). A critical epitope in CD147 facilitates memory CD4(+) T-cell hyper-activation in rheumatoid arthritis. *Cellular & Molecular Immunology*, *16*(6), 568–579.

Guo, J., Zhang, T., Cao, H., Li, X., Liang, H., Liu, M., et al. (2019). Sequencing of the MHC region defines HLA-DQA1 as the major genetic risk for seropositive rheumatoid arthritis in Han Chinese population. *Annals of the Rheumatic Diseases*, *78*(6), 773–780.

Han, M., Li, Y., Liu, S., Jiang, S., Yuan, L., Xia, L., et al. (2018). Elevation of serum IL-35 in patients with primary Sjogren's syndrome. *Journal of Interferon & Cytokine Research, 38*(10), 452–456.

Han, X., Wang, Y., Zhang, X., Qin, Y., Qu, B., Wu, L., et al. (2016). MicroRNA-130b ameliorates murine lupus nephritis through targeting the type I interferon pathway on renal mesangial cells. *Arthritis & Rhematology, 68*(9), 2232–2243.

Han, J. W., Zheng, H. F., Cui, Y., Sun, L. D., Ye, D. Q., Hu, Z., et al. (2009). Genome-wide association study in a Chinese Han population identifies nine new susceptibility loci for systemic lupus erythematosus. *Nature Genetics, 41*(11), 1234–1237.

He, J., Chen, Q. L., & Li, Z. G. (2006). Antibodies to alpha-fodrin derived peptide in Sjogren's syndrome. *Annals of the Rheumatic Diseases, 65*(4), 549–550.

He, J., Guo, J. P., Ding, Y., Li, Y. N., Pan, S. S., Liu, Y., et al. (2011). Diagnostic significance of measuring antibodies to cyclic type 3 muscarinic acetylcholine receptor peptides in primary Sjogren's syndrome. *Rheumatology (Oxford), 50*(5), 879–884.

He, J., Qiang, L., Ding, Y., Wei, P., Li, Y. N., Hua, H., et al. (2012). The role of muscarinic acetylcholine receptor type 3 polypeptide (M3RP205-220) antibody in the saliva of patients with primary Sjogren's syndrome. *Clinical and Experimental Rheumatology, 30*(3), 322–326.

He, J., Tsai, L. M., Leong, Y. A., Hu, X., Ma, C. S., Chevalier, N., et al. (2013). Circulating precursor CCR7(lo)PD-1(hi) CXCR5(+) CD4(+) T cells indicate Tfh cell activity and promote antibody responses upon antigen reexposure. *Immunity, 39*(4), 770–781.

He, D., Wang, J., Yi, L., Guo, X., Guo, S., Guo, G., et al. (2014). Association of the HLA-DRB1 with scleroderma in Chinese population. *PLoS One, 9*(9), e106939.

He, P., Wu, L. F., Bing, P. F., Xia, W., Wang, L., Xie, F. F., et al. (2019). SAMD9 is a (epi-) genetically regulated anti-inflammatory factor activated in RA patients. *Molecular and Cellular Biochemistry, 456*(1-2), 135–144.

He, J., Zhang, X., Wei, Y., Sun, X., Chen, Y., Deng, J., et al. (2016). Low-dose interleukin-2 treatment selectively modulates CD4(+) T cell subsets in patients with systemic lupus erythematosus. *Nature Medicine, 22*(9), 991–993.

He, J., Zhao, J., & Li, Z. (2008). Mucosal administration of alpha-fodrin inhibits experimental Sjogren's syndrome autoimmunity. *Arthritis Research & Therapy, 10*(2), R44.

Higgs, B. W., Liu, Y., Guo, J., Sebastian, Y., Morehouse, C., Zhu, W., et al. (2017). High-throughput RNA sequencing reveals distinct gene signatures in active IgG4-related disease. *Scientific Reports*, 7(1), 17567.

Hocevar, A., Ambrozic, A., Rozman, B., Kveder, T., & Tomsic, M. (2005). Ultrasonographic changes of major salivary glands in primary Sjogren's syndrome. Diagnostic value of a novel scoring system. *Rheumatology (Oxford), 44*(6), 768–772.

Hou, S., Qi, J., Liao, D., Zhang, Q., Fang, J., Zhou, Y., et al. (2013). Copy number variations of complement component C4 are associated with Behçet's disease but not with ankylosing spondylitis associated with acute anterior uveitis. *Arthritis and Rheumatism, 65*(11), 2963–2970.

Hou, S., Yang, Z., Du, L., Jiang, Z., Shu, Q., Chen, Y., et al. (2012). Identification of a susceptibility locus in STAT4 for Behçet's disease in Han Chinese in a genome-wide association study. *Arthritis and Rheumatism, 64*(12), 4104–4113.

Hu, F., Liu, H., Liu, X., Zhang, X., Xu, L., Zhu, H., et al. (2017). Pathogenic conversion of regulatory B10 cells into osteoclast-priming cells in rheumatoid arthritis. *Journal of Autoimmunity, 76*, 53–62.

Hu, F., Mu, R., Zhu, J., Shi, L., Li, Y., Liu, X., et al. (2014). Hypoxia and hypoxia-inducible factor-1alpha provoke toll-like receptor signalling-induced inflammation in rheumatoid arthritis. *Annals of the Rheumatic Diseases, 73*(5), 928–936.

Hu, C. J., Song, G., Huang, W., Liu, G. Z., Deng, C. W., Zeng, H. P., et al. (2012). Identification of new autoantigens for primary biliary cirrhosis using human proteome microarrays. *Molecular & Cellular Proteomics, 11*(9), 669–680.

Hu, F., Zhang, W., Shi, L., Liu, X., Jia, Y., Xu, L., et al. (2018). Impaired CD27(+)IgD(+) B cells with altered gene signature in rheumatoid arthritis. *Frontiers in Immunology*, *9*, 626.

Huang, C. C., Chiou, C. H., Liu, S. C., Hu, S. L., Su, C. M., Tsai, C. H., et al. (2019). Melatonin attenuates TNF-alpha and IL-1beta expression in synovial fibroblasts and diminishes cartilage degradation: Implications for the treatment of rheumatoid arthritis. *Journal of Pineal Research*, *66*(3), e12560.

Huang, J., Yuan, Q., Zhu, H., Yin, L., Hong, S., Dong, Z., et al. (2017). IL-17C/IL-17RE augments T cell function in autoimmune hepatitis. *Journal of Immunology*, *198*(2), 669–680.

Hui, M., Zhao, J., Tian, Z., Wang, J., Qian, J., Yang, X., et al. (2019). Red blood cell distribution width as a potential predictor of survival of pulmonary arterial hypertension associated with primary Sjogren's syndrome: A retrospective cohort study. *Clinical Rheumatology*, *38*(2), 477–485.

Jia, L., Shan, K., Pan, L. L., Feng, N., Lv, Z., Sun, Y., et al. (2017). Clostridium butyricum CGMCC0313.1 protects against autoimmune diabetes by modulating intestinal immune homeostasis and inducing pancreatic regulatory T cells. *Frontiers in Immunology*, *8*, 1345.

Jia, W., Wu, W., Yang, D., Xiao, C., Huang, M., Long, F., et al. (2018). GATA4 regulates angiogenesis and persistence of inflammation in rheumatoid arthritis. *Cell Death & Disease*, *9*(5), 503.

Jiang, H., Xiao, R., Lian, X., Kanekura, T., Luo, Y., Yin, Y., et al. (2012). Demethylation of TNFSF7 contributes to CD70 overexpression in CD4+ T cells from patients with systemic sclerosis. *Clinical Immunology*, *143*(1), 39–44.

Jiang, Z., Yang, P., Hou, S., Du, L., Xie, L., Zhou, H., et al. (2010). IL-23R gene confers susceptibility to Behçet's disease in a Chinese Han population. *Annals of the Rheumatic Diseases*, *69*(7), 1325–1328.

Jiang, L., Yin, J., Ye, L., Yang, J., Hemani, G., Liu, A. J., et al. (2014). Novel risk loci for rheumatoid arthritis in Han Chinese and congruence with risk variants in Europeans. *Arthritis & Rhematology*, *66*(5), 1121–1132.

Jiang, M., Yu, Y., Luo, J., Gao, Q., Zhang, L., Wang, Q., et al. (2017). Bone marrow-derived mesenchymal stem cells expressing thioredoxin 1 attenuate bleomycin-induced skin fibrosis and oxidative stress in scleroderma. *The Journal of Investigative Dermatology*, *137*(6), 1223–1233.

Jiao, Z., Wang, W., Hua, S., Liu, M., Wang, H., Wang, X., et al. (2014). Blockade of Notch signaling ameliorates murine collagen-induced arthritis via suppressing Th1 and Th17 cell responses. *The American Journal of Pathology*, *184*(4), 1085–1093.

Jin, S., Chen, H., Li, Y., Zhong, H., Sun, W., Wang, J., et al. (2018). Maresin 1 improves the Treg/Th17 imbalance in rheumatoid arthritis through miR-21. *Annals of the Rheumatic Diseases*, 77(11), 1644–1652.

Kolbinger, F., Loesche, C., Valentin, M. A., Jiang, X., Cheng, Y., Jarvis, P., et al. (2017). Beta-defensin 2 is a responsive biomarker of IL-17A-driven skin pathology in patients with psoriasis. *The Journal of Allergy and Clinical Immunology*, *139*(3), 923–932 e928.

Li, Z., An, Y., Su, H., Li, X., Xu, J., Zheng, Y., et al. (2018). Tofacitinib with conventional synthetic disease-modifying antirheumatic drugs in Chinese patients with rheumatoid arthritis: Patient-reported outcomes from a phase 3 randomized controlled trial. *International Journal of Rheumatic Diseases*, *21*(2), 402–414.

Li, M., Dai, B., Tang, Y., Lei, L., Li, N., Liu, C., et al. (2019). Altered bacterial-fungal interkingdom networks in the guts of ankylosing spondylitis patients. *mSystems*, *4*(2), e00176-18.

Li, G. Q., Fang, Y. X., Liu, Y., Meng, F. R., Wu, X., Zhang, C. W., et al. (2019). MALAT1-driven inhibition of Wnt signal impedes proliferation and inflammation in fibroblast-like synoviocytes through CTNNB1 promoter methylation in rheumatoid arthritis. *Human Gene Therapy*, *30*(8), 1008–1022.

Li, Y. H., Gao, Y. P., Dong, J., Shi, L. J., Sun, X. L., Li, R., et al. (2018). Identification of a novel autoantibody against self-vimentin specific in secondary Sjogren's syndrome. *Arthritis Research & Therapy*, *20*(1), 30.

Li, C. L., He, J., Li, Z. G., Zheng, L. W., & Hua, H. (2013). Effects of total glucosides of paeony for delaying onset of Sjogren's syndrome: An animal study. *Journal of Cranio-Maxillo-Facial Surgery*, *41*(7), 610–615.

Li, Z., He, J., & Yu, D. (2017). The rise of IL-2 therapy—A picture beyond Treg cells. *Nature Reviews Rheumatology*, *13*(6), 386.

Li, Q. Y., Li, H. Y., Fu, G., Yu, F., Wu, Y., & Zhao, M. H. (2017). Autoantibodies against C-reactive protein influence complement activation and clinical course in lupus nephritis. *Journal of the American Society of Nephrology*, *28*(10), 3044–3054.

Li, Z. G., Mu, R., Dai, Z. P., & Gao, X. M. (2005). T cell vaccination in systemic lupus erythematosus with autologous activated T cells. *Lupus*, *14*(11), 884–889.

Li, C., Mu, R., Guo, J., Wu, X., Tu, X., Liu, X., et al. (2014). Genetic variant in IL33 is associated with susceptibility to rheumatoid arthritis. *Arthritis Research & Therapy*, *16*(2), R105.

Li, C., Mu, R., Lu, X. Y., He, J., Jia, R. L., & Li, Z. G. (2014). Antilymphocyte antibodies in systemic lupus erythematosus: Association with disease activity and lymphopenia. *Journal of Immunology Research*, *2014*, 672126.

Li, N., Shi, S., Yang, F., Wang, H., Su, J., Huang, F., et al. (2018). A polysaccharide from Eclipta prostrata alleviates experimental autoimmune encephalomyelitis through inhibiting Th17 cells. *Carbohydrate Polymers*, *201*, 608–614.

Li, Y., Singer, N. G., Whitbred, J., Bowen, M. A., Fox, D. A., & Lin, F. (2017). CD6 as a potential target for treating multiple sclerosis. *Proceedings of the National Academy of Sciences of the United States of America*, *114*(10), 2687–2692.

Li, R., Sun, J., Ren, L. M., Wang, H. Y., Liu, W. H., Zhang, X. W., et al. (2012). Epidemiology of eight common rheumatic diseases in China: A large-scale cross-sectional survey in Beijing. *Rheumatology (Oxford)*, *51*(4), 721–729.

Li, Y. J., Yang, C. S., Lei, L., Wu, K. F., Yang, P. T., & Xiao, W. G. (2014). Serum nerve grow factor and brain-derived neurotrophic factor profiles in Sjogren's syndrome concomitant with interstitial lung disease. *Clinical Rheumatology*, *33*(8), 1161–1164.

Li, Y., Zhang, K., Chen, H., Sun, F., Xu, J., Wu, Z., et al. (2013). A genome-wide association study in Han Chinese identifies a susceptibility locus for primary Sjogren's syndrome at 7q11.23. *Nature Genetics*, *45*(11), 1361–1365.

Li, R., Zhao, J. X., Su, Y., He, J., Chen, L. N., Gu, F., et al. (2016). High remission and low relapse with prolonged intensive DMARD therapy in rheumatoid arthritis (PRINT): A multicenter randomized clinical trial. *Medicine (Baltimore)*, *95*(28), e3968.

Lian, X., Xiao, R., Hu, X., Kanekura, T., Jiang, H., Li, Y., et al. (2012). DNA demethylation of CD40l in CD4+ T cells from women with systemic sclerosis: A possible explanation for female susceptibility. *Arthritis and Rheumatism*, *64*(7), 2338–2345.

Liang, B., Ge, C., Lonnblom, E., Lin, X., Feng, H., Xiao, L., et al. (2019). The autoantibody response to cyclic citrullinated collagen type II peptides in rheumatoid arthritis. *Rheumatology (Oxford)*, *58*(7), 1623–1633.

Liang, J., Li, X., Zhang, H., Wang, D., Feng, X., Wang, H., et al. (2012). Allogeneic mesenchymal stem cells transplantation in patients with refractory RA. *Clinical Rheumatology*, *31*(1), 157–161.

Liang, H., Peng, B., Dong, C., Liu, L., Mao, J., Wei, S., et al. (2018). Cationic nanoparticle as an inhibitor of cell-free DNA-induced inflammation. *Nature Communications*, *9*(1), 4291.

Liang, J., Zhang, H., Kong, W., Deng, W., Wang, D., Feng, X., et al. (2018). Safety analysis in patients with autoimmune disease receiving allogeneic mesenchymal stem cells infusion: A long-term retrospective study. *Stem Cell Research & Therapy*, *9*(1), 312.

Liao, C. Y., Chien, S. T., Wang, C. C., Chen, I. H., Chiu, H. W., Liu, M. Y., et al. (2015). Sjogren's syndrome associated with protein losing gastroenteropathy manifested by intestinal lymphangiectasia successfully treated with prednisolone and hydroxychloroquine. *Lupus*, *24*(14), 1552–1556.

Liao, T. L., Hsieh, S. L., Chen, Y. M., Chen, H. H., Liu, H. J., Lee, H. C., et al. (2018). Rituximab may cause increased hepatitis C virus viremia in rheumatoid arthritis patients through declining exosomal microRNA-155. *Arthritis & Rhematology*, *70*(8), 1209–1219.

Lin, Z., Bei, J. X., Shen, M., Li, Q., Liao, Z., Zhang, Y., et al. (2011). A genome-wide association study in Han Chinese identifies new susceptibility loci for ankylosing spondylitis. *Nature Genetics*, *44*(1), 73–77.

Lin, T., & Gong, L. (2015). Topical fluorometholone treatment for ocular dryness in patients with Sjogren syndrome: A randomized clinical trial in China. *Medicine (Baltimore)*, *94*(7), e551.

Lin, X., Rui, K., Deng, J., Tian, J., Wang, X., Wang, S., et al. (2015). Th17 cells play a critical role in the development of experimental Sjogren's syndrome. *Annals of the Rheumatic Diseases*, *74*(6), 1302–1310.

Liu, Z., Dong, Z., Liang, X., Liu, J., Xuan, L., Wang, J., et al. (2017). Health-related quality of life and psychological status of women with primary Sjogren's syndrome: A cross-sectional study of 304 Chinese patients. *Medicine (Baltimore)*, *96*(50), e9208.

Liu, F., Feng, X. X., Zhu, S. L., Huang, H. Y., Chen, Y. D., Pan, Y. F., et al. (2018). Sonic hedgehog signaling pathway mediates proliferation and migration of fibroblast-like synoviocytes in rheumatoid arthritis via MAPK/ERK signaling pathway. *Frontiers in Immunology*, *9*, 2847.

Liu, J., Huang, X., Hao, S., Wang, Y., Liu, M., Xu, J., et al. (2018). Peli1 negatively regulates noncanonical NF-kappaB signaling to restrain systemic lupus erythematosus. *Nature Communications*, *9*(1), 1136.

Liu, J. J., Li, R., Gan, Y. Z., Zhang, R. J., Li, J., Cai, Y. M., et al. (2019). Clinical deep remission and related factors in a large cohort of patients with rheumatoid arthritis. *Chinese Medical Journal*, *132*(9), 1009–1014.

Liu, R., Li, X., Zhang, Z., Zhou, M., Sun, Y., Su, D., et al. (2015). Allogeneic mesenchymal stem cells inhibited T follicular helper cell generation in rheumatoid arthritis. *Scientific Reports*, *5*, 12777.

Liu, Y., Liao, X., Wang, Y., Chen, S., Sun, Y., Lin, Q., et al. (2017). Autoantibody to MDM2: A potential serological marker of primary Sjogren's syndrome. *Oncotarget*, *8*(9), 14306–14313.

Liu, Y., Mu, R., Gao, Y. P., Dong, J., Zhu, L., Ma, Y., et al. (2016). A cytomegalovirus peptide-specific antibody alters natural killer cell homeostasis and is shared in several autoimmune diseases. *Cell Host & Microbe*, *19*(3), 400–408.

Liu, J., Pu, W., Li, Y., Ma, Y., Zhu, Q., Wan, W., et al. (2019). Genetic association of non-MHC region with ankylosing spondylitis in a Chinese population. *Annals of the Rheumatic Diseases*, *78*(6), 852–853.

Liu, R., Su, D., Zhou, M., Feng, X., Li, X., & Sun, L. (2015). Umbilical cord mesenchymal stem cells inhibit the differentiation of circulating T follicular helper cells in patients with primary Sjogren's syndrome through the secretion of indoleamine 2,3-dioxygenase. *Rheumatology (Oxford)*, *54*(2), 332–342.

Liu, Z., Wang, J., Lai, J., Wang, Q., Zhao, J., Huang, C., et al. (2018). Is it possible to apply the treat-to-target strategy in primary Sjogren's syndrome-associated pulmonary arterial hypertension? *Clinical Rheumatology*, *37*(11), 2989–2998.

Liu, M., Wu, X., Liu, X., He, J., Su, Y., Guo, J., et al. (2015). Contribution of dendritic cell immunoreceptor (DCIR) polymorphisms in susceptibility of systemic lupus erythematosus and primary Sjogren's syndrome. *Human Immunology*, *76*(11), 808–811.

Liu, Z., Yang, X., Tian, Z., Qian, J., Wang, Q., Zhao, J., et al. (2018). The prognosis of pulmonary arterial hypertension associated with primary Sjogren's syndrome: A cohort study. *Lupus*, *27*(7), 1072–1080.

Liu, W., Zhang, Y., Zhu, W., Ma, C., Ruan, J., Long, H., et al. (2018). Sinomenine inhibits the progression of rheumatoid arthritis by regulating the secretion of inflammatory cytokines and monocyte/macrophage subsets. *Frontiers in Immunology*, *9*, 2228.

Lu, L. J., Bao, C. D., Dai, M., Teng, J. L., Fan, W., Du, F., et al. (2009). Multicenter, randomized, double-blind, controlled trial of treatment of active rheumatoid arthritis with T-614 compared with methotrexate. *Arthritis and Rheumatism*, *61*(7), 979–987.

Lu, X., Guo, J., Zhou, X., Li, R., Liu, X., Zhao, Y., et al. (2011). Deletion of LCE3C_LCE3B is associated with rheumatoid arthritis and systemic lupus erythematosus in the Chinese Han population. *Annals of the Rheumatic Diseases*, *70*(9), 1648–1651.

Lu, Y., Li, L., Lin, Z., Wang, L., Lin, L., Li, M., et al. (2018). A new treatment modality for rheumatoid arthritis: Combined photothermal and photodynamic therapy using Cu7.2 S4 nanoparticles. *Advanced Healthcare Materials*, 7(14), e1800013.

Luan, J., Zhao, Y., Zhang, Y., Miao, J., Li, J., Chen, Z. N., et al. (2017). CD147 blockade as a potential and novel treatment of graft rejection. *Molecular Medicine Reports*, *16*(4), 4593–4602.

Luo, H., Li, X., Liu, J., Andrew, F., & George, L. (2012). Chinese herbal medicine in treating primary Sjogren's syndrome: A systematic review of randomized trials. *Evidence-based Complementary and Alternative Medicine*, *2012*, 640658.

Luo, J., Xu, S., Lv, Y., Huang, X., Zhang, H., Zhu, X., et al. (2019). Clinical features and potential relevant factors of renal involvement in primary Sjogren's syndrome. *International Journal of Rheumatic Diseases*, *22*(2), 182–190.

Lv, Q. W., Zhang, W., Shi, Q., Zheng, W. J., Li, X., Chen, H., et al. (2015). Comparison of Tripterygium wilfordii hook F with methotrexate in the treatment of active rheumatoid arthritis (TRIFRA): A randomised, controlled clinical trial. *Annals of the Rheumatic Diseases*, *74*(6), 1078–1086.

Miao, M., Hao, Z., Guo, Y., Zhang, X., Zhang, S., Luo, J., et al. (2018). Short-term and low-dose IL-2 therapy restores the Th17/Treg balance in the peripheral blood of patients with primary Sjogren's syndrome. *Annals of the Rheumatic Diseases*, 77(12), 1838–1840.

Mo, W. X., Yin, S. S., Chen, H., & Zhang, X. (2018). Amino-bisphosphonates, gammadeltaT cells, and their roles in rheumatoid arthritis. *Annals of the Rheumatic Diseases*, 77(9), e58.

Mo, W. X., Yin, S. S., Chen, H., Zhou, C., Zhou, J. X., Zhao, L. D., et al. (2017). Chemotaxis of Vdelta2 T cells to the joints contributes to the pathogenesis of rheumatoid arthritis. *Annals of the Rheumatic Diseases*, *76*(12), 2075–2084.

Mok, M. Y., & Lau, C. S. (1997). Protein losing enteropathy and primary Sjogren's syndrome. *Clinical and Experimental Rheumatology*, *15*(6), 705.

Nie, H., Zheng, Y., Li, R., Guo, T. B., He, D., Fang, L., et al. (2013). Phosphorylation of FOXP3 controls regulatory T cell function and is inhibited by TNF-alpha in rheumatoid arthritis. *Nature Medicine*, *19*(3), 322–328.

Pan, W., Zhu, S., Dai, D., Liu, Z., Li, D., Li, B., et al. (2015). MiR-125a targets effector programs to stabilize Treg-mediated immune homeostasis. *Nature Communications*, *6*, 7096.

Pang, Y., Tan, Y., Li, Y., Zhang, J., Guo, Y., Guo, Z., et al. (2016). Serum A08 C1q antibodies are associated with disease activity and prognosis in Chinese patients with lupus nephritis. *Kidney International*, *90*(6), 1357–1367.

Perry, H. D., Solomon, R., Donnenfeld, E. D., Perry, A. R., Wittpenn, J. R., Greenman, H. E., et al. (2008). Evaluation of topical cyclosporine for the treatment of dry eye disease. *Archives of Ophthalmology*, *126*(8), 1046–1050.

Qi, Y. Y., Zhou, X. J., Nath, S. K., Sun, C., Wang, Y. N., Hou, P., et al. (2018). A rare variant (rs933717) at FBXO31-MAP1LC3B in Chinese is associated with systemic lupus erythematosus. *Arthritis & Rhematology*, *70*(2), 287–297.

Qiu, F., Tang, R., Zuo, X., Shi, X., Wei, Y., Zheng, X., et al. (2017). A genome-wide association study identifies six novel risk loci for primary biliary cholangitis. *Nature Communications*, *8*, 14828.

Qu, S., Du, Y., Chang, S., Guo, L., Fang, K., Li, Y., et al. (2017). Common variants near IKZF1 are associated with primary Sjogren's syndrome in Han Chinese. *PLoS One*, *12*(5), e0177320.

Ren, H., Wang, W. M., Chen, X. N., Zhang, W., Pan, X. X., Wang, X. L., et al. (2008). Renal involvement and followup of 130 patients with primary Sjogren's syndrome. *The Journal of Rheumatology*, *35*(2), 278–284.

Shao, M., He, J., Zhang, R., Zhang, X., Yang, Y., Li, C., et al. (2019). Interleukin-2 deficiency associated with renal impairment in systemic lupus erythematosus. *Journal of Interferon & Cytokine Research*, *39*(2), 117–124.

Shen, Y., Xie, J., Lin, L., Li, X., Shen, P., Pan, X., et al. (2017). Combination cyclophosphamide/glucocorticoids provide better tolerability and outcomes versus glucocorticoids alone in patients with Sjogren's associated chronic interstitial nephritis. *American Journal of Nephrology*, *46*(6), 473–480.

Shi, J., Sun, X., Zhao, Y., Zhao, J., & Li, Z. (2008). Prevalence and significance of antibodies to citrullinated human papilloma virus-47 E2345-362 in rheumatoid arthritis. *Journal of Autoimmunity*, *31*(2), 131–135.

Song, I. W., Chen, H. C., Lin, Y. F., Yang, J. H., Chang, C. C., Chou, C. T., et al. (2016). Identification of susceptibility gene associated with female primary Sjogren's syndrome in Han Chinese by genome-wide association study. *Human Genetics*, *135*(11), 1287–1294.

Su, Y., Jia, R. L., Han, L., & Li, Z. G. (2007). Role of anti-nucleosome antibody in the diagnosis of systemic lupus erythematosus. *Clinical Immunology*, *122*(1), 115–120.

Sun, J., Li, R., Guo, J., Jia, Y., Sun, X., Liu, Y., et al. (2012). Superior molecularly altered influenza virus hemagglutinin peptide 308-317 inhibits collagen-induced arthritis by inducing CD4+ Treg cell expansion. *Arthritis and Rheumatism*, *64*(7), 2158–2168.

Sun, X. Y., Shi, J., Han, L., Su, Y., & Li, Z. G. (2008). Anti-histones antibodies in systemic lupus erythematosus: Prevalence and frequency in neuropsychiatric lupus. *Journal of Clinical Laboratory Analysis*, *22*(4), 271–277.

Sun, L., Wang, D., Liang, J., Zhang, H., Feng, X., Wang, H., et al. (2010). Umbilical cord mesenchymal stem cell transplantation in severe and refractory systemic lupus erythematosus. *Arthritis and Rheumatism*, *62*(8), 2467–2475.

Sun, X., Xiao, Y., Zeng, Z., Shi, Y., Tang, B., Long, H., et al. (2018). All-trans retinoic acid induces CD4+CD25+FOXP3+ regulatory T cells by increasing FOXP3 demethylation in systemic sclerosis CD4+ T cells. *Journal of Immunology Research*, *2018*, 8658156.

Szabo, K., Papp, G., Barath, S., Gyimesi, E., Szanto, A., & Zeher, M. (2013). Follicular helper T cells may play an important role in the severity of primary Sjogren's syndrome. *Clinical Immunology*, *147*(2), 95–104.

Tang, R., Wei, Y., Li, Y., Chen, W., Chen, H., Wang, Q., et al. (2018). Gut microbial profile is altered in primary biliary cholangitis and partially restored after UDCA therapy. *Gut*, *67*(3), 534–541.

Tzioufas, A. G., & Moutsopoulos, H. M. (2008). Ultrasonography of salivary glands: An evolving approach for the diagnosis of Sjogren's syndrome. *Nature Clinical Practice. Rheumatology*, *4*(9), 454–455.

Wang, H. Y., Cui, T. G., Hou, F. F., Ni, Z. H., Chen, X. M., Lu, F. M., et al. (2008). Induction treatment of proliferative lupus nephritis with leflunomide combined with prednisone: A prospective multi-centre observational study. *Lupus*, *17*(7), 638–644.

Wang, J., Dai, M., Cui, Y., Hou, G., Deng, J., Gao, X., et al. (2018). Association of abnormal elevations in IFIT3 with overactive cyclic GMP-AMP synthase/stimulator of interferon genes signaling in human systemic lupus erythematosus monocytes. *Arthritis & Rhematology*, *70*(12), 2036–2045.

Wang, J. R., Gao, W. N., Grimm, R., Jiang, S., Liang, Y., Ye, H., et al. (2017). A method to identify trace sulfated IgG N-glycans as biomarkers for rheumatoid arthritis. *Nature Communications*, *8*(1), 631.

Wang, J., Guo, X., Yi, L., Guo, G., Tu, W., Wu, W., et al. (2014). Association of HLA-DPB1 with scleroderma and its clinical features in Chinese population. *PLoS One*, *9*(1), e87363.

Wang, Y., Shu, Y., Xiao, Y., Wang, Q., Kanekura, T., Li, Y., et al. (2014). Hypomethylation and overexpression of ITGAL (CD11a) in CD4(+) T cells in systemic sclerosis. *Clinical Epigenetics*, *6*(1), 25.

Wang, T., Sun, X., Zhao, J., Zhang, J., Zhu, H., Li, C., et al. (2015). Regulatory T cells in rheumatoid arthritis showed increased plasticity toward Th17 but retained suppressive function in peripheral blood. *Annals of the Rheumatic Diseases*, *74*(6), 1293–1301.

Wang, J., Wang, C., Liang, Y., Pan, H., Jiang, Z., Li, Z., et al. (2019). Serum IgG N-glycans act as novel serum biomarkers of ankylosing spondylitis. *Annals of the Rheumatic Diseases*, *78*(5), 705–707.

Wang, Q., Xiao, Y., Shi, Y., Luo, Y., Li, Y., Zhao, M., et al. (2015). Overexpression of JMJD3 may contribute to demethylation of H3K27me3 in CD4+ T cells from patients with systemic sclerosis. *Clinical Immunology*, *161*(2), 396–399.

Wang, Y., Xiao, Y., Zhong, L., Ye, D., Zhang, J., Tu, Y., et al. (2014). Increased neutrophil elastase and proteinase 3 and augmented NETosis are closely associated with beta-cell autoimmunity in patients with type 1 diabetes. *Diabetes*, *63*(12), 4239–4248.

Wang, C. H., Yao, H., Chen, L. N., Jia, J. F., Wang, L., Dai, J. Y., et al. (2012). CD147 induces angiogenesis through a vascular endothelial growth factor and hypoxia-inducible transcription factor 1alpha-mediated pathway in rheumatoid arthritis. *Arthritis and Rheumatism*, *64*(6), 1818–1827.

Wang, Q., Zhou, X., Zhao, Y., Xiao, J., Lu, Y., Shi, Q., et al. (2018). Polyphyllin I ameliorates collagen-induced arthritis by suppressing the inflammation response in macrophages through the NF-kappaB pathway. *Frontiers in Immunology*, *9*, 2091.

Wen, T., Li, Y., Wu, M., Sun, X., Bao, X., Lin, Y., et al. (2012). Therapeutic effects of a novel tylophorine analog, NK-007, on collagen-induced arthritis through suppressing tumor necrosis factor alpha production and Th17 cell differentiation. *Arthritis and Rheumatism*, *64*(9), 2896–2906.

Wen, W., Liu, Y., Zhao, C., Sun, X., Zhang, C., & Li, Z. (2015). Clinical and serologic features of primary Sjogren's syndrome concomitant with autoimmune hemolytic anemia: A large-scale cross-sectional study. *Clinical Rheumatology*, *34*(11), 1877–1884.

Wen, C., Zheng, Z., Shao, T., Liu, L., Xie, Z., Le Chatelier, E., et al. (2017). Quantitative metagenomics reveals unique gut microbiome biomarkers in ankylosing spondylitis. *Genome Biology*, *18*(1), 142.

Wen, L., Zhu, C., Zhu, Z., Yang, C., Zheng, X., Liu, L., et al. (2018). Exome-wide association study identifies four novel loci for systemic lupus erythematosus in Han Chinese population. *Annals of the Rheumatic Diseases*, 77(3), 417.

Weng, X., Liu, Y., Cui, S., & Cheng, B. (2018). The role of RORalpha in salivary gland lesions in patients with primary Sjogren's syndrome. *Arthritis Research & Therapy*, *20*(1), 205.

Wu, G. L., Li, T. Y., Fan, Y. S., Yu, G. Y., & Chen, J. (2013). Effect of Chinese herbal medicine for nourishing yin, supplementing qi, and activating blood on the Th1/Th2 immune balance in peripheral blood in patients with primary Sjogren's syndrome. *Chinese Journal of Integrative Medicine*, *19*(9), 696–700.

Wu, G. L., Pu, X. H., Yu, G. Y., & Li, T. Y. (2015). Effects of total glucosides of peony on AQP-5 and its mRNA expression in submandibular glands of NOD mice with Sjogren's syndrome. *European Review for Medical and Pharmacological Sciences*, *19*(1), 173–178.

Wu, L., Qin, Y., Xia, S., Dai, M., Han, X., Wu, Y., et al. (2016). Identification of cyclin-dependent kinase 1 as a novel regulator of type I interferon signaling in systemic lupus erythematosus. *Arthritis & Rhematology*, *68*(5), 1222–1232.

Wu, R., Zeng, J., Yuan, J., Deng, X., Huang, Y., Chen, L., et al. (2018). MicroRNA-210 overexpression promotes psoriasis-like inflammation by inducing Th1 and Th17 cell differentiation. *The Journal of Clinical Investigation*, *128*(6), 2551–2568.

Xiang, Y. J., & Dai, S. M. (2009). Prevalence of rheumatic diseases and disability in China. *Rheumatology International*, *29*(5), 481–490.

Xiao, F., Lin, X., Tian, J., Wang, X., Chen, Q., Rui, K., et al. (2017). Proteasome inhibition suppresses Th17 cell generation and ameliorates autoimmune development in experimental Sjogren's syndrome. *Cellular & Molecular Immunology*, *14*(11), 924–934.

Xu, L., Liu, X., Liu, H., Zhu, L., Zhu, H., Zhang, J., et al. (2017). Impairment of Granzyme B-producing regulatory B cells correlates with exacerbated rheumatoid arthritis. *Frontiers in Immunology*, *8*, 768.

Xu, Y., Mo, N., Jiang, Z., Lu, S., Fu, S., Wei, X., et al. (2019). Human leukocyte antigen (HLA)-DRB1 allele polymorphisms and systemic sclerosis. *Modern Rheumatology*, 1–8. Epub ahead of print.

Xu, X., Su, G., Hu, H., Wang, Y., Hong, X., Shi, H., et al. (2017). Effects of regions of interest methods on apparent coefficient measurement of the parotid gland in early Sjogren's syndrome at 3T MRI. *Acta Radiologica*, *58*(1), 27–33.

Xu, J., Wang, D., Liu, D., Fan, Z., Zhang, H., Liu, O., et al. (2012). Allogeneic mesenchymal stem cell treatment alleviates experimental and clinical Sjogren syndrome. *Blood*, *120*(15), 3142–3151.

Xu, Y., Wang, W., Tian, Y., Liu, J., & Yang, R. (2016). Polymorphisms in STAT4 and IRF5 increase the risk of systemic sclerosis: A meta-analysis. *International Journal of Dermatology*, *55*(4), 408–416.

Xu, L., Xia, M., Guo, J., Sun, X., Li, H., Xu, C., et al. (2016). Impairment on the lateral mobility induced by structural changes underlies the functional deficiency of the lupus-associated polymorphism FcgammaRIIB-T232. *The Journal of Experimental Medicine*, *213*(12), 2707–2727.

Xuan, J., Wang, Y., Xiong, Y., Qian, H., He, Y., & Shi, G. (2018). Investigation of autoantibodies to SP-1 in Chinese patients with primary Sjogren's syndrome. *Clinical Immunology*, *188*, 58–63.

Yan, S., Li, M., Wang, H., Yang, X., Zhao, J., Wang, Q., et al. (2018). Characteristics and risk factors of pulmonary arterial hypertension in patients with primary Sjogren's syndrome. *International Journal of Rheumatic Diseases*, *21*(5), 1068–1075.

Yan, S. M., Zhao, Y., Zeng, X. F., Zhang, F. C., & Dong, Y. (2008). Lung involvement of primary Sjogren's syndrome. *Zhonghua Jie He He Hu Xi Za Zhi*, *31*(7), 513–516.

Yang, Y., Chen, L., Jia, Y., Liu, Y., Wen, L., Liang, Y., et al. (2018). Monoclonal gammopathy in rheumatic diseases. *Clinical Rheumatology*, *37*(7), 1751–1762.

Yang, M., Deng, J., Liu, Y., Ko, K. H., Wang, X., Jiao, Z., et al. (2012). IL-10-producing regulatory B10 cells ameliorate collagen-induced arthritis via suppressing Th17 cell generation. *The American Journal of Pathology*, *180*(6), 2375–2385.

Yang, X., Lin, K., Ni, S., Wang, J., Tian, Q., Chen, H., et al. (2017). Serum connective tissue growth factor is a highly discriminatory biomarker for the diagnosis of rheumatoid arthritis. *Arthritis Research & Therapy*, *19*(1), 257.

Yang, X. K., Liu, J., Chen, S. Y., Li, M., Zhang, M. M., Leng, R. X., et al. (2019). UBASH3A gene polymorphisms and expression profile in rheumatoid arthritis. *Autoimmunity*, *52*(1), 21–26.

Yang, M., Sun, L., Wang, S., Ko, K. H., Xu, H., Zheng, B. J., et al. (2010). Novel function of B cell-activating factor in the induction of IL-10-producing regulatory B cells. *Journal of Immunology*, *184*(7), 3321–3325.

Yang, H. X., Wang, J., Wen, Y. B., Fei, Y. Y., Jiang, M. D., Zhou, M. Y., et al. (2018). Renal involvement in primary Sjogren's syndrome: A retrospective study of 103 biopsy-proven cases from a single center in China. *International Journal of Rheumatic Diseases*, *21*(1), 223–229.

Ye, W., Chen, S., Huang, X., Qin, W., Zhang, T., Zhu, X., et al. (2018). Clinical features and risk factors of neurological involvement in Sjogren's syndrome. *BMC Neuroscience*, *19*(1), 26.

Ye, H., Su, Y., Li, R., Zhao, J., Liu, X., Mei, Y., et al. (2016). Comparison of three classification criteria of rheumatoid arthritis in an inception early arthritis cohort. *Clinical Rheumatology*, *35*(10), 2397–2401.

Ye, H., Zhang, J., Wang, J., Gao, Y., Du, Y., Li, C., et al. (2015). CD4 T-cell transcriptome analysis reveals aberrant regulation of STAT3 and Wnt signaling pathways in rheumatoid arthritis: Evidence from a case-control study. *Arthritis Research & Therapy*, *17*, 76.

Ye, Z., Zhang, N., Wu, C., Zhang, X., Wang, Q., Huang, X., et al. (2018). A metagenomic study of the gut microbiome in Behçet's disease. *Microbiome*, *6*(1), 135.

Yin, X., Lin, Y., Shen, C., Wang, L., Zuo, X., Zheng, X., et al. (2017). Integration of expression quantitative trait loci and pleiotropy identifies a novel psoriasis susceptibility gene, PTPN1. *The Journal of Gene Medicine*, *19*(1–2), e2939.

Yu, D. F., Chen, Y., Han, J. M., Zhang, H., Chen, X. P., Zou, W. J., et al. (2008). MUC19 expression in human ocular surface and lacrimal gland and its alteration in Sjogren syndrome patients. *Experimental Eye Research*, *86*(2), 403–411.

Yuan, Y., Qiu, J., Lin, Z. T., Li, W., Haley, C., Mui, U. N., et al. (2019). Identification of novel autoantibodies associated with psoriatic arthritis. *Arthritis & Rheumatology*, *71*(6), 941–951.

Yue, J., Griffith, J. F., Xiao, F., Shi, L., Wang, D., Shen, J., et al. (2017). Repair of bone Erosion in rheumatoid arthritis by denosumab: A high-resolution peripheral quantitative computed tomography study. *Arthritis Care & Research (Hoboken)*, *69*(8), 1156–1163.

Zeng, Q. Y., Chen, R., Darmawan, J., Xiao, Z. Y., Chen, S. B., Wigley, R., et al. (2008). Rheumatic diseases in China. *Arthritis Research & Therapy*, *10*(1), R17.

Zeng, S. Y., Gong, Y., Zhang, Y. P., Chen, S. B., Chen, J. Y., Lin, C. Q., et al. (2015). Changes in the prevalence of rheumatic diseases in Shantou, China, in the past three decades: A COPCORD study. *PLoS One*, *10*(9), e0138492.

Zeng, T., & Tan, L. (2018). 14-3-3eta protein: A promising biomarker for rheumatoid arthritis. *Biomarkers in Medicine*, *12*(8), 917–925.

Zhang, F., Bae, S. C., Bass, D., Chu, M., Egginton, S., Gordon, D., et al. (2018). A pivotal phase III, randomised, placebo-controlled study of belimumab in patients with systemic lupus erythematosus located in China, Japan and South Korea. *Annals of the Rheumatic Diseases*, *77*(3), 355–363.

Zhang, X. W., Li, C., Ma, X. X., Zhao, J. X., An, Y., Liu, S., et al. (2014). Short-interval lower-dose intravenous cyclophosphamide as induction and maintenance therapy for lupus nephritis: A prospective observational study. *Clinical Rheumatology*, *33*(7), 939–945.

Zhang, X., Mu, R., Wang, X., Xu, C., Duan, T., An, Y., et al. (2015). The impact of rheumatoid arthritis on work capacity in Chinese patients: A cross-sectional study. *Rheumatology (Oxford)*, *54*(8), 1478–1487.

Zhang, N. Z., Shi, C. S., Yao, Q. P., Pan, G. X., Wang, L. L., Wen, Z. X., et al. (1995). Prevalence of primary Sjogren's syndrome in China. *The Journal of Rheumatology*, *22*(4), 659–661.

Zhang, R., Sun, T., Song, L., Zuo, D., & Xiao, W. (2014). Increased levels of serum galectin-3 in patients with primary Sjogren's syndrome: Associated with interstitial lung disease. *Cytokine*, *69*(2), 289–293.

Zhang, W., Zhang, C., Chen, P., Yang, C., Gan, X., Hussain, M., et al. (2016). Circulation autoantibody against Lamin A/C in patients with Sjogren's syndrome. *Oncotarget*, 7(49), 80252–80261.

Zhang, X., Zhang, S., He, J., Hu, F., Liu, H., Li, J., et al. (2015). Ultrasonographic evaluation of major salivary glands in primary Sjogren's syndrome: Comparison of two scoring systems. *Rheumatology (Oxford)*, *54*(9), 1680–1687.

Zhang, X., Zhang, D., Jia, H., Feng, Q., Wang, D., Liang, D., et al. (2015). The oral and gut microbiomes are perturbed in rheumatoid arthritis and partly normalized after treatment. *Nature Medicine*, *21*(8), 895–905.

Zhang, X., Zhang, F., Wu, D., Bao, C., Zhu, P., Zhang, X., et al. (2013). Safety of infliximab therapy in rheumatoid arthritis patients with previous exposure to hepatitis B virus. *International Journal of Rheumatic Diseases*, *16*(4), 408–412.

Zhang, J., Zhang, L., Zhang, Y., Yang, J., Guo, M., Sun, L., et al. (2015). Gene-based meta-analysis of genome-wide association study data identifies independent single-nucleotide polymorphisms in ANXA6 as being associated with systemic lupus erythematosus in Asian populations. *Arthritis & Rhematology*, *67*(11), 2966–2977.

Zhang, P., Zhao, M., Liang, G., Yin, G., Huang, D., Su, F., et al. (2013). Whole-genome DNA methylation in skin lesions from patients with psoriasis vulgaris. *Journal of Autoimmunity*, *41*, 17–24.

Zhao, J., Ma, J., Deng, Y., Kelly, J. A., Kim, K., Bang, S. Y., et al. (2017). A missense variant in NCF1 is associated with susceptibility to multiple autoimmune diseases. *Nature Genetics*, *49*(3), 433–437.

Zhao, J., Su, Y., Li, R., Ye, H., Zou, Q., Fang, Y., et al. (2014). Classification criteria of early rheumatoid arthritis and validation of its performance in a multi-centre cohort. *Clinical and Experimental Rheumatology*, *32*(5), 667–673.

Zhao, M., Tan, Y., Peng, Q., Huang, C., Guo, Y., Liang, G., et al. (2018). IL-6/STAT3 pathway induced deficiency of RFX1 contributes to Th17-dependent autoimmune diseases via epigenetic regulation. *Nature Communications*, *9*(1), 583.

Zhao, S., Wang, Y., Liang, Y., Zhao, M., Long, H., Ding, S., et al. (2011). MicroRNA-126 regulates DNA methylation in CD4+ T cells and contributes to systemic lupus erythematosus by targeting DNA methyltransferase 1. *Arthritis and Rheumatism*, *63*(5), 1376–1386.

Zhao, W., Zhang, C., Shi, M., Zhang, J., Li, M., Xue, X., et al. (2014). The discoidin domain receptor 2/annexin A2/matrix metalloproteinase 13 loop promotes joint destruction in arthritis through promoting migration and invasion of fibroblast-like synoviocytes. *Arthritis & Rhematology*, *66*(9), 2355–2367.

Zhao, M., Zhou, Y., Zhu, B., Wan, M., Jiang, T., Tan, Q., et al. (2016). IFI44L promoter methylation as a blood biomarker for systemic lupus erythematosus. *Annals of the Rheumatic Diseases*, *75*(11), 1998–2006.

Zheng, N., Guo, C., & Wu, R. (2018). Iguratimod is effective in refractory rheumatoid arthritis patients with inadequate response to methotrexate-cyclosporin A-hydroxychloroquine-prednisone. *Scandinavian Journal of Rheumatology*, *47*(5), 422–424.

Zheng, M., Zhang, L., Yu, H., Hu, J., Cao, Q., Huang, G., et al. (2016). Genetic polymorphisms of cell adhesion molecules in Behçet's disease in a Chinese Han population. *Scientific Reports*, *6*, 24974.

Zhou, X. J., Lu, X. L., Nath, S. K., Lv, J. C., Zhu, S. N., Yang, H. Z., et al. (2012). Gene-gene interaction of BLK, TNFSF4, TRAF1, TNFAIP3, and REL in systemic lupus erythematosus. *Arthritis and Rheumatism*, *64*(1), 222–231.

Zhou, Y., Wang, X., An, Y., Zhang, X., Han, S., Li, X., et al. (2018). Disability and health-related quality of life in Chinese patients with rheumatoid arthritis: A cross-sectional study. *International Journal of Rheumatic Diseases*, *21*(9), 1709–1715.

Zhou, C., You, Y., Shen, W., Zhu, Y. Z., Peng, J., Feng, H. T., et al. (2016). Deficiency of sorting nexin 10 prevents bone erosion in collagen-induced mouse arthritis through promoting NFATc1 degradation. *Annals of the Rheumatic Diseases*, *75*(6), 1211–1218.

Zhu, H., Li, R., Da, Z., Bi, L., Li, X., Li, Y., et al. (2018). Remission assessment of rheumatoid arthritis in daily practice in China: A cross-sectional observational study. *Clinical Rheumatology*, *37*(3), 597–605.

Zhu, S., Pan, W., Song, X., Liu, Y., Shao, X., Tang, Y., et al. (2012). The microRNA miR-23b suppresses IL-17-associated autoimmune inflammation by targeting TAB2, TAB3 and IKK-alpha. *Nature Medicine*, *18*(7), 1077–1086.

Zhu, H., Wu, L. F., Mo, X. B., Lu, X., Tang, H., Zhu, X. W., et al. (2019). Rheumatoid arthritis-associated DNA methylation sites in peripheral blood mononuclear cells. *Annals of the Rheumatic Diseases*, *78*(1), 36–42.

Zou, Y., Xu, S., Xiao, Y., Qiu, Q., Shi, M., Wang, J., et al. (2018). Long noncoding RNA LERFS negatively regulates rheumatoid synovial aggression and proliferation. *The Journal of Clinical Investigation*, *128*(10), 4510–4524.

CHAPTER EIGHT

Understanding tumor-infiltrating lymphocytes by single cell RNA sequencing

Xianwen Ren*, Zemin Zhang
Beijing Advanced Innovation Centre for Genomics, Peking-Tsinghua Centre for Life Sciences, Biomedical Pioneering Innovation Center (BIOPIC), School of Life Sciences, Peking University, Beijing, China
*Corresponding author: e-mail address: renxwise@pku.edu.cn

Contents

Abstract

The clinical success of immune checkpoint blockade provides great hope for curing cancers. However, the patient responses are not even. Precise understanding of tumor immunity is necessary to improving the current cancer immunotherapies and to developing new treatment options. Here we applied full-length single cell RNA-seq (scRNA-seq) to three cancer types and provide a comprehensive single T cell data resource for understanding various characteristics of tumor-infiltrating T cells. We also developed an analytical framework named as STARTRAC to quantitatively characterize the dynamic properties of various T cell subsets including tissue preference, clonal expansion, migration, and state transitions from the scRNA-seq snapshots of tumor immune microenvironments. Conserved and cancer type-specific T cell subsets and developmental patterns were revealed, and detailed molecular portrait of the tumor immunity-relevant T cell clusters were provided, shedding lights into the cellular and molecular mechanisms underlying the composition, heterogeneity, and formation of tumor immune microenvironments. Important genes such as LAYN and IGFLR1 also provided new options for future development of cancer therapeutics.

Advances in Immunology, Volume 144
ISSN 0065-2776
https://doi.org/10.1016/bs.ai.2019.08.004

1. Introduction

The success of cancer immunotherapy has dramatically altered the oncological research and treatment landscape over the past decade (Sharma & Allison, 2015). Therapies represented by checkpoint blockade lead to remarkable clinical responses (Topalian, Drake, & Pardoll, 2015; Topalian, Taube, Anders, & Pardoll, 2016), but currently the benefits cannot be extended to all patients or cancer types. Understanding the underlying mechanisms of tumor immunity with/without immunotherapies is therefore paramount to identify robust bio-markers predicting responses of current therapies and to develop new therapies to benefit cancer patients not responding to current treatments. Several critical factors including mutational loads, tumor-infiltrating lymphocytes (TILs), and the expression levels of drug targets have provided valuable metrics to predict patient responses for anti-CTLA4 or anti-PD1 therapies (Brahmer et al., 2012; Topalian et al., 2015, 2016, 2012). However, these metrics are far from to be precisely and uniformly applied to practical clinical uses. Thorough understanding of tumor-resident immune cells, particularly T cells, is critical to the development of new response predictors and novel cancer immunotherapies. The rapid development of single-cell sequencing technologies allows detailed characterization of tumor-infiltrating immune cells with unprecedented resolution. In 2016, single-cell transcriptome analysis has been applied to cancerous and immune cells from melanoma patients, revealing the immune status of tumor microenvironment and opening the avenue for understanding tumor microenvironment at the single-cell level (Tirosh et al., 2016). Illuminating the single-cell immune characteristics of other cancer types has been a pressing task to advance the development of cancer immunotherapy. Here we focused on hepatocellular carcinoma (HCC), non-small cell lung cancer (NSCLC), and colorectal cancer (CRC), applied full-length scRNA-seq technology SMART-seq2 (Picelli et al., 2014), and gave a comprehensive and detailed portrait of tumor-infiltrating T cells (Fig. 1) (Guo et al., 2018; Zhang et al., 2018; Zheng et al., 2017a). In particular, we proposed a novel analytical framework for single T cell analysis by RNA-seq and TCR tracking (named as STARTRAC) (Zhang et al., 2018), based on which dynamic features of tumor-infiltrating T cells including clonal expansion, migration and state transition were quantitatively characterized, providing critical insights into the immune microenvironment of tumors (Fig. 2).

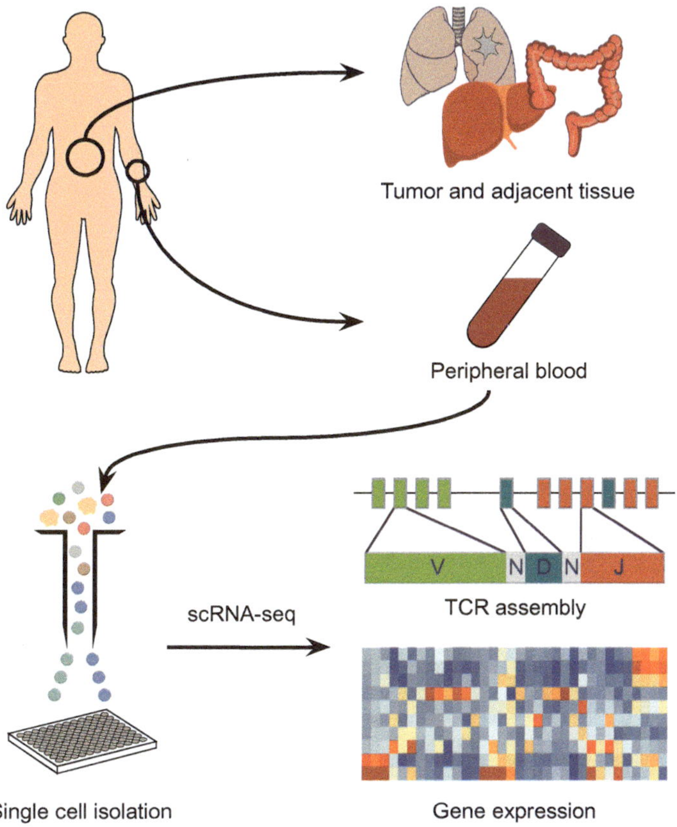

Fig. 1 Understanding tumor-infiltrating T cells by scRNA-seq. HCC, NSCLC and CRC were addressed by SMART-seq2, with tumor, adjacent normal tissue, and peripheral blood from the same patents obtained for comparison. Single cells were sorted by FACS and then sent for SMART-seq2-based sequencing. Gene expression profiles and TCR sequences were analyzed from the sequencing results to characterize the properties of tumor-infiltrating T cells.

2. A brief survey of single-cell sequencing technology and related data analysis

Single-cell sequencing technologies have been improved considerably since the initial proof-of-principle studies (Tang et al., 2009). Modification of the underlying chemistry of single-cell library preparation has provided diverse approaches to obtain and amplify single-cell nucleic acids for subsequent high-throughput sequencing, allowing investigation of tumor microenvironment with granular resolution (Ren, Kang, & Zhang, 2018).

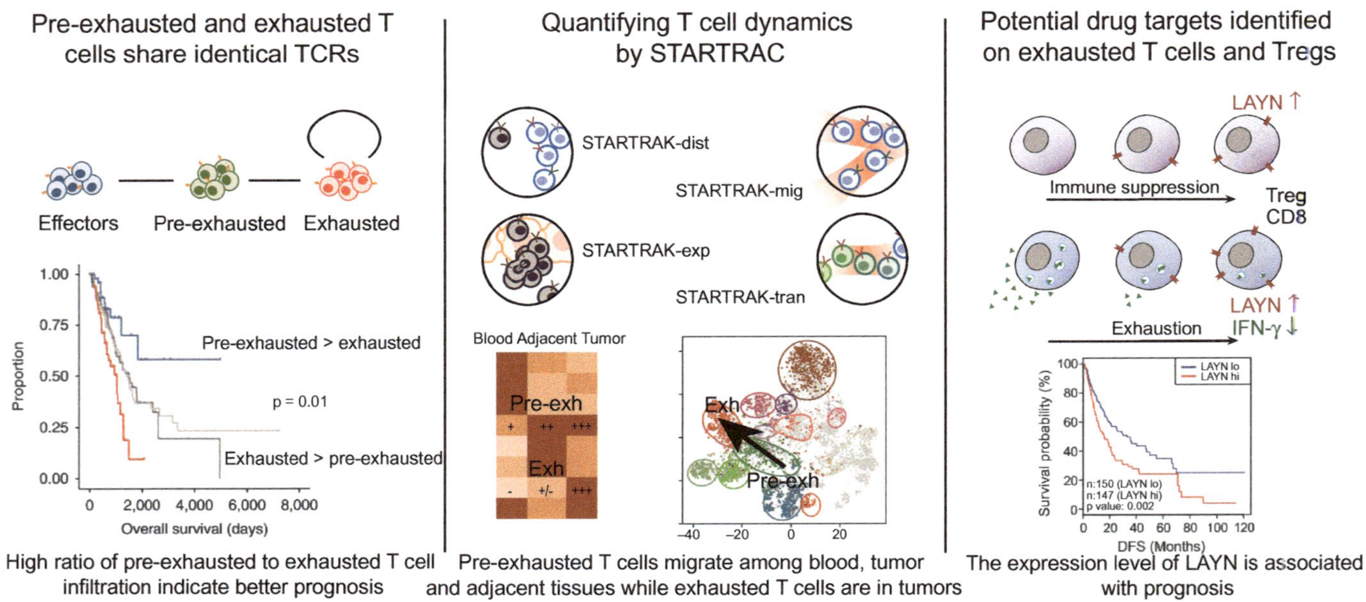

Fig. 2 Conserved patterns were observed across three cancer types. Identical TCRs were observed along blood-enriched effector T cells, tumor and adjacent normal-enriched effector memory T cells (pre-exhausted, characterized by GZMK+), and tumor-enriched exhausted T cells. The ratio of pre-exhausted to exhausted T cells in tumor is associated with patient survival. STARTRAC analysis further characterized the properties quantitatively and revealed the transitions between pre-exhausted and exhausted T cells in tumor. Molecules such as LAYN were found specifically expressed in T cells exerting immune suppression functions including Tregs and exhausted T cells, and are associated with patient survival, providing potential novel drug targets.

Because an individual cancer cell typically contains only ~6–12 pg of DNA and 10–50 pg of total RNA (depending on the cell types and status) (Livesey, 2003), amplification is essential for single-cell library preparation to fulfill the sequencing input requirements, forming a critical aspect to discriminate single cell sequencing techniques (Navin, 2014). Another important feature in evaluating single cell sequencing methods is the cell throughput. Various methods based on flow cytometry, droplet-based microfluidics, and combinatorial indexing have been proposed to improve the cell throughput in a single experiment. According to the differences in amplification methods and cell throughput, different single-cell DNA and RNA sequencing, epigenomic sequencing, and simultaneous sequencing of the genome, transcriptome, epigenome, and epitopes of the same single cell have been available, facilitating detailed exploration of tumor microenvironments (Ren et al., 2018). For RNA sequencing, SMART-seq2 (Picelli et al., 2014) and droplet-based 10X Genomics (Zheng et al., 2017b) become two representative methods frequently used in studies of tumor microenvironments, with SMART-seq2 providing full-length mRNA coverage, high sensitivity to lowly-expressed genes but low cell throughput while 10X Genomics providing 3′ tagging of mRNAs and high cell throughput. As SMART-seq2 also allows transcript assembly, we applied it to studies of tumor-infiltrating T cells of HCC (Zheng et al., 2017a), NSCLC (Guo et al., 2018) and CRC (Zhang et al., 2018).

Accompanying to the tremendous progress of experimental single-cell sequencing technologies, specialized bioinformatics and algorithmic approaches have also been developed to best interpret the obtained single-cell data while reducing the potential technological noise and biases. A typical analytical pipeline of single-cell RNA-seq data includes quality control (removing low-quality reads and cells), imputation of dropout events, normalization and correction of batch effects, clustering for identification of cell types, identification of differentially expressed genes among clusters, inference of potential cell developmental trajectories, and data visualization (Ren et al., 2018). Progresses of algorithms, software, and reference databases in this broad area provide various tools for uncovering the mystery of tumor immune complexity at the single-cell resolution.

Despite the dramatic advances, substantial limitations and challenges still exist in single-cell dissection of tumor immune microenvironment. The first challenge lies in the notable technological dropouts introduced during the amplification step. In single-cell RNA sequencing, lowly expressed genes, although they may encode proteins with important regulatory or signaling functions, are prone to be dropped out and susceptible to technological noise even when detected. Difficulties may arise due to dropouts of critical surface markers or transcription factors that can indicate the cell identity. The second challenge is how to interpret those cell clusters identified on the transcriptional level as developmentally and functionally distinct immune cell subsets. While scRNA-seq can reveal the expression levels of biomarkers specific to predefined immune cell types by conventional immune methods, the unprecedented single-cell resolution has revealed much more complicated biomarker combinations. Accurate inference the developmental lineage and functional state of observed single cells is still a pivotal question in single-cell-based immune studies, the ultimate resolution of which may require the integration of both computational and experimental methods.

Spatial information of single cells in patient bodies and even fine-grained within specific tissues is also critical to interpret single cell sequencing data of immune cells but is often lost during the cell isolation step before library preparation. It is urgently needed to identify how cells are organized to implement the concerted function within a tissue of interest. While many experimental techniques have been developed to keep or restore the spatial information of sequenced single cells such as fluorescence in situ hybridization (FISH), single-molecule fluorescence in situ hybridization (smFISH), laser capture microdissection, laser scanning microscopy, including two-photon laser scanning microscopy, and fluorescence in situ sequencing, there still exists great gap between these technologies and single cell sequencing (Ren et al., 2018). For example, FISH-based technologies can map the spatial distribution of a set of selected genes upon which the identity of single cells can be inferred based on RNA-seq data. However, the methods are limited to two dimensions and the number of spatially-resolved genes is limited to tens to hundreds. Laser capture microdissection can simultaneously record the spatial information of single cells subject to sequencing. However, the cellular throughput of such methods is extremely limited due to the great operation difficulties, and the biological interpretation of the recorded spatial positions are confined as adjacent cells generally cannot be properly dissected for scRNA-seq.

Despite of the aforementioned difficulties when applying scRNA-seq to dissecting tumor immune microenvironment, we proposed a framework named as STARTRAC (Single T cell Analysis by RNA-seq and TCR tracking) to derive the dynamic properties of tumor-infiltrating T cells including cell identity, tissue preference, migration, clonal expansion, and state transitions (Zhang et al., 2018), and applied this analytical framework to scRNA-seq data of tumor microenvironments of HCC (Zheng et al., 2017a), NSCLC (Guo et al., 2018) and CRC (Zhang et al., 2018).

3. STARTRAC: A computational framework to quantify dynamics of T cells from snapshot scRNA-seq data

Noticing the difficulties when applying scRNA-seq to studying tumor immune microenvironment, we present STRATRAC as a framework, defined by four indices, to analyze different dynamic aspects of tumor-infiltrating T cells based on paired scRNA-seq of tumor, adjacent normal tissue and peripheral blood with TCR assembly. By adding experimental designs of adjacent normal tissues and peripheral blood for scRNA-seq analysis, it becomes possible to quantify tissue preference and migrations across tissues of T cells with unique TCR sequences as tags to indicate the lineages of T cells.

The life cycle of T cells involves immune and non-immune organs, with different T cells having different tissue preference. To quantify the T cell preference, we designed STARTRAC-dist (STARTRAC-distribution) to measure the enrichment of T cell clusters across tissues from random expectation. Given a contingency table of T cell clusters by tissues, we first apply Chi-squared test to evaluate whether the distribution of T cell clusters across tissues significantly deviates from random expectations. We then calculate the STARTRAC-dist index for each combination of T cell clusters and tissues according the following formula:

$$I_{\text{dist}}^{\text{STARTRAC}} = R_{o/e} = \frac{\text{Observed}}{\text{Expected}}$$

where $R_{o/e}$ is the ratio of observed cell number over the expected cell number of a given combination of T cell cluster and tissue. The expected cell number for each combination of T cell clusters and tissues were obtained from the Chi-squared test. Different from the Chi-squared values, which are defined as $(\text{Observed} - \text{Expected})^2/\text{Expected}$ and can only indicate the divergence of observations from random expectations, $I_{\text{dist}}^{\text{STARTRAC}}$ defined by $R_{o/e}$ can indicate whether cells of a certain T cell cluster are enriched or depleted in a specific tissue. For examples, if $R_{o/e} > 1$, it suggests that cells of the given T cell cluster are more frequently observed than random expectations in the specific tissue, i.e., enriched. If $R_{o/e} < 1$, it suggests that cells of the given T cell cluster are observed with less frequency than random expectations in the specific tissue, i.e., depleted. By calculating the STARTRAC-dist indices via $R_{o/e}$, we can quantify the tissue preference of T cell clusters efficiently.

The other three STARTRAC indices, STARTRAC-expa (STARTRAC-expansion), STARTRAC-migr (STARTRAC-migration) and STARTRAC-tran (STARTRAC-transition), are designed to measure the degree of clonal expansion, migration across tissues, and state transitions of T cell clusters upon TCR tracking, respectively. For STARTRAC-expa, we first adopted the normalized Shannon entropy to calculate the evenness of the TCR repertoire of the given T cell cluster and then defined the STARTRAC-expa index as $1 - \text{evenness}$. Mathematically, the STARTRAC-expa index of a specific cluster with N clonotypes was defined by the following formula:

$$I_{\text{expa}}^{\text{STARTRAC}} = 1 - \text{eveness} = 1 - \frac{-\sum_{i=1}^{N} p_i \log_2 p_i}{\log_2 N}$$

where p_i is the cell frequency of clonotype i in the cluster and a clonotype is defined by identical, full-length, paired α and β TCR chains. Although the definition of STARTRAC-expa is mathematically identical to the clonality scores frequently used in bulk TCR repertoire sequencing studies, two distinctions exist. First, STARTRAC-expa is defined for T cell clusters while the traditional TCR clonality is defined for specific specimens. A T cell cluster in STARTRAC framework can consist of T cells from multiple tissues and patients, but the specimens subject to bulk TCR repertoire sequencing are typically from a unique tissue and patient. Second, STARTRAC-expa uses a more stringent clonotype definition. For traditional bulk TCR sequencing studies, clonotypes are generally defined based on identical CDR3 (the third complementarity-determining region) sequences of TCR α or β chains due to technological limitations. However, STARTRAC-expa is defined using the strictest clonotype definition, which requires both the full-length α and β chains of TCRs are identical at the nucleotide level. Thus, although STARTRAC-expa has identical mathematical formula as the traditional TCR clonality definition, they have distinct biological meanings. STARTRAC-expa ranges from 0 to 1, with 0 indicating no clonal expansion for each clonotype while 1 indicating that the cluster is composed of only one clonally expanded clonotype. If a cluster is composed of multiple clonotypes and each clonotype is subject to distinct extent of clonal expansion, STARTRAC-expa will be between 0 and 1, with high STARTRAC-expa indicating high clonality.

For cells with identical TCRs, even if they are present in different tissues or in different development states, logically they originated from the same ancestry cell and have migrated across tissues or undergone state transitions. Based on this principle, we define STARTRAC-migr and STARTRAC-tran to evaluate the extent of tissue migration and state transition of each clonotype, respectively. For each clonotype, given its distribution across tissues (peripheral blood, adjacent normal mucosa and tumor), we define its STARTRAC-migr index I^t_{migr} as:

$$I^t_{\text{migr}} = -\sum_{j=1}^{J} p^t_j \log_2 p^t_j$$

where p^t_j is the ratio of the number of cells with TCR t in tissue j to the total number of cells with TCR t and $\sum_{J=1}^{J} p^t_j = 1$. Similarly, its STARTRAC-tran index I^t_{tran} can be defined as:

$$I^t_{\text{tran}} = -\sum_{k=1}^{K} p^t_k \log_2 p^t_k$$

where p^t_k is the ratio of the number of cells with TCR t in cluster k to the total number of cells with TCR t, $\sum_{k=1}^{K} p^t_k = 1$ and K is the total number of cell clusters. Although both definitions use Shannon entropy for calculation, they are distinct from the measurement of TCR clonality in bulk TCR repertoire sequencing. As described above, the traditional TCR clonality is defined at the sample level; however, STARTRAC-migr and STARTRAC-tran are defined primarily at the clonotype level. Given one clonotype, the evenness or diversity of its TCR repertoire will always be zero because all the cells have identical TCRs, while the STARTRAC-migr and STARTRAC-tran indices will be non-trivial because cells of the same clonotype can migrate across tissues or change their transcriptional states due to a combination of internal and external factors. And thus, the inputs of the formulas of STARTRAC-migr and STARTRAC-tran are also different from the traditional TCR clonality measure and STARTRAC-expa. The input of STARTRAC-migr is the observed cell frequency across tissues of a certain clonotype, while the input of STARTRAC-tran is the observed cell frequency across cell clusters of a certain clonotype. By contrast, the input of STARTRAC-expa is the observed cell frequency across clonotypes of a certain cell cluster, and the input for the traditional TCR clonality measure is the observed sequence frequency across a TCR repertoire of a given sample.

After the extent of tissue migration of each clonotype is quantified by STARTRAC-migr, given a cluster with total T clonotypes, the STARTRAC-migr index at the cluster level $I_{\text{migr}}^{\text{STARTRAC}}$ can be defined as the weighted average of TCR clonotype level migration indices of all the clonotypes contained in the cluster:

$$I_{\text{migr}}^{\text{cls}} = \sum_{t=1}^{T} p_{\text{cls}}^{t} I_{\text{migr}}^{t}$$

where p_{cls}^{t} is the ratio of the number of cells with clonotype t in cluster cls to the total number of cells in cluster cls.

Similarly, when the extent of state transition of each clonotype is quantified by STARTRAC-tran, given a cluster with total T clonotypes, the STARTRAC-tran index at the cluster level can be defined as the weighted average of the clonotype level state transition indices of all the clonotypes contained in the cluster:

$$I_{\text{tran}}^{\text{cls}} = \sum_{t=1}^{T} p_{\text{cls}}^{t} I_{\text{tran}}^{t}$$

where p_{cls}^{t} is the ratio of the number of cells with clonotype t in cluster cls to the total number of cells in cluster cls.

Of note, both STARTRAC-migr and STARTRAC-tran are defined at two different levels (clonotypes and clusters), with the clonotype-level definitions describing the extent of migration and state transition of a given clonotype, and the cluster-level definitions depicting the summarization of such properties of all clonotypes within a cluster.

Besides the overall evaluation of the extents of migration and state transitions by STARTRAC-migr and STARTRAC-tran, we also define pairwise STARTRAC-migr (pSTARTRAC-migr) and STARTRAC-tran (pSTARTRAC-tran) indices for precise quantification. For example, given a clonotype t and two tissue types (e.g., blood and tumor), the pSTARTRAC-migr index ${}_{p}I_{\text{migr}}^{t}$ is calculated by the following formula:

$${}_{p}I_{\text{migr}}^{t} = -\sum_{j=1}^{2} p_{j}^{t} \log_2 p_{j}^{t}$$

where p_{j}^{t} is the ratio of the number of cells with TCR t in tissue j to the total number of cells with TCR t in tissues 1 and 2 (i.e., blood and tumor), and $\sum_{j=1}^{2} p_{j}^{t} = 1$. In other words, pSTARTRAC-migr uses the same formula as

STARTRAC-migr but limits the number of tissues to two and the frequencies of cells between two specified tissues are re-calculated. Likewise, given a clonotype t and two T cell clusters (e.g., T_{em} and T_{ex}), the pSTARTRAC-tran index ${}_pI^t_{tran}$is calculated by the following formula:

$$ {}_pI^t_{\text{tran}} = -\sum_{k=1}^{2} p^t_k \log_2 p^t_k $$

where p^t_k is the ratio of the number of cells with TCR t in cluster k to the total number of cells with TCR t in clusters 1 and 2 (i.e., T_{em} and T_{ex}), and $\sum_{k=1}^{2} p^t_k = 1$. Thus, pSTARTRAC-tran uses the same formula as STARTRAC-tran but limits the number of clusters to two and the frequencies of cells between the two specified clusters are re-calculated. Once pairwise STARTRAC-migr and STARTRAC-tran for clonotypes are obtained, the corresponding indices for clusters are calculated via weighted average according to their clonotype composition. As all STARTRAC-migr and STARTRAC-tran indices are defined by Shannon entropy, high values indicate high migration and state transition, respectively.

With the development of STARTRAC, dissection of tumor microenvironment by scRNA-seq not only can reveal the T cell composition and transcriptional characteristics, but also allows the quantification of various dynamic properties including clonal expansion, migration across tissues, and transitions between various developmental states. The applications of scRNA-seq and STARTRAC to HCC, NSCLC and CRC revealed critical cellular and molecular characteristics of their immune microenvironments.

4. Characteristics of tumor-infiltrating T cells in hepatocellular carcinoma

HCC is one of the leading causes of cancer-related death worldwide (El-Serag, 2011) and chronic hepatitis B virus (HBV) infection is assumed to be the major cause of HCC in China. Limited treatment options and clinical success in immunotherapies (Prieto, Melero, & Sangro, 2015) raise urgent need to understanding the immune properties of HCC and the contributions of HBV in the progress of HCC and the response to immunotherapies. While HCC tumors were demonstrated to harbor abundant TILs (Kasper, Drebber, Stippel, Dienes, & Gillessen, 2009), the underlying mechanism of their inefficacy of eliminating tumor cells is still elusive. Hence, HBV-infected HCC tumors provide an appealing model to characterize the dysfunction of TILs at the crossroad of tumor and chronic infection. Smart-seq2-based scRNA-seq analyses of >5000 single T cells isolated from HBV-positive HCC patients provided us a global snapshot of the molecular and cellular biological scenarios of T cells. Eleven transcriptionally distinct T cell subsets were identified, covering a wide spectrum of T cells including naïve, effector, memory and exhausted T cells. TCR sequences assembled from the scRNA-seq data also allowed and the revelation of potential developmental paths of these subsets. Genes specifically expressed in exhausted CD8+ T cells and tumor-specific regulatory T cells (Tregs), for example, layilin (LAYN), provide important biomarkers to indicate the immune suppression status of tumor microenvironment and potential therapeutic targets. We found that over-expressing LAYN in primary CD8+ T cells resulted in inhibition of interferon (IFN)-g production, suggesting the regulatory role of LAYN in CD8+ T cells.

We performed bulk exome- and RNA-seq for six treatment-naive HCC patients. Copy-number variation and somatic mutations of the tumor samples of these patients were consistent with known HCC genomic patterns, confirming the clinical and pathological diagnosis of these patients as HCCs. The presence of infiltrating T lymphocytes in tumor tissues was confirmed using immunohistochemistry (IHC) with antibodies against CD3, CD4, CD8, and FOXP3, indicating the possibility of applying scRNA-seq to study the immune characteristics of HCC tumors. Opal multicolor IHC staining revealed that CD8+ T cells, but not FOXP3+ Tregs, were much lower in the core of tumors than in the outer cortex, indicating the inefficiency of CD8+ T cell infiltration into tumor cores. Then CD3+ CD4+ CD25−, CD3+ CD4+ CD25^{high} and CD3+ CD8+ T cells from single-cell suspensions prepared from tumor, tumor-adjacent normal tissue, and peripheral blood were then sorted to enrich helper, regulatory, and effector T cells. The percentage of CD4+ CD25^{high} T cells within all CD4+ T cells isolated from tumor tissues was much higher than those in normal tissues and peripheral blood, suggesting enrichment of Tregs in the tumor microenvironment. A total of 5063 individual T cells had successfully undergone scRNA-seq with an average of 1.29 million uniquely mapped read pairs per cell.

Unsupervised clustering of the 5063 T cell expression profiles using the spectral clustering method implemented in SC3 (Kiselev et al., 2017) revealed 11 stable clusters, including five clusters for CD8+ and six clusters for CD4+ cells. The CD8+ cluster C1_CD8-LEF1 was dominant in peripheral blood and specifically expressed naïve T cell marker genes including LEF1 and CCR7. C2_CD8-CX3CR1 was characterized by the high expression of CX3CR1, FCGR3A, and FGFBP2, associated with effector T cell signatures. C3_CD8-SLC4A10 was characterized by specific expression of SLC4A10, ZBTB16, and RORC, associated with mucosal-associated invariant T cells (MAIT), which were confirmed by predominantly bearing semi-invariant TCR alpha chains with TRAV1-2/TRAJ33, TRAV1-2/TRAJ20, or TRAV1-2/TRAJ12. C4_CD8-LAYN, predominantly composed of cells from tumor tissues, expressed high levels of exhausted T cell markers CTLA4, PDCD1, and HAVCR2. The remaining CD8+ cells, falling into the fifth cluster, C5_CD8-GZMK, shared a few common genes with cluster 4, such as PDCD1 and DUSP4 but with high expression of GZMK that was absent in C4_CD8-LAYN.

The distribution of CD8+ T clusters was similar among patients, with naïve T cells (high CCR7 expression) and effector memory T cells (high CX3CR1) prevalent in peripheral blood while MAIT cells were prevalent in non-tumor adjacent liver tissue. Exhausted CD8+ T cells were exclusively enriched in tumor samples. Compared with adjacent normal tissues, MAIT cells were significantly reduced in HCC tumors, consistent with the finding in the TCGA HCC cohort in which the expression of the MAIT marker gene SLC4A10 in HCC tumors was significantly lower ($P=0.003$, paired Wilcoxon test) than paired normal samples. Survival analysis suggested that lower SLC4A10 expression in HCC was associated with poor prognosis in the TCGA cohort ($P=0.037$, log rank test), suggesting potential roles of MAIT cells in the HCC tumor immunity.

Similarly, six major CD4+ T cell clusters can be identified. C6_CD4-CCR7 cells, mostly derived from blood, comprised of mainly naïve CD4+ T cells with high expression of SELL, TCF7, and CCR7. Both C7_CD4-FOXP3 and C8_CD4-CTLA4 were FOXP3+, indicating the nature of Tregs, with C7_CD4-FOXP3 mainly from peripheral blood and C8_CD4-CTLA4 from tumors. Cells from C10_CD4-CXCL13 and C11_CD4-GNLY were primarily T helper cells from normal and tumor tissues and were characterized by high expression of GZMA and CCL5. C10_CD4-CXCL13 specifically expressed CXCL13, PDCD1, CTLA4, and TIGIT, consistent with signatures of exhausted CD4 T cells. C11_CD4-GNLY exhibited high expression of cytotoxic molecules including NKG7, GNLY, and GZMB, indicative of the nature of cytotoxic CD4 T cells.

Comparison of tumor-infiltrating Tregs with blood-derived Tregs identified 401 genes specifically expressed in tumor-infiltrating Tregs (adjusted

$P<0.01$,limma (Ritchie et al., 2015) moderated t test, and $\geq$2-fold changes), including FOXP3, CTLA4, TNFRSF18, TNFRSF4, and CCR8. These genes significantly overlapped with those identified by three previous studies in melanoma, breast, colon, and lung cancers ($P<2e-85$, hypergeometric test) (De Simone et al., 2016; Plitas et al., 2016; Tirosh et al., 2016). Among the 33 common Treg signature genes from these three studies, 31 genes were also recapitulated. The two missed genes CRADD and IL32 also showed significantly higher expression (adjusted $P<6e-12$, limma moderated t test) in tumor-specific infiltrating Tregs but with slightly lower fold changes. Therefore, scRNA-seq based on relatively limited patient samples could robustly provide detailed portraits of tumor-infiltrating lymphocytes. 146 genes that uniquely enriched in this dataset include RGS1, STAT3, and PTPN22, which were previously reported to be associated with Treg function regulations (Fousteri et al., 2014; Goode et al., 2013; Pallandre et al., 2007). The identification of these tumor Treg-specific genes may provide important clues for investigating the molecular mechanisms of tumor immune suppression and for future development of cancer immunotherapy.

Tumor-infiltrating exhausted CD8+ T cells demonstrated 82 specifically expressed genes compared with nonexhausted tumor-infiltrating CD8+ T cells. Multiple known exhaustion markers including HAVCR2, PDCD1, ENTPD1, CTLA4, TIGIT and TNFRSF9 were top-ranked. Several genes such as MYO7A, WARS, and CXCL13 were also reported in the scRNA-seq study of melanoma (Tirosh et al., 2016) while a few genes including LAYN, PHLDA1, and SNAP47 were reported to be associated with T cell exhaustion for the first time. Notably, 22 of these exhaustion-related genes including CTLA4 and TIGIT were also highly expressed in tumor-infiltrating Tregs. Exhaustion status evaluated with such exhaustion-specific gene signature revealed that patients at the late stage exhibited significantly higher exhaustion level than other patients ($P=0.02$, Student's t test). Switching to the TCGA HCC cohort, higher expression of PHLDA1 and SNAP47 were both associated with poor prognosis of HCC patients.

LAYN, encoding layilin, was previously reported to be highly expressed in Tregs isolated from lung and colon tumors (De Simone et al., 2016). Our data revealed that LAYN was specifically expressed in both tumor Tregs (C8_CD4-CTLA4) and exhausted CD8+ T cells (C4_CD8-LAYN). The TCGA HCC survival data also suggested that higher expression of LAYN was associated with reduced disease-free survival ($P=0.002$, log rank test) after normalizing T cell infiltration levels with CD3. On the protein level, LAYN was not detected on blood-derived resting CD14+ myeloid cells, B cells, CD4+ T cells, Tregs, or CD8+ T cells. However, after T cells activation by anti-CD3 and anti-CD28 antibodies for 2 days, LAYN presence on >30% Tregs and CD8+ T cells can be detected. Further examination suggested that LAYN was preferentially upregulated in FOXP3+ Helios+ Tregs than FOXP3+ Helios− Tregs, suggesting that LAYN expression may be associated with the repressive function of Tregs. In vitro stimulation experiments revealed that the expression of LAYN in CD8+ T cells can be observed 1 day after stimulation and persists even 6 days after activation. Interestingly, the expression of LAYN might be mutually exclusive with LAG3 while independent on PDCD1. Overexpression of LAYN in CD8+ T cells by retroviral vectors can significantly reduce the expression level of gamma interferon, suggesting the regulatory role of LAYN in CD8+ T cells.

The full-length scRNA-seq data also allowed assembly of TCRs, which can be further used to indicate the developmental lineages of T cells. In total, we obtained paired productive full-length TCR sequences for 94% (3792/4032) T cells (including both of the α and β chains). While the TCR sequences were unique for most of the cells, identical TCRs were detected in a fraction of T cells. Clonal T cells that have identical TCRs were significantly enriched in tumor-infiltrating CD8+ T cells and Tregs. Compared with ~10% clonal CD8+ T cells observed in blood and normal liver tissues, tumor tissues showed a much higher percentage at ~30% ($P<0.05$, Student's t test). Similar patterns were also observed in tumor-infiltrating Tregs, with blood-derived Tregs showing little clonal expansion while tumor Tregs being highly clonally expanded STARTRAC analysis indicated that tumor exhausted CD8+ T cells and Tregs show relatively low migration properties across tumor, adjacent normal tissue and peripheral blood, indicating the possibility of local proliferation of exhausted CD8+ T cells and Tregs after antigen-stimulation. As these patients were also HBV-positive, the clonal expansion may also be attributed to chronic viral antigen stimulation. However, the low extent of T cell clonal expansion in tumor-adjacent normal liver may reduce the possibility of viral antigen stimulation.

Developmental trajectory inference by Monocle2 (Trapnell et al., 2014), confirmed by EMBEDDR (Campbell, Ponting, & Webber, 2015), SCORPIUS (Schlitzer et al., 2015) and TSCAN (Ji & Ji, 2016) arranged different CD8+ T clusters in a pseudo-time process beginning with C1_CD8-LEF1 cells (naïve CD8+ T cells), then C2_CD8-CX3CR1 (effector memory

CD8+ T cells) and C5_CD8-GZMK, and ending with C4_CD8-LAYN cells (exhausted CD8+ T cells). In the predicted developmental trajectory, C5_CD8-GZMK appeared to be an intermediate state between effector and exhausted T cells. This expression-based finding was independently supported by the TCR-based clonal analysis. Of the total 61 TCR pairs shared by cells from at least two different clusters, 30 were shared between C2_CD8-CX3CR1 and C5_CD8-GZMK and 20 were shared between C5_CD8-GZMK and C4_CD8-LAYN. By contrast, no more than five TCR pairs were shared between other clusters, supporting the development transitions from effector T cells to C5_CD8-GZMK and then to exhausted cells.

CD4+ T helper cells showed a slightly different differentiation trajectory, with the C6_CD4-CCR7 naive T cells and C9_CD4-GZMA T helper cells primarily forming the trajectory backbone while C10_CD4-CXCL13 (exhausted CD4+ T cells) and C11_CD4-GNLY (cytotoxic CD4+ T cells) cells were located in different directions. Shared TCRs were frequently observed between C9_CD4-GZMA and C10_CD4-CXCL13 or between C9_CD4-GZMA and C11_CD4-GNLY. Few shared TCRs were observed between C10_CD4-CXCL13 and C11_CD4-GNLY, suggesting low possibility of direct transitions from C11_CD4-GNLY to C10_CD4-CXCL13. Both the trajectory and TCR analyses suggested that exhausted CD4 and CD8 T cells were more developmentally linked to the intermediate populations marked by GZMA and GZMK signatures than the effector populations. The intermediate C5_CD8-GZMK and C9_CD4-GZMA may provide important therapeutic targets of which preventing the transition to exhausted cells may promote tumor immunity. STARTRAC analysis suggested that these two intermediate clusters had the highest state transition potentials.

In addition to CD4+ Tregs, a small number of exhausted CD8+ T cells also expressed the Treg marker FOXP3, some of which shared the same TCRs with FOXP3^{-} exhausted CD8+ T cells based on TCR analysis, suggesting the same developmental origins. The presence of these CD8+ FOXP3+ regulatory T cells in HCC was further confirmed by multicolor IHC. The expression profiles of these cells were characterized by both Treg and cytolytic signatures, with high expression of Treg hallmarks including FOXP3, CTLA4, TNFRSF18, and TNFRSF9 and cytolytic-related genes PRF1, GZMA, and NKG7, indicating the potential presence of both suppressive and cell-killing characteristics. As no CD8+ FOXP3+ T cells were detected in either blood or adjacent normal tissues, these CD8+ FOXP3+ T cells seem to be specifically associated with the HCC tumor microenvironment. And the origin and function of CD8+ FOXP3+ T cells will be a critical question in tumor immunity.

STARTRAC analysis suggested that tumor-infiltrating Tregs (C8_CD4-CTLA4) shared a relatively small number of TCRs with exhausted CD8+ T cells, indicating that the possible developmental origins of inducible tumor Tregs from CD4+ helper T cells. However, the vast majority (71/87) of the tumor-specific Treg TCRs were exclusive to themselves, in contrast to tumor-associated exhausted CD8+ T cells that share a higher number of common TCRs with other clusters of CD8 T cells in tumor.

5. Characteristics of tumor-infiltrating T cells in lung cancer

NSCLC is the leading cause of cancer-related mortality and accounts for ~85% of lung cancers (Herbst, Heymach, & Lippman, 2008). Compared to HCC, NSCLC is reported to have better response to immune checkpoint blockade (Brahmer et al., 2012; Hellmann et al., 2017; Topalian et al., 2015, 2016). NSCLC tumors typically harbor extensive genomic alterations (Collisson et al., 2014), with high mutation load linking to the better response to immunotherapy (Rizvi et al., 2015). To dissect the molecular and cellular landscape of T cells in NSCLC tumor microenvironment, we applied the same scRNA-seq protocols on T cells isolated from tumor, adjacent normal tissues and peripheral blood for 14 treatment-naïve NSCLC patients, including 11 adenocarcinomas and three squamous cell carcinomas. A total of 12,346 cells were obtained with an average sequencing depth of 1.04 million uniquely-mapped read pairs (Guo et al., 2018).

Similar to analysis in HCC scRNA-seq T cell data, unsupervised clustering based on t-SNE (van der Maaten & Hinton, 2008) and densityClust (Rodriguez & Laio, 2014) revealed seven CD8 and nine CD4 clusters, covering clusters of CD8+ (naïve, effector, resident memory or exhausted), conventional CD4+ (naïve, central memory, effector or exhausted) cells, and CD4+ Tregs. STARTRAC analysis suggested these clusters had distinct tissue preferences. For example, CD8-C1-LEF1 and CD4-C1-CCR7, representing naïve CD8+ and CD4+ T cells, contained mostly cells from blood, whereas CD8-C6-LAYN (CD8+ exhausted T cells) and CD4-C9-CTLA4 (CD4+ Tregs) were exclusively populated within tumors. In contrast, the two effector T cell clusters, CD8-C3-CX3CR1 and CD4-C3-GNLY, preferred to both blood and the adjacent normal tissue. These two clusters were characterized by high expression of chemokine receptor CX3CR1 and genes associated with cytotoxicity, including PRF1, GZMA and GZMB and low expression of T cell exhaustion markers such as PDCD1, CTLA4 and HAVCR2.

TCR assembly based on TraCeR (Stubbington et al., 2016) revealed that a sizable fraction of clonally expanded cells were distributed across tissues. STARTRAC analysis revealed that naïve T cell clusters CD8-C1-LEF1 and CD4-C1-CCR7 displayed negligible clonal expansion while effector T cell clusters CD8-C3-CX3CR1 and CD4-C3-GNLY not only had the highest proportions of clonal cells, consistent with previous HCC findings. The STARTRAC migration indices indicated that CD8-C1-LEF1 and CD4-C1-CCR7 were blood-preferred but CD8-C3-CX3CR1 and CD4-C3-GNLY showed the highest migration potential across tissues. The high migration potential was consistent with genes involved in the "focal adhesion", "cell adhesion molecules (CAMs)", "leukocyte trans-endothelial migration" and "regulation of actin cytoskeleton" pathways which were highly expressed in the corresponding clusters CD8-C3-CX3CR1 and CD4-C3-GNLY.

9% (158 out of 1669) CD8+ T cell clones were found in at least two clusters, suggesting that the transcriptionally distinct CD8+ T cell clusters were also developmentally connected. Developmental trajectory inference based on gene expression profiles by Monocle (Trapnell et al., 2014) suggested a branched structure, with CD8-C6-LAYN exhaustion cluster positioned at the opposite end of both CD8-C1-LEF1 naïve and CD8-C3-CX3CR1 effector clusters while CD8-C2-CD28, CD8-C4-GZMK and CD8-C5-ZNF683 were located in between. STARTRAC analysis not only indicated that the expression-based trajectory was consist with TCR analysis, with neighboring clusters along the trajectory shared significantly more TCRs than distant clusters but also that clusters in the intermediate part of the trajectory had high state transition scores. Mapping T cell naïveness, cytotoxicity, and exhaustion gene signatures (Tirosh et al., 2016) on the predicted trajectory revealed that Monocle component 1 was highly associated with T cell exhaustion whereas component 2 was positively associated with cytotoxicity and negatively associated with naïveness, indicating that two distinct processes, i.e., the inherent T cell developmental program and tumor-induced T cell exhaustion, together shaped the states of CD8+ T cells in NSCLC.

Differential expression analysis revealed 90 genes highly expressed in tumor-infiltrating exhausted CD8+ T cells compared with other T cells in tumor. The 90 signature genes showed significant overlaps with exhaustion-related genes identified in scRNA-seq studies of HCC

(Zheng et al., 2017a) and melanoma (Tirosh et al., 2016). These human tumor-based studies contained a common set of 23 genes, 14 of which (CXCL13, SIRPG, ENTPD1, MYO7A, SARDH, IGFLR1, CD27, PARK7, ITM2A, VCAM1, SNAP47, TPI1, CCND2 and TNFRSF1B) were absent in the mouse study of T cell exhaustion induced by chronic lymphocytic choriomeningitis virus infection (Crawford et al., 2014), representing human-specific exhaustion markers.

CD8-C4-GZMK and CD8-C5-ZNF683, having high STARTRAC transition scores, showed lower exhaustion scores than CD8-C6-LAYN, suggestive of a possible "pre-exhaustion" state. CD8-C4_GZMK could also be detected in HCC tumors, but CD8-C5-ZNF683 cells were significantly more abundant in NSCLC tumors, suggesting their specific functions in NSCLC immunity. Interestingly, analyses of the independent lung adenocarcinoma (LUAD) cohort from TCGA indicated that patients with high expression of the signature genes of CD8-C5-ZNF683 and low CD8-C6-LAYN signal (after normalizing for T cell fractions by CIBERSORT) showed significantly better overall survival compared to those with a low CD8-C5-ZNF683 to CD8-C6-LAYN signal ratio ($P=0.01$, Cox regression). Such survival differences could also be seen for patients with low vs high CD8-C4-GZMK to CD8-C6-LAYN signal ratios ($P=0.006$, Cox regression). Thus, the ratio of "pre-exhausted" to exhausted T cells was associated with a favorable prognosis in LUAD. However, such a pattern cannot be extended the lung squamous cell carcinomas cohort of TCGA, indicating potential differences between lung cancer types.

The developmental trajectory of conventional CD4+ T helpers also exhibited a branched structure, with CD4-C2-ANXA1, CD4-C4-CD69, CD4-C5-EOMES and CD4-C6-GZMA bridging naïve CD4-C1-CCR7, effector CD4-C3-GNLY and exhausted CD4-C7-CXCL13 clusters. CD4-C7-CXCL13 was characterized by high expression of T cell exhaustion markers PDCD1, CTLA4, HAVCR2 and TIGIT and T follicular helper (T_{FH})-like features including high BCL6, IL21, CXCL13 and ICOS together with low expression of CXCR5. Similar to CD8+ T cells, Monocle component 1 was associated with T cell cytotoxicity and negatively associated with naïveness, whereas component 2 was associated with exhaustion.

CD4-C8-FOXP3 was predominantly blood-derived Tregs whereas CD4-C9-CTLA4 was Tregs present mostly in tumors. STARTRAC analysis indicated that CD4-C9-CTLA4 had high clonal expansion scores, low migration scores and intermediate state transition index, indicating local clonal expansion of suppressive tumor-resident Tregs. Close examination of this suppressive Treg cluster CD4-C9-CTLA4 revealed a considerable degree of heterogeneity based on genes associated with Treg functions, particularly TNFRSF9 (4-1BB), a known activation marker for antigen-specific Tregs. A striking bimodal expression distribution within CD4-C9-CTLA4 cells was observed according to the expression level of TNFRSF9, probably delineating Tregs recently activated within tumors from resting ones. Compared to the TNFRSF9—population, TNFRSF9 + Tregs highly expressed a set of 260 genes (False Discovery Rate < 0.01, fold change ≥ 2), including genes associated with immunosuppressive functions such as REL and LAYN. Survival analysis of the TCGA LUAD dataset showed that the 260-gene signature was predictive of worse patient prognosis ($P = 0.0005$, Cox regression). In particular, the expression of IL1R2 significantly correlated with poor prognosis of TCGA LUAD patients ($P = 0.0005$, Cox regression).

6. Characteristics of tumor-infiltrating T cells in colorectal cancer

For CRC, recent clinical trials have demonstrated that patients with microsatellite instability (MSI) respond better to the immune-checkpoint blockade of PD-1 than those with microsatellite-stable (MSS) phenotypes (Le et al., 2015). However, the underlying mechanisms are not fully understood. Application of scRNA-seq may reveal the immune differences between MSI and MSS CRCs and shed light on the mechanisms of responses to immune checkpoint blockade. By dissecting the single T cell landscape of colorectal carcinoma, adjacent normal mucosa and peripheral blood, we obtained transcriptome data for 11,138 single T cells from 12 patients with CRC, including 4 MSI and 8 MSS patients, with an average of 1.25 million uniquely mapped read pairs (Zhang et al., 2018). 10,805 cells remained after quality control, of which 91.4% had at least one pair of full-length productive α and β chains assembled. A total of 7274 clonotypes with unique productive α–β chain paired TCRs were found, of which 870 had two or more cells and resulted in 3474 clonal T cells.

Unsupervised clustering analysis revealed 8 CD8+ and 12 CD4+ T cell clusters, covering naive, central memory, effector memory, recently activated effector memory or effector, MAIT, regulatory, and exhausted, and conventional helper T cells. In contrast to HCC and NSCLC datasets,

CRC-specific T cell subsets including Th17 (CD4_C08-IL23R), follicular T helper cells (CD4_C06-CXCR5), follicular T regulatory cells (CD4_C11-IL10), CD8_C05-CD6 and CD8_C06-CD160 were found. The latter two clusters highly expressed CD69 and ITGAE, known markers of tissue-resident memory T cells, with CD8_C05-CD6 probably representing lamina propria T cells and CD8_C06-CD160 as intraepithelial lymphocytes (IELs) based on the highly expressed natural killer cell markers.

STARTRAC-dist revealed the distinct tissue preference of the T cell clusters. For CD8+ T cells, naive, central memory, and recently activated effector memory cells were predominantly enriched in blood. Exhausted T cells were enriched specifically in tumors while the two resident memory subsets were frequently found in normal mucosa. Likewise, among CD4+ subtypes, naive and effector-like cells were enriched in blood, follicular T helper cells were enriched in normal mucosa, and two IFNG+ Th1-like subsets and Th17 were enriched in tumors. Three FOXP3+ Treg cell clusters, CD4_C10-FOXP3, CD4_C11-IL10 and CD4_C12-CTLA4, were enriched in blood, normal mucosa and tumors, respectively.

STARTRAC-expa revealed that exhausted and recently activated effector memory CD8+ T cells were clusters with the highest degree of clonal expansion followed by IELs. Exhausted CD8+ T cells also enriched with MKI67^{high} cells which were characterized by proliferation-related pathways as confirmed by IHC, indicating ongoing proliferation. Most clonotypes of the proliferating exhausted T cells (40 out of 46) also covered exhausted T cells with low proliferative activity suggesting the same antigenicity. Similar to observations in HCC and NSCLC, exhausted T cells in CRC were observed to express higher levels of effector molecules such as IFNG, GZMB, GZMH and PRF1 than other CD8+ T cells. Transcription factors preferentially expressed in CD8+ exhausted T cells include PRDM1, BATF, RBPJ, TOX and BHLHE40, with the latter three less characterized in literature.

Similar to observations in HCC and NSCLC, the STARTRAC-migr analysis of CD8+ clusters revealed that recently activated effector memory T cells characterized by CX3CR1 had the highest mobility, followed by effector memory T cells characterized by high expression of GZMK. Pairwise STARTRAC-migr analyses revealed that recently activated effector memory T cells can migrate among blood, normal mucosa and tumors and GZMK+ effector memory T cells prefer to migration between mucosa and tumors. In contrast, exhausted T cells exhibited tumor exclusivity. These findings by STARTRAC-migr analyses were supported by the expression patterns of genes related to chemokine receptors, integrin and other trafficking-related molecules such as S1P receptors. For example, CX3CR1+ recently activated effector memory T cells highly expressed S1PR1, S1PR5 and ITGB7, supporting their capability to circulate in the periphery and home to normal mucosa and tumors.

STARTRAC-tran analysis indicated that both CX3CR1+ recently activated effector memory and exhausted T cell clusters were developmentally associated with GZMK+ effector memory T cells, similar to the observations in HCC and NSCLC. Close examination revealed that GZMK+ effector memory T cells were also connected to normal mucosa-enriched resident memory T cells with a moderate degree. Trajectory analysis based on the expression profiles by Monocle revealed similar observations.

Among 124 expanded clonotypes of CX3CR1+ recently activated effector memory T cells, 24 clonotypes had clonal cells of the same cluster located inside tumors, 55 were linked to tumor-infiltrating GZMK+ effector memory cells, and 7 were associated with blood GZMK+ effector memory cells, supporting the migration of this cell type and the developmental transitions to tumor effector memory T cells. Notably, tumor effector memory T cell clones linked to blood CX3CR1+ T cells were mutually exclusive with those linked to tumor exhausted T cells, suggesting that antigen stimulation may play important roles in determining the developmental trajectories of tumor-infiltrating T cells. The transition from effector memory to exhausted T cells may predominantly occur in tumors based on their tissue distribution and TCR overlaps.

In contrast to CD8+ cells, CD4+ helper T cells exhibited low clonal expansion overall. Among all CD4+ T helper clusters, CD4_C03-GNLY exhibited the highest clonal expansion according to STARTRAC-expa analysis. This cluster highly expressed genes including NKG7, PRF1, GNLY and GZMH, a signature that is profoundly similar to that of CD8+ recently activated effector memory T cells. Notably, the CD4_C03-GNLY cluster also showed high migration comparable to those of CD8+ recently activated effector memory T cells and was characterized by CX3CR1. Similarly, CD4_C03-GNLY was developmentally linked to the CD4+ effector memory T cell populations in normal mucosa and tumors.

Different from conventional T helper cells whose clonal expansion was mainly found in peripheral blood, tumor-infiltrating Treg cells showed more clonal expansion than those in blood. Most (88%) of the clonal tumor-infiltrating Treg cells belonged to TCR clonotypes exclusively within tumors, similar to observations in HCC and NSCLC. Inducible Treg cells were also found in tumors, which shared TCRs with helper T cells in tumors. STARTRAC-tran analysis suggested that these inducible Treg cells were developmentally linked to T H 17 and CXCL13+ BHLHE40+ Th1-like cells.

By comparing MSI and MSS tumors, a specific Th1-like CXCL13+ BHLHE40+ cluster was found predominantly enriched in MSI tumor microenvironments, whereas MSS tumors enriched with Th17 cells. Consistently, the CXCL13+ BHLHE40+ Th1-like cell signature was highly expressed in the MSI-high patients of the TCGA CRC cohort, whereas the Th17 signature was enriched in the MSS patients. While GZMK+ Th1-like cells were also characterized by IFNG+ TBX21+, similar to the CXCL13+ BHLHE40+ Th1-like cell cluster, no significant differences were observed between the enrichment of this cluster in MSI and MSS tumors. Notably, IFNγ-regulating transcription factors EOMES and RUNX3 24 were preferentially expressed in GZMK+ Th1 cells, whereas BHLHE40 was selectively expressed in CXCL13+ BHLHE40+ Th1-like cells, suggesting that distinctive transcriptional controls exist for T helper cells within tumors. Indeed, BHLHE40 not only regulates IFNγ but also represses IL-10 production, partially explaining the response of MSI CRC patients to immune checkpoint blockade. Furthermore, STARTRAC analyses revealed that CXCL13+ BHLHE40+ Th1-like cells were clonally expanded and enriched in MSI patients, with ongoing proliferation observed in tumors. Moreover, these cells exhibited developmental connections with the GZMK+ Th1-like cells, indicating the potential inter-conversion between these two IFNG+ subsets.

These CXCL13+ BHLHE40+ Th1-like cells in tumors showed high expression of CXCR3, HAVCR2, PDCD1, ICOS and TIGIT. Notably, a less-characterized gene, IGFLR1, was also upregulated in these cells. IGFLR1 belongs to the TNFR superfamily and has three potential ligands, with IGFL1 and IGFL3 showing high-affinity interactions. IGFLR1 was also upregulated in exhausted CD8+ T cells and Treg cells. In vitro experiments suggested that suboptimal T cell activation was sufficient to upregulate IGFLR1 in memory CD4+ T cells, with IGFL3 enhancing CD25 induction and IFNγ secretion in CD4+ T cells under this condition. The degree of IFNγ induction in total CD4+ T cells was correlated with the induction of IGFLR1 in memory T cells, and the IGFL3-augmented CD25 expression was observed only in IGFLR1+ memory T cells but not in the IGFLR1—cells in the same cultures. The synergistic effect by IGFL3 stimulation could be specifically blocked by an anti-IGFLR1 antibody.

For CD8+ T cells stimulated chronically and with a low degree, the addition of IGFL3 synergized the TCR-induced HAVCR2 expression, which could be blocked by an anti-IGFLR1 antibody.

7. Discussions and conclusions

Dissecting the heterogeneity of tumor-infiltrating T cells and their relationship with T cells in the adjacent tissues and peripheral blood is pivotal to understanding the status of tumor immunity and the associated local and systemic immune responses. Transcriptomic analyses based on scRNA-seq provided unprecedented resolution to characterize the properties of tumor immune microenvironment. We applied full-length scRNA-seq to three cancer types including liver, lung, and colorectal cancers, and developed an analytical framework named as STARTRAC to quantify the dynamic properties of T cell subsets from snapshots of the T cell transcriptomes. The comprehensive transcriptome data along with the dynamic characteristics revealed by STARTRAC dissected the heterogeneous tumor-infiltrating T cells into transcriptionally discriminating subsets, characterized their molecular signatures, tissue preference, clonality, migration and state transition, and indicated their associations with tumor immunity. Comparisons between cancer types revealed both conserved patterns and cancer type-specific T cell subsets, making implications for future cancer patient stratification, prediction of immunotherapy responses, and development of novel therapeutics.

The first remarkable commonality among the three cancer types is the high clonal expansion of both exhausted CD8+ T cells and Tregs in the tumor microenvironment. While CD8+ T cells are assumed to be the main players during tumor eradication, the exhaustion status may compromise their tumor-killing potential, resulting in unbalanced tumor immunity and finally tumor progression out of control. The high clonal expansion of exhausted CD8+ T cells and their ongoing proliferation observed in the tumor microenvironments of all three cancer types indicated their antigen-experiencing nature, and the high expression of effector molecules including IFNG, GZMB and PRF1 may indicate their effector function. But these highly expanded and cytotoxic CD8+ T cells simultaneously had the characteristics of T cell exhaustion, raising the question how the exhaustion status is induced and how it is related to antigen stimulation in tumor microenvironment. Close examination of the expression profiles of markers indicating T cell exhaustion suggested that the extent of exhaustion of tumor-infiltrating T cells varied greatly. How the degree of T cell exhaustion is determined molecularly should be explored with more efforts and these comprehensive scRNA-seq data may provide critical information. Surprisingly, Tregs, which exert the immune suppression function, showed similar patterns of clonal expansion to those of cytotoxic CD8+ T cells. Different from CD8+ T cells in tumor microenvironment, which shared identical TCRs with CD8+ effector memory T cells characterized by GZMK+ in both tumor and adjacent normal tissues, Tregs mainly shared TCRs with themselves in tumor. Only a small fraction of Tregs were found to share TCRs with conventional T helpers. It is of urgent need to unravel how the cytotoxic CD8+ T cells and Tregs interact in the tumor microenvironment and to what extent the molecular characteristics of each cell type contributes to the induction and recruitment of the other cell type. The plenty information of scRNA-seq data may provide important clues for these questions.

The second notable commonality among the three cancer types lies in the existence of a group of GZMK+ effector memory CD8+ T cells. STARTRAC analysis revealed that, for all the three cancer types, this group of T cells were abundant in both tumors and adjacent tissues, clonally expanded, and with high migration potentials and state transition possibility with exhausted CD8+ T cells in tumor. The bimodal distribution of PDCD1 in this groups of T cells and the shared TCRs with exhausted T cells suggested that this T cell group may be pre-exhausted T cells. The survival analysis finding that high ratios of pre-exhausted to exhausted T cells are associated with better prognosis in lung cancers suggests that this group of T cells may be critical targets of future cancer immunotherapy. Deep investigation of the biological and medical implications of this group of T cells is of extreme importance as it is also the key to understanding the contribution of systemic immune responses to tumor immunity.

While conventional CD4+ T cells were found in all the three cancer types, this group of T cells showed great heterogeneity among cancer types and even between patients with the same cancer types. In particular, a subgroup of conventional CD4+ T cells characterized by CXCL13+ BHLHE40+ was found significantly enriched in MSI CRC patients which have better responses to immune checkpoint blockade than those of MSS CRC patients. This finding is consistent with observations in mouse models that conventional CD4+ T cells play important roles in mediating systemic responses to immune checkpoint blockade (Spitzer et al., 2017). It is notable that the developmental trajectories of conventional CD4+ are also similar to those of CD8+ T cells, with a group of GZMK+ conventional CD4+ T cells being the intermediates from blood naïve/effector T cells to tumor exhausted T cells. However, the extent of clonal expansion of CD4+ conventional T cells is weaker than that of CD8+ T cells, with few TCRs observed to be shared among different subsets, raising the question of how conventional CD4+ T cells orchestrate with the function of CD8+ T cells. The observation of inducible Tregs that have identical TCRs with conventional CD4+ T cells also highlighted the importance to investigate how conventional CD4+ T cells contribute to the function of Tregs. Taken together, the heterogeneity of conventional CD4+ T cells and the complexity of their relationship with CD8+ T cells and Tregs suggest that conventional CD4+ T cells may form the major cell type that interprets the heterogeneity of cancer patients and predicts the responses of cancer immunotherapies.

In addition to T cell subsets mentioned above that were observed in all the three cancer types, T cell subsets including MAIT, CD8+ ZNF683+ T cells and CD8+ CD160+ T cells were preferentially enriched in the scRNA-seq data of HCC, NSCLC and CRC, respectively, reflecting the contribution of tissue-specific immunity. Compared to adjacent normal tissues, MAIT cells were significantly depleted in HCC and CD8+ CD160+ T cells were depleted in CRC. CD8+ ZNF683+ T cells showed enrichment in both tumors and adjacent normal tissues of NSCLC patients and shared TCRs with exhausted CD8+ T cells. The contributions of these tissue-specific T cell subsets to tumor immunity need further evaluations to develop cancer-specific immunotherapies. The identification of CD8+ Tregs in HCC also raises the question of how exhausted T cells convert with Tregs, which may provide critical implications for reversing the immune suppression state of tumor microenvironment.

On the molecular level, the comprehensive scRNA-seq data gave a nearly panoramic depiction of the various T cell subsets identified. The signature genes of exhausted T cells and Tregs provide important candidate targets to improve the current immunotherapies and even develop new therapies. In particular, LAYN is found to be specifically expressed in highly exhausted CD8+ T cells and Tregs, and is associated with poor prognosis of HCC patients. The regulatory function of LAYN was validated by in vitro overexpression of LAYN in blood-derived human CD8+ T cells which resulted in significantly reduced production of IFN-g, supporting that LAYN may be a plausible target for future cancer immunotherapies. Similarly, we also confirmed the function of IGFLR1, which was highly expressed in exhausted CD4+ and CD8+ T cells and Tregs, to be a costimulatory receptor and thus pivotal to the effector functions. The diverse expression patterns of these genes provide a rich resource for understanding the precise function and relationship of tumor-infiltrating cells and developing precision medicine for cancers.

In conclusion, we applied full-length scRNA-seq to three cancer types and provide a comprehensive single T cell data resource for understanding the various characteristics of tumor-infiltrating T cells. The development of STARTRAC allowed quantitative depiction of the dynamic properties of various T cell subsets including tissue preference, clonal expansion, migration and state transitions. The conserved and cancer type-specific T cell subsets and developmental patterns and the detailed molecular portrait of each cluster provide new insights into the composition, heterogeneity, and potentially formation of tumor immune microenvironments, and new options for future development of cancer therapeutics.

Acknowledgments

This project was supported by Beijing Advanced Innovation Centre for Genomics at Peking University, Key Technologies R&D Program (2016YFC0900100), and National Natural Science Foundation of China (31530036 and 91742203).

Competing interests

The authors declare no competing interests.

References

Brahmer, J. R., et al. (2012). Safety and activity of anti-PD-L1 antibody in patients with advanced cancer. *New England Journal of Medicine*, *366*, 2455–2465.

Campbell, K., Ponting, C. P., & Webber, C. (2015). Laplacian eigenmaps and principal curves for high resolution pseudotemporal ordering of single-cell RNA-seq profiles. *bioRxiv*, *511*, 027219.

Collisson, E. A., et al. (2014). Comprehensive molecular profiling of lung adenocarcinoma. *Nature*, *511*, 543–550.

Crawford, A., et al. (2014). Molecular and transcriptional basis of CD4(+) T cell dysfunction during chronic infection. *Immunity*, *40*, 289–302.

De Simone, M., et al. (2016). Transcriptional landscape of human tissue lymphocytes unveils uniqueness of tumor-infiltrating T regulatory cells. *Immunity*, *45*, 1135–1147.

El-Serag, H. B. (2011). Current concepts hepatocellular carcinoma. *New England Journal of Medicine*, *365*, 1118–1127.

Fousteri, G., et al. (2014). The protein tyrosine phosphatase PTPN22 controls forkhead box protein 3 T regulatory cell induction but is dispensable for T helper type 1 cell polarization. *Clinical and Experimental Immunology*, *178*, 178–189.

Goode, E. L., et al. (2013). Inherited variants in regulatory T cell genes and outcome of ovarian cancer. *PLos One*, *8*, e53903.

Guo, X., et al. (2018). Global characterization of T cells in non-small-cell lung cancer by single-cell sequencing. *Nature Medicine*, *24*, 978.

Hellmann, M. D., et al. (2017). Nivolumab plus ipilimumab as first-line treatment for advanced non-small-cell lung cancer (CheckMate 012): Results of an open-label, phase 1, multicohort study. *Lancet Oncology*, *18*, 31–41.

Herbst, R. S., Heymach, J. V., & Lippman, S. M. (2008). Molecular origins of cancer: Lung cancer. *New England Journal of Medicine*, *359*, 1367–1380.

Ji, Z., & Ji, H. (2016). TSCAN: Pseudo-time reconstruction and evaluation in single-cell RNA-seq analysis. *Nucleic Acids Research*, *44*, e117.

Kasper, H.-U., Drebber, U., Stippel, D. L., Dienes, H. P., & Gillessen, A. (2009). Liver tumor infiltrating lymphocytes: Comparison of hepatocellular and cholangiolar carcinoma. *World Journal of Gastroenterology*, *15*, 5053–5057.

Kiselev, V. Y., et al. (2017). SC3: Consensus clustering of single-cell RNA-seq data. *Nature Methods*, *14*, 483.

Le, D. T., et al. (2015). PD-1 blockade in tumors with mismatch-repair deficiency. *New England Journal of Medicine*, *372*, 2509–2520.

Livesey, F. J. (2003). Strategies for microarray analysis of limiting amounts of RNA. *Briefings in Functional Genomics & Proteomics*, *2*, 31–36.

Navin, N. E. (2014). Cancer genomics: One cell at a time. *Genome Biology*, *15*, 452.

Pallandre, J.-R., et al. (2007). Role of STAT3 in CD4(+)CD25(+)FOXP3(+) regulatory lymphocyte generation: Implications in graft-versus-host disease and antitumor immunity. *Journal of Immunology*, *179*, 7593–7604.

Picelli, S., et al. (2014). Full-length RNA-seq from single cells using Smart-seq2. *Nature Protocols*, *9*, 171–181.

Plitas, G., et al. (2016). Regulatory T cells exhibit distinct features in human breast cancer. *Immunity*, *45*, 1122–1134.

Prieto, J., Melero, I., & Sangro, B. (2015). Immunological landscape and immunotherapy of hepatocellular carcinoma. *Nature Reviews Gastroenterology & Hepatology*, *12*, 681–700.

Ren, X. W., Kang, B. X., & Zhang, Z. M. (2018). Understanding tumor ecosystems by single-cell sequencing: Promises and limitations. *Genome Biology*, *19*, 14.

Ritchie, M. E., et al. (2015). limma powers differential expression analyses for RNA-sequencing and microarray studies. *Nucleic Acids Research*, *43*, e47.

Rizvi, N. A., et al. (2015). Mutational landscape determines sensitivity to PD-1 blockade in non-small cell lung cancer. *Science*, *348*, 124–128.

Rodriguez, A., & Laio, A. (2014). Clustering by fast search and find of density peaks. *Science*, *344*, 1492–1496.

Schlitzer, A., et al. (2015). Identification of cDC1- and cDC2-committed DC progenitors reveals early lineage priming at the common DC progenitor stage in the bone marrow. *Nature Immunology*, *16*, 718.

Sharma, P., & Allison, J. P. (2015). Immune checkpoint targeting in cancer therapy: Toward combination strategies with curative potential. *Cell*, *161*, 205–214.

Spitzer, M. H., et al. (2017). Systemic immunity is required for effective cancer immunotherapy. *Cell*, *168*, 487.

Stubbington, M. J. T., et al. (2016). T cell fate and clonality inference from single-cell transcriptomes. *Nature Methods*, *13*, 329–332.

Tang, F., et al. (2009). mRNA-Seq whole-transcriptome analysis of a single cell. *Nature Methods*, *6*, 377–U386.

Tirosh, I., et al. (2016). Dissecting the multicellular ecosystem of metastatic melanoma by single-cell RNA-seq. *Science*, *352*, 189–196.

Topalian, S. L., Drake, C. G., & Pardoll, D. M. (2015). Immune checkpoint blockade: A common denominator approach to cancer therapy. *Cancer Cell*, *27*, 450–461.

Topalian, S. L., Taube, J. M., Anders, R. A., & Pardoll, D. M. (2016). Mechanism-driven biomarkers to guide immune checkpoint blockade in cancer therapy. *Nature Reviews. Cancer*, *16*, 275–287.

Topalian, S. L., et al. (2012). Safety, activity, and immune correlates of anti-PD-1 antibody in cancer. *New England Journal of Medicine*, *366*, 2443–2454.

Trapnell, C., et al. (2014). The dynamics and regulators of cell fate decisions are revealed by pseudotemporal ordering of single cells. *Nature Biotechnology*, *32*, 381–U251.

van der Maaten, L., & Hinton, G. (2008). Visualizing data using t-SNE. *Journal of Machine Learning Research*, *9*, 2579–2605.

Zhang, L., et al. (2018). Lineage tracking reveals dynamic relationships of T cells in colorectal cancer. *Nature*, *564*, 268.

Zheng, C., et al. (2017a). Landscape of infiltrating T cells in liver cancer revealed by single-cell sequencing. *Cell*, *169*, 1342.

Zheng, G. X. Y., et al. (2017b). Massively parallel digital transcriptional profiling of single cells. *Nature Communications*, *8*, 14049.

FSC
www.fsc.org
MIX
Papier | Fördert
gute Waldnutzung
FSC® C083411

Kolibri 360 GmbH
Ferdinand-Jühlke-Straße 7
99095 Erfurt, Deutschland
produktsicherheit@kolibri360.de